CHILD HEALTH
and
DISEASE

CHILD HEALTH
and
DISEASE

A SHORT TEXTBOOK OF CLINICAL PAEDIATRICS

Bijon Kr Chakraborty

MBBS, DCH (Cal.), FRCP (Edin.), DCH (Lond.), FIAGP

New Central Book Agency (P) Ltd

LONDON

DELHI KOLKATA PUNE HYDERABAD ERNAKULAM

REGD. OFFICE
8/1 Chintamoni Das Lane, Kolkata 700 009, India
email: ncbapvtltd@eth.net
OVERSEAS
27 Catherine Court, Chase Road, Southgate, London, N14 4RB
EXPORT
212 Shahpur Jat, New Delhi 110 049
email: ncbaexp@ncbapvtltd.com
BRANCHES
4262/3 1st Floor, Flat Nos. 105 & 106
Ansari Road, Daryaganj, New Delhi 110 002
email: ncbadel@ncbapvtltd.com

House No. 3-1-315, 1st Floor
Nimboliadda, Kachiguda, Hyderabad 500 027
email: ncbahydb@ncbapvtltd.com

Shop Nos. 3 & 4, Vinayak Towers
681/B Budhwar Peth, Appa Balwant Chowk
Pune 411 002
email: ncbapune@ncbapvtltd.com

GSS Shopping Complex, 1st Floor
Opposite College Post Office, Convent Road
Ernakulam 682 035
email: ncbaernk@ncbapvtltd.com

Child Health and Disease

First Published: 1986
Reprinted: 2010

PUBLISHER AND TYPESETTER
New Central Book Agency (P) Ltd
8/1 Chintamoni Das Lane, Kolkata 700 009

PRINTER
New Central Book Agency (P) Ltd
Web-Offset Division, Dhulagarh, Sankrail, Howrah

COVER-PRINTER
Biswanath Studio, Kolkata

COVER DESIGNER
Prasanta Sur

TECHNICAL EDITOR
Dr Mita Sen MBBS

ISBN: 978-81-7381-570-6

Price: Rs 235.00 [Rupees Two Hundred and Thirty-five]

PREFACE

I am inspired to write this book specially for my undergraduate students when Calcutta University started the semester system of teaching both in pre-clinical and clinical curriculum. The students in their very short stay in Paediatric studies in clinical stage, become very much disturbed and puzzled to learn the technique, how to deal with their little clients. Moreover, paediatrics is now established itself as a separate discipline in Medicine both from the point of passing examination and furthermore to take post-graduate studies, may even to cater health care as young doctors in the community where more than 40% of our population belong to this age group.

This book will be helpful specially for the undergraduates, even post-graduate students of D.C.H. and M.D. (Paediatrics). Moreover, to the large general practitioners, in their busy schedule to accumulate preventive and curative aspect of paediatric teaching and management. The chapters are specially written for the vast majority of students and practitioners include neonatal care, nutrition and feeding, respiratory problems and last but not the least, paediatric emergencies. At last, I acknowledge my sincere thanks to all my colleagues, students and my little clients with their parents, whom I disturbed too much sometimes to get more informations for the benefit of future healthy generation and prosperous India.

Bijon Chakraborty.

Dedicated
to
my mother
whose immortal touch always I feel,
to
my father for his blessing and
to
my wife and children
who gave me inspiration when I am tired.

CONTENTS

PREFACE

CONTENTS

CONTENTS

LIST OF FIGURES

LIST OF FIGURES

CHAPTER – ONE

INTRODUCTION

Principles of Paediatric teaching in the basic level with preventive approach.

Medical education today is attracting the serious attention of medical educationist all over the world as it represents a collosal problem with an obvious impact of nation-wide consciousness for readjustment to the present and the future needs of the country. Medicine is dynamic and things which begin at the beginning are continuously changing. Paediatrics in modern dynamic medicine is a fundamental discipline and not just a matter of few ailments of infants and children. However the realization that Child Health needed top priority, was evident all the time, may be illustrated through a few quotes from the Bhore Committee report (1946) – "Nearly one half of total deaths at all ages take place among children under 10 years. Of these, approximately half is among infants under one year". The medical student must be equipped with sufficient knowledge to enable him to discharge his responsibilities as a paediatrician. Paediatrics is not an accretion to a curriculum already heavily loaded but, an essential component of a programme extending from pre-clinical to post-graduate years. Recently there has been considerable introspection and rethinking regarding curricular contents and methodology in teaching at under-graduate and post-graduate levels.

Paediatrics, means the therapy in childhood ailments, is now recognised as a discipline which not only involves the diagnosis and treatment of sick children, but also includes the prevention of illness and the promotion of normal development and health in childhood.

Paediatric education today essentially needs training and education of the students in the home background, otherwise they will be trained to function in a setting where things are available to them which are unknown at home. Within medicine, a unified child health care which provides preventive care and early detection of handicap and disease, as well as palliative treatment, must be the objective. In a wider context there is a need for close co-operation between those who provide the educational, social and health services for children. In India, the priorities in child health service are very different, although the same principles may be applied as in the western countries. The type of paediatric service provided upon must be related to the economics of the country, the social benefits and customs of the community, which sometimes have definite scientific background, the level of education, geographical and climatic factors and the availability of medical personnel. Although our infantile mortality rate has dropped from 140 per thousand to 120, still in some urban and rural areas the mortality rate from combination of malnutrition and infectious diseases are very high among children below 6 years of age. It is not justified to say that till the economic conditions improve our child health care could not be improved. Instead it has been shown that appropriate paediatric care can, even in the presence of extreme poverty and in the absence of expensive capital resources, transform the pattern of childhood mortality and morbidity. This needs more training of available professional personnel to cater health services in the line of prevention. The paramedical staff including the social workers can infiltrate to the deeper societies, where need of health care and health education is much more. These poor mothers should be taught importance of breast feeding, timely introduction of weaning foods, good effects of immunisation, use of pure drinking water etc. Also they should realise the beneficial effect of family planning and plan for a smaller family with healthy children. Our rural population comprising more than 80% of our total population and only 20% medical personnel available to look after them, should receive the health services at their door-step with more of prevention of disease rather than when they will suffer from disease, which might exhaust their family budget — so intensification of primary health care, where mother in the house is the primary worker. Even though Government of India has accepted the Primary Health Care approach to reach the goal of health for all by the year 2000 A.D, there are 8 elements in the minimal definition of primary health care. Each of these element makes a substantial demand on the limited manpower and financial resources. The policy of prioritisation may therefore be relevant while developing MCH models. Based on the causation of high maternal, infant and pre-school mortality, the priorities for intervention would be (i) timely treatment of diarrhoeal disease (ii) timely treatment of acute respiratory disease (iii) prevention and care of low birth weight babies (iv) child spacing and population stabilisation (v) provision of adequate antenatal, intranatal and post natal care (vi) promotion of breast feeding (vii) prevention of neonatal tetanus and prevention and treatment of malnutrition and (viii) prevention of measles.

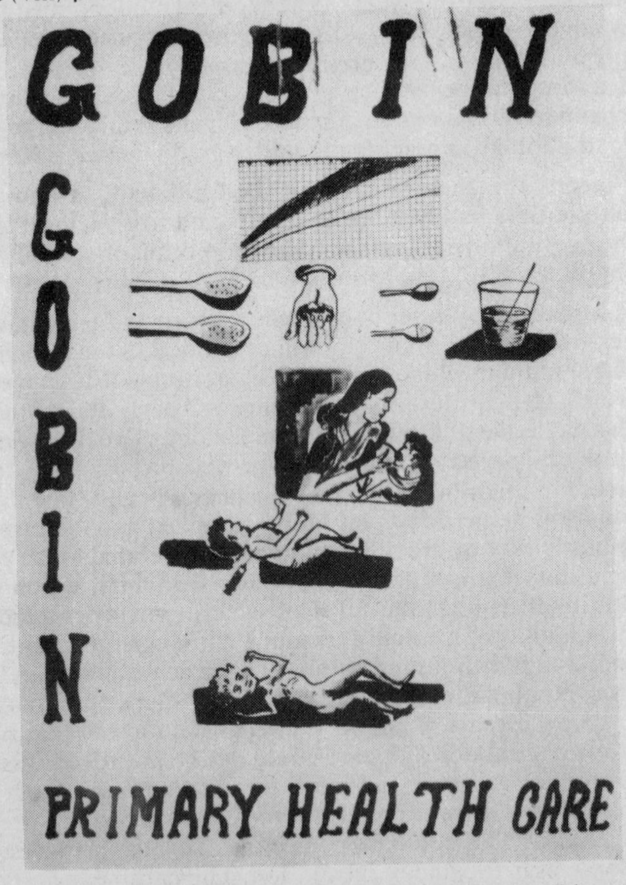

Fig.1.1 : GOBIN : G-growth; O-oral rehydration salts; B-breast feeding; I-immunization; N-nutrition

The interest and well being of children s the main concern of every welfare state and India being committed to the philosophy of social welfare of society, particular care has been taken to provide for protection, training, education, maintenance and rehabilitation of children.

Of a population of 730 million, 19.9% are concentrated in 3000 towns or urban places adjacent to the town or city and 80% are spread over five hundred thousand villages. Children under 14 years of age constitute 42.08 percent of total population in the country. It is interesting to know that 82% of children between 5-14 years of age live in villages. In recent years there has been a trend towards fall in crude death rate and expectation of life rising to the age of 50 years. However, the birth rate has not shown a corresponding decline because of continuing high mortality amongst children. The infant mortality varies from 100 to 125 in urban and rural areas respectively (1979). The second year mortality reveals the post infantile deaths during childhood. The pre-school mortality is almost one-third or 37.5% of mortality of all ages. It has been estimated that only 72% of all children born reach five years of age. In view of collosal loss of human potential, there has been a high birth 33.2 per 1,000 rate which has given a high growth rate of 1.67%. Majority of deaths are due to such preventable causes like malnutrition, diarrhoea and respiratory infections. One of the most important factor for such high mortality especially in pre-school age group and morbidity in general is the lack of preventive and curative medical services for the community in rural areas. Inspite of 80% of population living in rural area only about twenty percent of medical personnel of modern system of medicine are available and they do seldom penetrate beyond the primary health centres. The bulk of rural medical services is manned by indigenous practitioners or paramedicos. It is only in recent years that more rural people think diseases to have physical origin but quite a percentage still describe super-natural causation of illness. In the absence of basic concept of health and hygiene, infections are frequent and in the absence of prompt therapy high mortality results.

Examination of the newborn infant :

In countries where full medical services are available it is one part of continuing medical care and is undertaken in the light of an accurate account of the preceding pregnancy, birth and family history. In fact the routine examination of the new born takes place in three parts. The first is the responsibility of the doctor or midwife incharge of the birth and assesses the condition of the baby immediately after birth including the respiratory states or other appropriate system of measurement of vitality at the time of birth. For the great majority of infants, the immediate examinations show no abnormality. The infant can be given to the mother and the good news told to her. Where the first examination is normal and the infant has continued to show no abnormal symptoms or signs, the second part of the routine examination should take place some hours after birth but within the first 48 hours. The occasion of this examination, which may invite questions from mother because it is done in front of her, so that she can have a comprehensive guide and advice regarding further rearing up of her infant and to express any anxieties that she may feel.

Next routine examination should be done after 6 weeks in a well baby clinic where one should take account of the motor, manipulative, special sensory, intellectual and social aspects of development should be assessed. Here also the mothers should be advised regarding minor congenital abnormalities present in their children and their remedies arranged. Moreover, regarding the nutritional, immunisation advices and procedures should be taken up, specially the importance of breast feeding and prevention of infectious diseases by proper immunisation programme.

CHILD HEALTH SERVICES

In India under six clinics are now a proven method of reducing childhood mortality and morbidity. The objective is to provide low-cost curative and preventive care to as large a proportion of the population as possible. In this clinic mother is educated at each stage of the child's development. Such clinics are best run in conjunction with the antenatal and family planning services rendered from hospital, primary and subsidiary health centres. This clinic should supervise the following essential activities :

1. The supervision of the health of all children upto the age of six.
2. The prevention of malnutrition, malaria, measles, pertussis, tuberculosis, smallpox, poliomyelitis, diphtheria and tetanus.
3. The provision of simple treatment for diarrhoeas with or without dehydration, respiratory infections and other common childhood skin infections.

THE CARE OF SICK CHILDREN

History — 'taking' :

In paediatrics most of the history is commonly obtained from a third person, usually the mother. More so in our country the uneducated, shy mothers may not supply detail history but still through constant care of her child, is often a most reliable observer of minute physical changes due to disease. Moreover, in paediatrics, the young children also helpful in giving their discomfort and history of previous disease conditions.

Scheme of history — 'taking' :

This should follow a definite pattern. History taking and clinical examination in paediatrics, calls for skill and knowledge which cannot be taught through the written word. They can only be learned and then modified according to circumstances by continual and critical practice. This chapter dealing with history taking can only provide a guide.

Complaint : The reason for the consultation should be noted in non medical language, e.g., 'Breathing difficulties' and not dyspnoea.

Present illness : This is the most vital part of history. This part should be taken in detail giving the mode of onset, the main complaints and the additional symptoms giving the duration of various complaints in sequence of orders. Leading questions should be avoided as far as possible. Details of bowel habit, micturition, appetite, sleep, cough and gain in weight and height should be recorded.

Previous history : The development of a child ranges from conception; the findings of the present should be interpreted in the light of his past and of the progress he is making. Continuity in the history is often helpful.

Paediatric history : Special points under this heading is essential :

(a) Birth history :

i) Antenatal,
ii) Intranatal,
iii) Post-natal — immediate seven days post-natal period.

(b) Feeding history : Starting from early neonatal period upto five years.

(c) Mile-stones of development :

Both of physical growth and mental development with attaining performance skills.

(d) Immunisation histories :

From birth upto 5 years including BCG, Triple antigen, Polio, Measles, Typhoid and Cholera with primary and secondary boosters.

Family history :

The health of the other members of the family and people with whom the child is in close contact should be noted. Particular problems require detailed enquiry along particular lines.

School : Conditions of life at school are important. Is he well adjusted to it ? Is he teased ? Is his attendance regular ? Is his progress in learning satisfactory ?

Clinical examination :

This differs from adult examination because the physician will have to establish rapport with the baby before he is allowed to put his hand on his baby patient. So utilise the time of few minutes with talking to parents. Moreover in paediatrics, use of eyes has got prime importance to diagnosis than all other methods added together.

Head : Shape, size and circumference to be noted, with its sutures and fontanelles.

Eyes : The condition of the eyelids, conjunctiva, cornea, vitreous and fundus should be examined even with an ophthalmoscope. The blindness may be due to congenital cataract, congenital optic atrophy, congenital cerebral agenesis or acquired conditions such as retinoblastoma or retrolental fibroplasia, congenital abnormalities include ptosis, coloboma of the iris and BCM (Blinding corneal malnutrition) due to Vit.A deficiency.

Nose : Patency of the nasal airway should be checked and nasal septum examination, nasal discharge to be noted.

Ears : A defect of hearing may remain undetected in the early years of life unless special tests are made. Delay in talking or apparent backwardness and behaviour problems should always arouse suspicion.

Throat : After inspection of mouth, the next step is to see the throat clearly in a good light. As a rule, the oropharynx should be inspected by depressing the tongue with a spatula.

In paediatric examination, it is said that some are 'must examination' irrespective of disease conditions, e.g., ant-fontanelle — for state of intracranial tension and state of hydration, ears and nose for discharge, throat for any patch, body weight — for nutritional state and if chances available to see macroscopically a specimen of stool and a sample of urine microscopically for detection of pus cells. These examinations at bed side are essential for paediatric diagnosis and that's why they are 'Must' examinations in paediatrics.

Also in general examinations, one should look for colour of skin, mouth, lips, gums and teeth — appearance of dentition, carries, the cervical lymph glands etc. The neck region should be inspected both the lateral and central parts.

Chest : The shape of the thorax and of the spine should be noted by inspection and palpation. The percussion and auscultation in experienced ears may not be disturbed even in a crying child, moreover, this act of crying might help with more air inside the respiratory bronchus and alveoli.

Heart : The precordium, the visible apical impulse should be inspected. In comparison to adult the apex in a child is more up in the left 4th interspace and out on the nipple line due to shape of the heart and relative space in the thoracic cavity. The auscultation of accentuated and splitting P_2 is a normal phenomenon. Regarding observation of arterial pulsations, in all cardiac cases, the femoral pulses should be felt to start with.

Abdomen : The abdomen of the infant is normally full and rounded upto the age of four. The liver is also palpable below the right costal margin upto the age of six years. Rectal examination should always be done whenever an acute abdominal condition is present.

Legs and arms : The shape of legs and arms should be noted. The abnormal shortness of the arms and legs is present in achondroplasia. Congenital dislocation of the hip should be tested in new born period.

Nervous system : Examination of the nervous system requires much patience and the child's cooperation. First, the patient should be watched in movement, at play, then the limbs should be handled and the rest of the examination will follow. The tendon reflexes are obtained. The abnormal movements, the tone of the muscles should be tested and looked for. In patients under 12-18 months the plantar reflex may be equivocal and a quick upward movement is a normal finding. Hypotonia and incoordination should be noted when he handles toys, undresses and dresses or moves about in play to detect any incoordination or ataxia.

The testing of sensation is often not done in young children due to lack of coordination.

In conclusion, in paediatric examination, the examiner, may not get a chance of systematic approach of physical examination, so he or she should spend enough time to take the history and also use the eyes more than physical touch to get enough materials from his physically immature client.

Reference :

COURT, D & JACKSON, A. (1972) : Paediatrics in the Seventies : British Paediatric Association and Nuffield Provincial Hospitals Trust, London, Oxford University Press.

DRUGS AND CHILDREN

Introduction

Boreus mentioned that pharmacokinetics was a child of Paediatrics. A number of therapeutic accidents in new borns led paediatricians and clinical pharmacologists to study the effect of drugs in the perinatal period. Many of these theraphy related accidents could be elucidated and explained through pharmacokinetic investigations and deliberations. Three aspects which are of importance for the study of intoxication were elimination and cumulation, deep compartmentalisation and protein binding.

The process of elimination of drugs were less active in the newborn than in older children, drugs which were mainly excreted renally behaved accordingly e.g. penicillin and its derivative.

The greater proportion of enzymes which were involved in metabolic liver function and the elimination of drugs also exhibited only slight activity at the time of birth. The acetylation was slowed down in the fourth week of life. Conjugation with glucuronic acid exhibited reduced activity up to the second month of life while this was the case for conjugation with glutathione and aminoacids upto the third month. An important observation to remember was that some drugs, such as sulfonamides were mainly acetylated during the first days of life instead of being mainly glucuronated, as was the rule later on. The acetylation process matured more rapidly. A classic example of the danger to the newborn arising from ignorance of this behaviour was the so-called "Gray syndrome" due to chloramphenicol therapy in newborn period. The deep compartments one of which is amniotic fluid, is normally during treatment of the

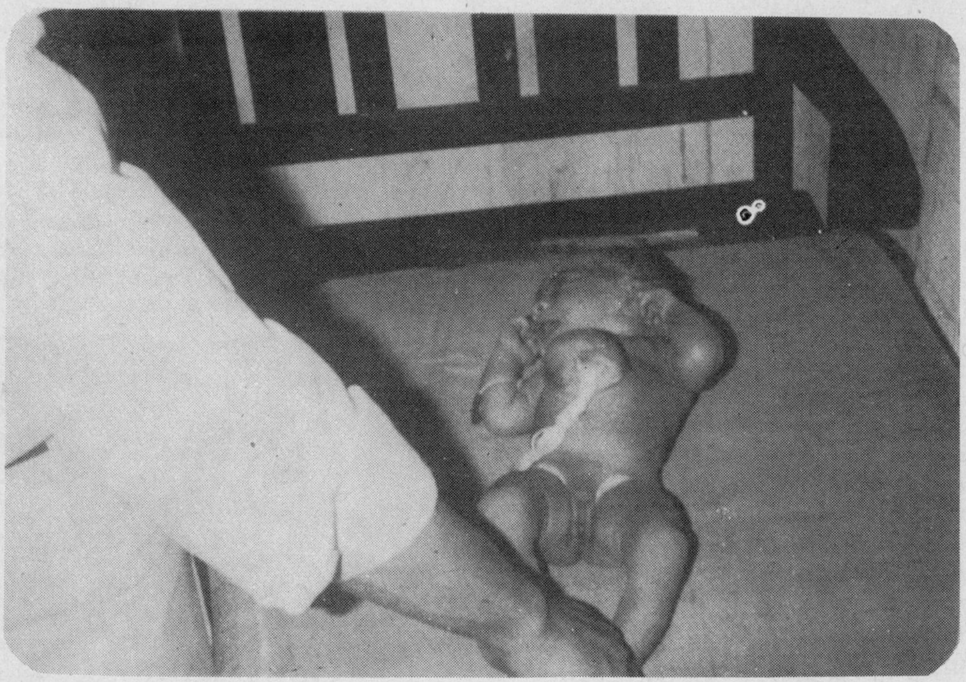

Fig.1.2 : Congenital malformation Omphalocele

pregnant woman, the fetus was part of the mother's distribution volume. The concentrations were almost identical. If however the fetus excreted the substance via the kidneys into the amniotic fluid and then took it again orally, this could result in a concentration which was much higher than that in the maternal organs. Moreover, because of the delayed elimination a measurable level could still be demonstrated in the newborn after birth for a longer period of time than in the mother. This applied, for example, to ampicillin, digitoxin and many other such substances and also to substances in question in drug dependent mother. For this reason, neonates for example exhibited the symptoms of withdrawal syndrome distinctly later than their mothers. After antibiotic treatment of their mothers, infants more frequently exhibited sepsis with organisms which were resistant to the drug used. Moreover if there was disturbance of flow even in the deep compartments, so even if the compartment was very small, the influence of this behaviour upon the development of the offending drugs be it ever so small, formed part of an anatomical structure which was particularly sensitive, such as the inner ear, toxic damage could occur, especially with long term therapy. Here in certain circumstances the concentration in the central compartment e.g. plasma and the deep compartment may no longer correspond.

Since a lower protein concentration and lesser binding capacity were frequently measured in the newborn than in the adult the danger caused by displacement of this binding was relatively great, especially in connection with hyperbilirubinaemia of the neonate. The sulfonamide, salicylates, phenytoin, caffeine, benzoate and other substances could displace bilirubin from albumin and kernicterus may result with relatively slight concentrations.

RELATION BETWEEN PHARMACOKINETICS AND CLINICAL EFFECTS IN THE NEWBORN.

The effect of the drug upon the neonate was dependant upon inter-individual fluctuations of two individuals — women during pregnancy and child birth and the newborn period. In this connection use of analgesics before delivery. After administration, both short term and long term effects may be observed in the newborn. The use of pethidine before delivery, might result immediately after birth, respiratory depression, become apparent. In addition there had been reports of longterm effects after pethidine and other Obstetric analgesics, such as abnormal neurological behaviour and depression of vital functions, which were observed by some authors upto four weeks after birth. The use of xanthine derivatives e.g. theophylline and caffeine as respiratory stimulant. It stimulates the central respiratory centres, the recovery of certain heart functions, dilatation of the blood vessels, no influence of cerebral blood vessels there by an increase intracranial pressure increase in renal blood flow. The toxic effects in the form of tachycardia, hyperglycemia and glucosuria had also been observed because of the reduced plasma protein-binding the concentration of the free drug was higher than the total concentration in the body.

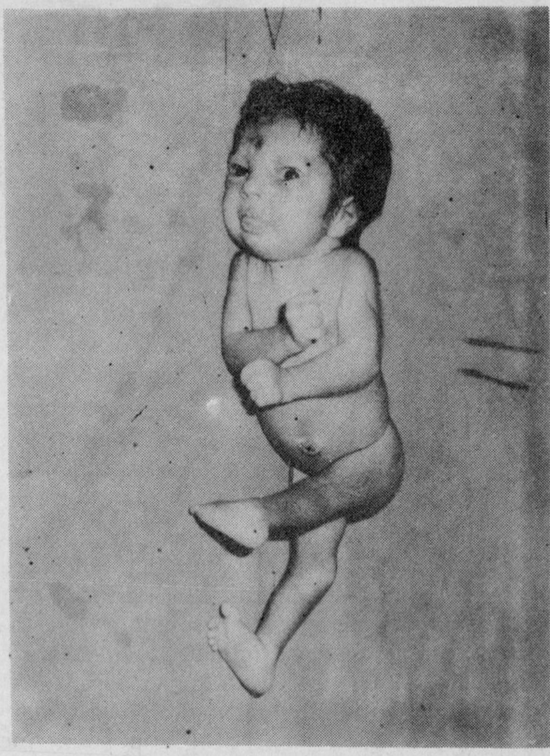

Fig.1.3 : Arthrogryposis Multiplex

The use of diuretics in the perinatal period were a good example with which to illustrate the risks to newborn babies when they could recieve an unknown amount of the drugs via the placenta or breast milk or may even itself receive a diuretic. The newborns and more immature, the infants due to half life of the drug is longer, if there is shorter duration of pregnancy the side effects are greater. The infants under influence of diuretics excreted more water and more sodium than normally. They had become dehydrated more and had therefore required an infusion more often. The nephrotoxicity of aminoglycosides increase through furosemide use, although the fluid and mineral losses had undoubtedly played a part. In some cases ototoxicity and thrombocytopaenia has been observed in the newborns. Finally protein binding was hampered and all diuretics displace bilirubin from albumen, as do other drugs such as sulphonamides. So that one must bear in mind the danger of Kernicterus.

The use of aminoglycosides in contrast to other antibiotics, did not seem more toxic in neonates than in adults, nevertheless, they should be used cautiously in order to avoid possible damage. In choosing an aminoglycoside, one should take into account the pathogen and its sensitivity, because differences in toxicity seem to be very subtle and not yet clearly demonstrated.

DRUGS USED IN PREGNANCY

Drugs are being increasingly used in clinical practice for treatment of various disease states in pregnant women. This list excludes vitamins, and minerals, anaesthetics agents, alcohol consumption, cigarette smoking or tobacco leaf chewing and exposure to environmental pollutants as an insecticides, and other chemicals. The drug effects of the foetus are in general undesireable and it is believed that 1-5% of congenital defects in the human are drug related. The problem of drug transfer from the mother to the foetus and the possibility of fetal/neonatal development disturbances, hence surfaces as and when medication is called for in pregnancy. However, the longterm probable effects of foetal drug exposure in utero and drug behaviour in maternal nutritional status on brain function of the neonate and future behaviour pattern are poorly understood. The embryonic period extends between 4th week to 8-9 weeks of pregnancy and the foetal period between 9th week till birth. The placenta becomes functional since the third week of gestation and assures its function till delivery. Some drugs believed to be nontoxic on the embryo but most probable effect of some other drugs in this period lead to death or severe damage of the embryo, with resultant abortion as for example cytotoxic drugs and antimalarials.

There is general agreement that embryonic period (4th to 9th week of gestation) is the critical period for drug induced congenital malformation, the dramatic example being thalidomide disaster. The teratogenicity not evident at birth may also manifest in later life as shown by the report of vaginal adenosis and cervical carcinoma of adolescent girls whose mother had received diethyl stilboestrol in early pregnancy. Some of the other teratogenic agents include besides hormones Progestin and androgens, folic acid antagonists, anticonvulsants, alkalytating agents. The drug exposure during fetal life period 8-9 weeks of gestation till birth may lead to prematurity and abortion or tissue injury. IUGR (intrauterine growth retardation) is the characteristic toxic effect of some drugs administered during the second half of pregnancy. Prenatal drugs administered to the mother may also compromise the newborn's immediate adaptation to extra uterine existence and provoke withdrawal signs, respiratory depression etc. The newborn's reaction to stress situation may also be impaired by intrauterine drug exposure. The longterm effects of perinatal drug impact on brain function and personality development and effects of multiple drug interaction during this period are poorly understood. It now appears that while envisaging therapy in pregnancy, and while weighing benefit/risk ratio to the baby, emphasis need to be shifted more towards doing no harm. All the same possibility of foetal therapy or correction of foetal disturbances through maternally delivered agents offers exciting prospects :

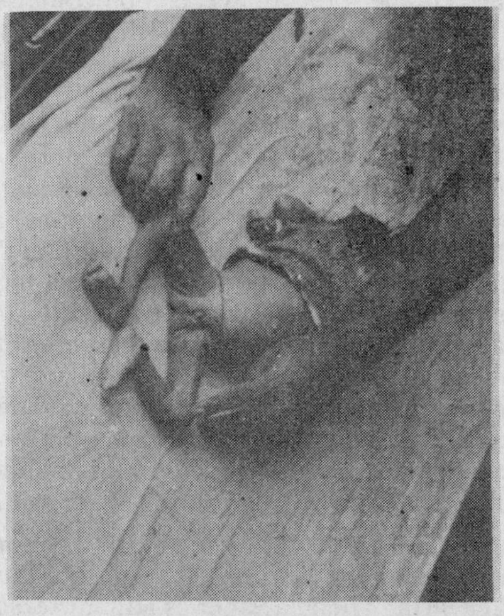

Fig.1.4 : Intersex problems (enlarged, hypertrophied clitoris)

SPECIFICITY OF PHARMACOLOGY FOR NEWBORN AND CHILDREN

Strangely enough, the differential pharmacology of children and adolescents is not yet well known, and the notions developed for adults one generally applied to children, with a correction of the doses in ratio to weight, body surface or volume of extra-cellular fluid. Much more is known about the specific aspects of the pharmacology of newborns and infants. In the past quarter century, various accidents occuring in newborns have been identified. The role of great concentration of oxygen in the development of retrolental fibroplasia (opacification of the transparent media of the eye behind the crystalline lens) in prematures demonstrated in 1952. Three years later, the haemolytic anaemia and icterus produced by the water soluble vitamin K_2 administration for the prevention of haemmorrhagic disease in newborns were described. The toxic effect of some sulphonamides, producting icterus in premature was revealed in 1956, and a similar fact was noted with Novobiocin in 1961. In 1959 chloramphenicol was shown to be toxic for newborns, and the name of "Gray Syndrome" was given to the anomalies often fatal which it may cause. The description showed a combination of pallor, circumoral grayness respiratory difficulties and cardiovascular collapse. Since 1961, we have learned to recognize the more benign side effects due to tetracycline, bulging of the fontanelle and yellowing of the teeth.

In newborns, renal excretion is limited, due to the immaturity of glomerular filtration and tubular secretion. The metabolic inactivities of foreign substances (and of natural steroids) by the enzymatic detoxication system linked with microsomal function of the liver cells is not effective at birth. These enzymes go through progressive maturation during the first days of life. But some substances such as phenobarbital or coramine may acclerate the maturation. The competition between non-conjugated bilirubin and various drugs for their bond with plasmatic albumin and the role of the PH. Haematin and the free fatty acids explain several of the accidents observed. The special affinity of the organs of the newborn, the momentaneous sensitivity of the immature tissue (retina : non-myelinized neurone, and erythrocytes) and last, the very different dilution volumes in newborns who have a higher total body fluid content and extra cellular intracellular fluid ratio than adults constitute other explanatory systems for the characteristics of drug metabotism in newborns and more specially in prematures. In recent years it has been noted that these difficulties may be cumulative as in the case of chloramphenicol — but they have a positive counter balancing effect for other drugs such as digoxin, theophylline or phenobarbital.

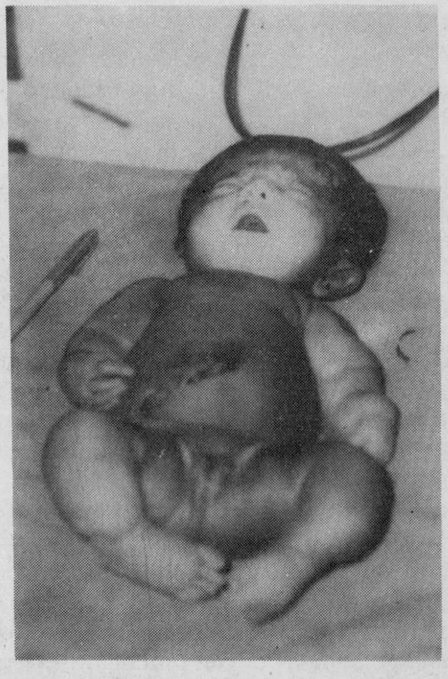

Fig.1.5 : Osteogenesis imperfecta (congenita)

When drugs are administered to the mother during the last day of her pregnancy or even during the delivery, they go into the foetal circulation and sometimes persists after birth. The anaesthetics administered to the mother during labour — the long-lived barbiturates are poorly metabolized and may produce prolonged sleep and respiratory depression in the newborns. It would seem that neonatal hypoglycemia has been observed in relation with the intake of certain sulphonamides or diuretics by the mother. Haemmorrhagic accidents have very recently been described in the offspring of mother taking aspirin by disordered clumping of platelets or phenobarbital by abnormal synthesis of certain coagulation factors. The study of Silverman etl (Paediatrics 18:614, 1956) showed that drug therapy in icteric newborn infants may be extremly hazardous. It was shown that drug with high affinity for albumin can displace bilirubin from the carrier protein resulting in Kernicterus. This has resulted in the exclusion of certain drugs with a high affinity for albumin from the list of potentially dangerous drugs because the maximal molar concentration of the drug in plasma proved to be very low e.g. digitoxin, diazepam and furosemide on the other hand many drugs with a relatively low affinity for albumin but with a high dosages in molar units cause a real risk e.g. cloxacillin, sulphonamides, large doses of carbancillin, aminoglycosides are the safest antibiotics in hyper-bilirubinimia.

The other social poisons coffee, alcohol, tobacco, narcotics are excreted by the mother's milk and may intoxicate newborns and infants. They should be prescribed by nursing women. In 1978 it was suspected that the very high concentrations of nicotine in the milk of mothers who are heavy smokers, play a role in the sudden death of some infants and even may give birth to premature delivery with low birth weight babies.

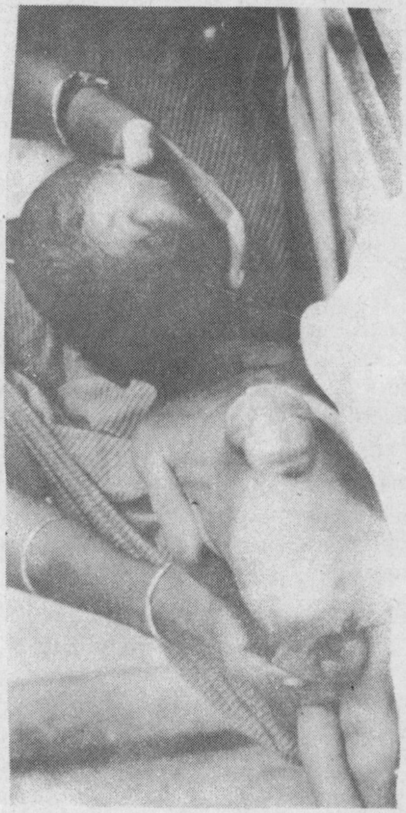

Fig.1.6 : Myelomeningocele (neural tube defect)

When an infant or child is malformed or mentally retarded the parents often blame themselves and attribute the child's problems to events that occured during pregnancy. The cause of about 40% of congential malformations is unknown. Several generalizations can be made about teratogenes. None are harmful to every exposed foetus, some drugs e.g. phenytoines and other maternal conditions (Radiation and infection) may cause only a 2-3 fold increase in the overall incidence of malformations. Since the increase caused by a teratogen may be relatively small, harmful effects may be difficult to demonstrate. In general, exposure during the 1st trimester of pregnancy is probably most harmful.

IMMUNIZATION AT RISK INFANTS

Small-pox vaccine is now considered unnecessary because the disease has been completely eradicated from the world map. In fact the government of India has also largely stopped manufacturing this vaccine since, June 1981. At present the risk of vaccination (2 to 3 deaths per 100-000 doses) is far greater than that of getting the disease. In recent times, considerable doubts have been expressed regarding the efficacy of BCG vaccination. The clinicians should, however be aware that the consensus at present, is still in favour of its continuance as it, definitely prevents severe and often fatal forms of tuberculosis viz. meningeal, miliary and disseminated types.

The children with known convulsive disorders or those who get a convulsion with the 1st dose of DPT vaccine, should not be given this vaccine. All such children should be immunized with DT (dual antigen) which does not contain pertussis vaccine.

The oral polio vaccine is a live attenuated vaccine and the virus is highly sensitive to effects of warm temperature. The duration of vaccine potency depends on the temperature at which the vaccine is stored. The following precautions must also be taken while using polio vaccine : (i) A sterile needle must be used to withdraw polio vaccine every time, otherwise the vaccine may be easily contaminated. (ii) The dose of the polio vaccine to be given must be checked from accompanying instructions. The different preparations contain different concentrations of polio virus and require different changes. (iii) The polio vaccine should be avoided during an episode of gastroenteritis (because of possibility of interference by other enteroviruses). It is also advisable to avoid this vaccine at the onset of a coryzal illness, as this may occasionally be a prodomal of natural polio infection. The vaccine should be discarded if it is discoloured or contains suspended particles.

The measles vaccine can produce reactions in about 25-30% of cases. The onset of reactions is usually 3—4 days after the measles vaccination. The cold, cough, fever, and erythematous rash can occur in all combinations. The fever may occasionally be high grade and may last for 3—5 days. In a small percentage of case all the symptoms may occur mimicking a mild episode of measles. The side effects of measles vaccine are due to the viremia itself and hence require only symptomatic management.

DRUG EFFECTS ON MALNUTRITION

The *malnutrition* is generally complex, and several deficiencies occur simultaneously, leading to functional and/or anatomic abnormalities in almost all organs and tissues. This result is a potentially modified state of response to drugs, depending on four situations; a change in the kinetics of the drugs, modifications in the tissular affinity, altered interactions between drugs and receptors, weakening of the immense defense system due to malnutrition. Some anomalies induced by malnutrition are conducive to a changed orientation in the absorption, metabolism and pharmacokinetics of certain drugs. Indeed several factors are considerably modified, the digestive absorption, the dilution volumes, the plasmatic and tissue proteins, the hepatic and cardiorenal functions. Digestive absorption may be defective due to anorexia, vomiting and diarrhoea, hypochlorhydia, atrophy of the intestinal mucosa, changes in peristalsis, intestinal dysfunctions and modification in the bacterial flora. A great variety of anomalies in the absorption of drugs has been observed in the malabsorption syndromes, particularly in the coeliac disease and pancreatic maldigestions such as mucoviscidosis. The changes in the volumes of the organisms are characterized by an increase in the extra and intracellular fluid, the plasmatic volume and the total body fluid. Plasmatic transport proteins are discussed, particularly albumin and the vector lipo-protein, where as the gammaglobulins are high. There is a decrease in tissue proteins especially the muscular ones and this may lower the tissue affinity. The functions of the liver cell may be altered, decreased synthesis of apoprotein, phospholipides, endoplasmic reticulum and decreased secretion of BSP. Little is known of the state of the hepatic system for an activating drugs. Reduced heat flow and lengthened circulation time along with some alterations in renal functioning, may be observed in severe malnutrition and affect excretion. In truth, these different factors may play in contradictory directions to modify the concentration of the free form of the drugs, increase in the dilution volume but decrease in the bonding plasmatic proteins, decreased and slowed digestive absorption, but the some effect or inactivation and excretion. It is therefore difficult to predict the actual anomalies.

DRUG INTERACTIONS

Drug interaction is commonly delivered as an increased or decreased effect of one or both drugs when two or more drugs are given simultaneously. The aforesaid definitions are usually confined to drug — drug interactions. But as a non-drug adverse reactions from a category by itself, drug-non-drug interactions are also important and relevant in clinical practice.

TYPES OF DRUG-NON-DRUG — INTERACTIONS

1. Drug — food interactions e.g MAO inhibitors and cheese
2. Drug — beverage interactions e.g. Metronidazol and alcohol
3. Durg — laboratory test interaction e.g. L-dopa and Uric acid
4. Drug — infusion fluid interaction e.g. ampicillin and glucose
5. Durg — disease interaction e.g. digoxin and renal failure
6. Durg — Parasitic interactions e.g. Herxhiemar reactions with penicillin
7. Drug — host interactions e.g age and barbiturates
8. Durg — sunlight e.g. phenothiazine and photo alleragy
9. Drug — chemical interactions e.g. DDT and induction of hepatic microsomal enzymes

CLINICAL MANIFESTATIONS ASSOCIATED WITH ALLERGIC REACTIONS TO DRUGS

Generalised reactions

Drug fever
Anaphylaxis

Respiratory tract

Rhinitis
Asthma

Haematological

Thrombocytopenia
Leucopenia
Agranulocytosis
Aplastic anemia

Dermatological

Urticaria
Eczema
Contact dermatitis
Fixed drug eruption
Photo sensitivity
Pruritus
Erythema multiforme & the stevens-johnson syndromes
Toxic epidermal necrolysis
Patchy erythema or morbilliform rash
Exfoliative dermatitis

SPECIFIC STRESSES OF ADOLESCENCE

Certain specific stresses will make the adolescent vulnerable, less likely to mature adequately and more likely either to choose inadequate solutions inappropriate for his potential or to break down. Whether such a break down should be called illness or not, the medical practitioner is likely to be called upon for help, for the incidence of adolescents at risk is high according to various authors although the number referred to psychiatrist remain low. Thus in one study in UK, it was found only 0.5 per cent of the adolescent population were referred. The special factors which contribute to adolescent break down can be grouped as follows. In the first category are factors derived from childhood. Birth injury not only produces specific syndromes such as minimal cerebral dysfunction (M C D) which persists into adolescence, but also makes the child more likely vulnerable to stress. The contribution factors, do seem contribute to some adolescent disturbances. The presence of Psychiatric disturbances in childhood makes the passage through adolesence more difficult. The physical illness and childhood deprivation creates dependency problems. The deprivation in childhood is a frequent finding in a disturbed adolescents.

Many youngsters take the drugs as an experiment or for kicks and soon cease. Those who take them to relieve anxiety or depression are more likely to run into trouble in so far as the drugs usually result in problem — avoiding rather than problem solving e.g forgetting about the need to study for examinations, as opposed to persisting at the task.

Many drugs posses the capacity to produce central nervous system stimulation, depression or hallucinations, or to produce distortions in perception, thinking or judgement. among commonly described drugs are alcohol, the hypnotics (down drugs) such as barbiturates and mandrex (methaqualone and diphenlydramine) stimulants (up drugs) such as amphetamine and cocaine hallucinatory drugs such as cannabis and lysergic acid diethylamine (L S D) and narcotics such as morphia (opium) and heroin. The drugs produce a temporary self-esteem while the ensuring depression is reduced by further drug abuse, at times leading to a vicious circle and drug addiction.

(1) Perinantal pharmacology — Risk of intoxication of the newborn : Neonatology excerpts from XVI International Congress of Paed. at Barcelona, September, 8-13th. 1980.

(2) Royer P : The pharmacology of the contagious Diseases in newborns and children in the developing countries — children in the tropics 1980.

(3) Drug interactions in clinical practice — Quaterly Medical Review, Raptakos, Brett & Co. Ltd, Vol 29 No. 2 April, 1978.

(4) Text Books of Paed — edited by John. O. Forfar; Gavin c, Arneil Churchill Livingstone, Edinburgh and Lond., 1973.

(5) Nelson text book of Paed, Behman — vungham/G AKU — SHON/SAUNDERS 1983.

CHAPTER – TWO

THE NEWBORN

Perinatal and Infant Mortality :

Late fetal deaths (intrauterine death after more than 28 weeks gestation) together with deaths occurring immediately after birth are combined as the perinatal mortality (combined late fetal deaths and infant deaths under seven days of age per 1000 total births) is 78 per thousand (1968-69). The mortality during the first four weeks of life (Neonatal mortality) constitutes almost 60 percent of infant mortality. Common causes of perinatal mortality and their prevention :-

THE FIVE MAJOR CAUSES OF PERINATAL MORTALITY ARE :

1. Low birth weight babies (L.B.W.) – About 30 to 40% babies in India are L.B.W. as opposed to about 5 to 7% of newborns in West and mortality in preterm as 17.9%.
2. Perinatal hypoxia and birth trauma, the mortality is 41.6%.
3. Neonatal infections is leading to morbidity of 10.6% and mortality of 4%. It is estimated that between 150,000 and 200,000 infants die due to neonatal tetanus each year.
4. Congenital malformation – the incidence is 3% in 1978 in Calcutta.
5. ABO and Rhesus iso-immunization – the incidence is low in India as compared to the western countries only 5 to 7 percent of the population in India is Rh negative.

In determining the cause of perinatal death it is necessary to consider not only the morbid anatomical findings and the abnormalities that may have existed in the intrauterine environment and during the process of birth but also medico-social factors such as the quality of antenatal care. Most LBW babies in the west are preterm. In our country about two-third of these are both at term but are small for dates. The mortality in preterm babies is higher than the neonatal mortality for term small for dates babies. The greatest impact on further reduction of perinatal mortality can be made by recognizing various factors that initiate normal labour and application of this knowledge for arrest of labour which starts before term. Early recognition and management of maternal disorders, provision of adequate food and nutritional supplements specially folic acid during the last trimester of pregnancy and overall improvement in the socio-economic status may improve the average birth weight by 100-150 gm. and chances of survival of the infant. To improve and prevent the natal and immediate postnatal mortality, it should be aimed to reduce the perinatal hypoxia, prompt measures to deliver the child with speed and safety are of fundamental importance. The border line cases of cephalopelvic disproportion and malpresentation should be decided with urgently and proper operative interference should be taken and all deliveries must be attended by a paediatrician who should be equipped and experience in resuscitation of asphyxiated babies at birth. The measures should be taken to prevent the neonatal infections. In this regard the pregnant mother should be immunized with Inj.Tetvac at 28,32 and 36 weeks of pregnancy respectively so that baby is protected by maternal transfer of antibodies through placental circulation from developing neonatal tetanus. All early rupture of membranes of more than 12 hours. the mothers will receive prophylactic antibiotics before the delivery and also after the delivery the neonates should also be prevented from infection by proper antibiotic prophylaxis in the immediate post-natal period. In the nurseries, the measure should be taken to minimize the colonisation of bacteria of the baby in the eyes, skin and umbilicus by following barrier techniques of prevention of infection in the nursery. The cleaning measures should be adopted for various equipment used in the nursery to prevent nosocomial infections by opportunistic organism which depends basically on various factors, the micro-organisms, the host, the hospital staff, visitors, instruments, attendants, fellow patients and the environment.

The majority of congenital malformations are not associated with any predisposing etiologic factors and are not preventable with the current state of our knowledge. During the first trimester of pregnancy all types of viral infections, medications and irradiation should be avoided as far as possible. Girls should be given rubella vaccine before they get married. The chromosomal and genetic disorders are more prevalent in mothers aged more than 35 years and also in consanguineous marriages respectively. The prophylactic utility of anti-D immunoglobulin for the prevention of rhesus iso-immunization has been confirmed during the recent years. The injection of anti-D immunoglobulin (250μg.) should be given to Rh negative non-immunized mother soon after the delivery of a Rh positive baby within 72 hours of delivery.

Gestational age group :

Preterm (immature, born early or 'Premature') infant is defined as a baby with a gestation of less than 37 weeks (upto 36 weeks). The term 'Premature' should preferably by avoided in view of its reference to the birth weight in the earlier definitions of prematurity.

Term : Babies with a gestational age between 37-41 weeks are called term babies.

Post term or Post mature :

Babies with a gestational age of 42 weeks or more are classified as post term babies.

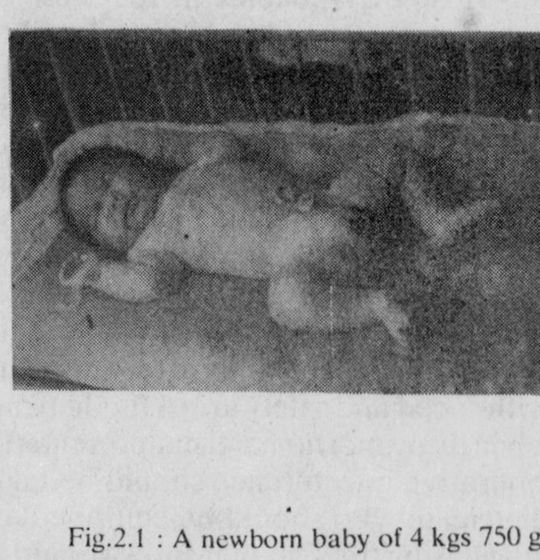

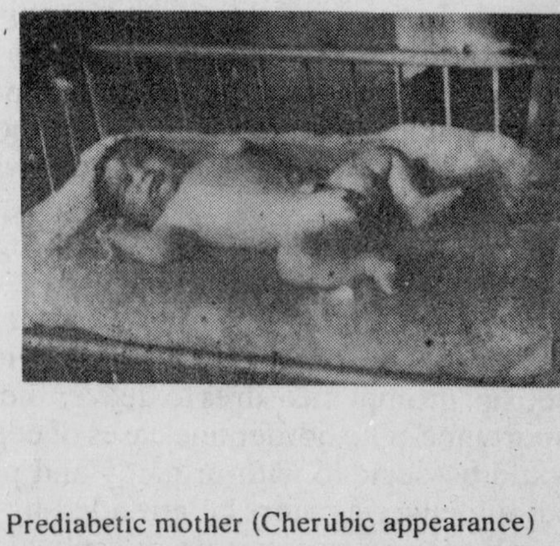

Fig.2.1 : A newborn baby of 4 kgs 750 gms of a Prediabetic mother (Cherubic appearance)

Birth weight : Low birth weight (LBW) — Babies with a birth weight of 2500 g. or less. These include preterm and small-for-dates term babies. In India, for purposes of special care, babies with a birth weight of 2200 g. or less are considered as high risk and are admitted to the special care nursery.

NEONATAL CARE

The present policy of 48 hours discharge of mothers and babies back to their own homes from maternity units provides an aided reason for the early comprehensive examination of all new born infants under this system, abnormalities in a few infants will be inevitably be undetected during the first 48 hours of life, but in practice only a small minority of infants need to be readmitted for hospital care. The birth weight, infant length and skull circumference should be recorded and after completion of the examination the estimated maturity of the infant at the time of birth should be noted.

The problems of neonates in the first few days of life about respiratory difficulty and malformations, advice may be sought. The multiple congenital abnormalities may be present in some infants, thus an infant with tracheo-eosophageal fistula may be found to have congenital heart disease and a renal abnormality. Infections are often

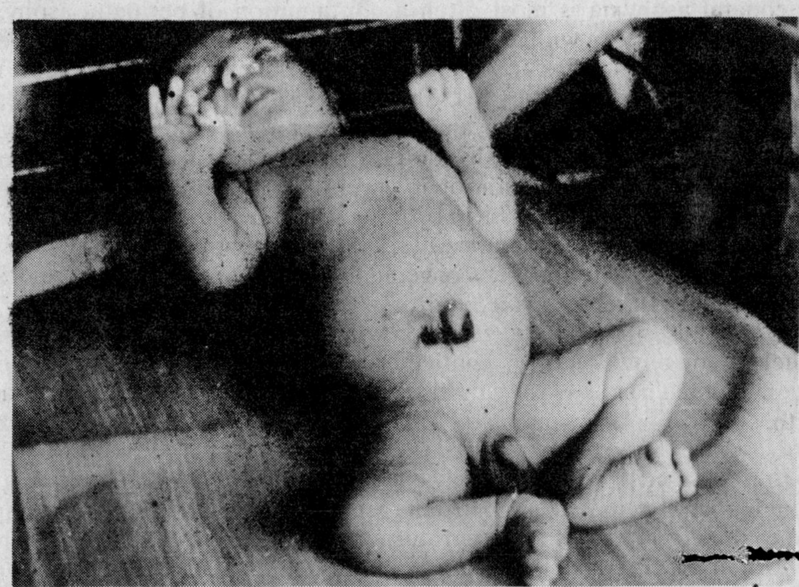

Fig.2.2 : Newborn baby with septicaemia from umbilical infection

septicaemic and multifocal rather than limited to the site of entry due to low level of immunoglobulins. In premature infants immaturity of many systems, temperature regulations, swallowing, respirations and hepatic handling of bilirubin may cause problems in the same infant. It was emphasised that anatomical disorders of the air way and malformations of the heart or lungs in addition to fetal and intranatal causes of asphyxia may prevent normal respiration after birth.

NEONATAL ASPHYXIA

The common problems after birth in the first week of life are —

1. Asphyxia
2. Birth trauma
3. Congenital malformations
4. Feeding problems

5. Haemorrhagic disease of newborn
6. Neonatal jaundice
7. Infections

Among the problems mentioned above, the important is neonatal asphyxia. In the delivery room, the newly born baby should be helped to establish independent breathing. During the foetal stages of development in utero, after the placenta is formed, it serves to transfer nutrition and oxygen from the mother and eliminates the fetal waste products. After seperation from the mother, the baby must breathe immediately or should be made to breathe, because within a few minutes of tying the cord the arterial oxygen tension falls. The birth asphyxia is the commonest medical emergency among newborn babies and is one of the leading causes of neonatal mortality in India.

The neonatal asphyxia is most often a continuation of perinatal asphyxia. The newborn needs to be born with an active respiratory centre and with good peripheral accessory respiratory muscles in order to carry out the vigorous movements required to initiate the first breath. Thus not only the existing perinatal asphyxia but also sedative drugs given to the mother and transferred across the placenta may depress the infant and lead to neonatal asphyxia. This is found in association with congenital cerebral malformation or infection or in cerebral damage caused by birth trauma. The obstruction of the airway at birth by mucus, blood or meconium is common and the establishment of an adequate airway remains the first essential procedure in the treatment of neonatal asphyxia. The congenital malformations which cause obstruction of the airway such as 'Pierre Robin Syndrome' and 'Laryngeal malformations' are rare but important causes of neonatal asphyxia which require immediate treatment. The others such as congenital diaphragmatic hernia — left side is much more common or severe congenital heart disease can also give rise to persistent neonatal asphyxia. After birth, once the baby is separated from his mother, he must breathe immediately or should be assisted to breathe because there are no sources of oxygen in the baby. About 5 to 10 percent of the babies may have difficulty in initiating breathing at birth. The infant is born wet, naked, and partially asphyxiated in a room whose temperature is geared to the comfort of the mother rather than the needs of the baby. Therefore, the newborn at birth tends to lose heat rapidly unless effectively dried, adequately covered and kept warm. The life threatening congenital malformations must be suspected at birth by quick clinical screening of the baby because their prognosis is directly related to the time taken to diagnose them. Establishment of breathing, maintenance of body temperature and early diagnosis of major malformations at birth, therefore, should override all other considerations of care in the labour room.

The overall management o erinatal asphyxia depends upon the clinical assessment of foetal asphyxial states during the active stages of foetal growth before the onset of labour by foetal monitoring and then during labour by Saling (1963) technique of blood sampling from capillary blood obtained by skin prick of the fetal scalp provides a reliable guide to the degree of fetal asphyxia. Then the asphyxial state of assessment of neonatal asphyxia are noted by five objective signs, one minute and five minutes after birth (Apgar) and scoring can be recorded, these are heart rate, respiratory effort, tone, response to catheter in nostril (tested after oropharynx is clear) and colour. There are varying degree of asphyxia neonatorum may be seen. In the mildest cases there may be minimal cyanosis of the extremities, whilst generalized cyanosis and ultimately an ashen pallor represent the more advanced stages. They lusty cry of the healthy newborn infant may be replaced by a weak cry whilst in severe cases the full picture of primary or secondary apnoea is already established. This variation in the degree of depression of respiratory movements reflects the extent to which the respiratory centre is itself depressed. It may be assumed that normal chemoreceptor mechanism are actively stimulating the respiratory centre; for this reason the priority must be to establish adequate oxygenation by positive pressure ventilation rather than by use of stimulant drugs.

The management of birth asphyxia needs after clamping the cord and after the first breath rather than immediately, except in babies with severe birth asphyxia, cord around the neck and rhesus iso-immunization.

The head should be kept low and baby received on a flat surface. The suction of oral cavity, oropharynx and nose should be done immediately by employing gentle intermittent negative pressure of 5-10 cm. of water. Excessive and forceful suction may lead to mucosal damage, bleeding and reflex bradycardia. If the infant does not then cry, followed by vigorous respiration, the pharynx must at once be sucked out with a sterile mucus catheter. Usually this will have the effect of stimulating normal respiration. When respiration still fails to occur, a doctor or a midwife experienced in the art of laryngeal intubation should immediately pass a laryngoscope to the back of the tongue in order to suck out the larynx and to intubate the upper trachea through an endotracheal tube, leaving the tube in place and subsequently the lungs can be ventilated by intermittent positive pressure ventilation, generating a positive pressure of 30 cm/H_2O pressure. It has become a routine practice in neonatal care but where there is no experienced hand, the doctor can carry out mouth-to-mouth respiration, one hand should be placed upon the infant's abdomen to reduce the tendency to inflate the stomach with air.

The other essentials are to maintain the body temperature of the newborn baby just after birth by well clothed, and by this process, environmental temperature of about 28° C. can be maintained. If facilities are available then incubator can be used with proper temperature, humidity and oxygen inhalation controls. The use of drugs do not help much, only when there is history of morphine or allied drugs given within 4 hours of birth, then with asphyxiated infant Nalorphine an antidote of morphine can be used in a dose of 0.1 mg/kg. of birth weight to the newborn or before labour to the mother (0.5 — 1.0 mg.) intramuscularly.

The management of other common neonatal problems have been discussed subsequently in the following chapters. The emphasis is given on the common medical problems in the second week of neonatal life, these are dyspnoea, cyanosis, jaundice and prolonged jaundice, etc.

The management of common medical problems after the 7th day of birth, such as dyspnoea cyanosis, jaundice, abnormal behaviour (CNS problems etc.) pallor, haemorrhage and purpura will have to be discussed. However, before going through the individual problem, let us recapitulate the importance of 2nd week of neonatal period.

There is no definite measures to diagnose a baby in the second week of neonatal period. But one may assess by looking at the umbilicus. The umbilical cord falls in between 6-8 days after birth. The raw surface become covered by a thin layer of skin, the wound is actually healed by 10-12 days.

There are other important land marks of 2nd week of neonatal period. The caloric requirement is 120-150 Cal/Kg/Day. The milk needed is 150-200 ml. of milk/kg/day. The haemodynamic adjustment occurs now, so disorders in relation to cardiovascular and respiratory tract may be exposed in this week. This week is very important for metabolic adjustment of various organic mineral, vitamins and effect of drugs used in the perinatal period leading on the jaundice, anaemia, vitamin and mineral deficiency convulsions and various drug effects, manifested as haemolytic jaundice, anaemia, haemorrhage etc. The baby in this week passes through relative deficiency of passive transported immunoglobulins and not very active IgM of its own leading to infective hazards. Moreover, due to adjustment of feeding in this week the baby develops complications related to gastro-intestinal tract in the way of vomiting, transition stools, kidney and excretory over load. Also there might be presence of thermal instability leading into hypothermia etc.

1. **Dysponea :**

The clinical diagnosis of dyspnoea or respiratory distress in the new born is suspected when the respiratory rate is more than 60 per minute in a quite resting baby and there are inspiratory costal recession or expiratory grunt. The dyspnoea in a newborn with a depressed respiratory centre may be absent despite severe cyanosis. The other infants with active respiratory centre may show severe respiratory distress with or without clinical cyanosis.

Among the neonatal pneumonias, the inhalation or aspiration pneumonia occurs after 7 days of birth, if the infant vomits and inhales a feed. The trache-oesophageal fistula without atresia invariably leads to aspiration pneumonia. In the management of an infant with tracheo-oesophageal fistula, it must be remembered that associated congenital defects are common and that in particular, there may be associated atresia of the small intestine. The broncho pneumonia may follow as a complication after perinatal asphyxia, particularly when areas of primary atelectasis persists. It may also occur as a part of a generalised neonatal septicaemia or as part of the cold injury syndrome. It is common in preterm newborns. The clinical respiratory signs of pneumonia may be absent or minimal in the newborn. It is suspected when the infant is listless and reluctant to feed and the rectal temperature is subnormal. On such slight doubt, chest x-ray, blood count and blood culture should be obtained and proper antibiotic to be used. The combination of Gentamycin and Penicillin is the best. The pulmonary haemorrhage with sudden respiratory distress may occur particularly in low birth weight small for dates often in association with hypoglycaemia commonly occur on 3rd day but may occur after one week or on 7th day can be suspected when blood stained mucus accumulates in the oropharynx.

2. **Cyanosis :**

One should doubt cyanotic and acyanotic congenital heart disease in any new born infant after one week, who develops respiratory distress or cyanosis and sudden development of heart failure.

The recognition of heart failure may at times be difficult due to similarities between the clinical features of cardiac failure and respiratory distress due to pulmonary origin as well as difficulties in the evaluation of cardiac size and jugular venous pressure in a newborn. The useful clinical signs of cardiac failure in the newborn includes tachypnoea, tachycardia, hepatomegaly with or without splenomegaly, oedema — puffiness of face or generalised oedema and rapid weight gain of more than 100 gms. per day, cardio-megaly by ECG and echocardiogram and also auscultatory findings. There might be presence of unexplained vomiting, sweating (VSD) and creps on both bases of the lungs are additional features suggestive of cardiac failure. A severe congenital heart disease can be extremely deceptive at birth. There may be no cyanosis in the first few days of life and the auscultatory signs are normal; insiduously during the next week generalised cyanosis develops with tachycardia and signs of congestive cardiac failure in which progressive enlargement and tender liver predominates. The cardiac murmurs may become evident and creps appear in both lung bases. It should be noted that two cyanotic congenital heart diseases most likely to present with cyanosis in the neonatal period are transposition of great vessels and pulmonary valve atresia are not usually associated with murmurs.

3. **Haemorrhage :**

Due to defective coagulation factors such as prothrombin, factor VII, IX and X deficiency, specially in preterm newborns may lead to bleeding from gastrointestinal tract, umbilical cord stump, circumcision site, nose, subaponeurotic bleeding under the scalp, sub-capsular bleeding in liver and also internal haemorrhages in viscerae. The hepatic insufficiency may be associated with hepatitis and metabolic disorders — galactosemia, fructosemia, inspissated bile syndrome in Rhesus isoimmunisation may lead to haemorrhage in the second week. These are associated with jaundice, purpuric spots etc. An inherited deficiency of coagulation factors rarely present in the neonatal period as haemorrhage in haemophilia, Christmas disease and afibrinogenimia (see also in the chapter of Haematology).

4. **Purpura :**

The critical level of thrombocytopaenia in newborn period is below 100,000 per cmm. It might lead to development of clinical purpura in the second week. The main causes of neonatal thrombocytopaenia are maternal idiopathic thrombocytopaenia, the megakaryocyte depression in bone marrow due to intra-uterine viral and bacterial infection in mothers leading to neonatal hepatitic syndrome and maternal medication in the perinatal period such as salicylates, anticoagulants and diuretics etc. Some hereditary disorders may present very rarely as purpura such as Wiskott-Aldrich syndrome. Due to sequestration of platelet leading to relative thrombocytopaenia in Giant haemangioma and big size cephal-haematoma (See also in the chapter of Haematology).

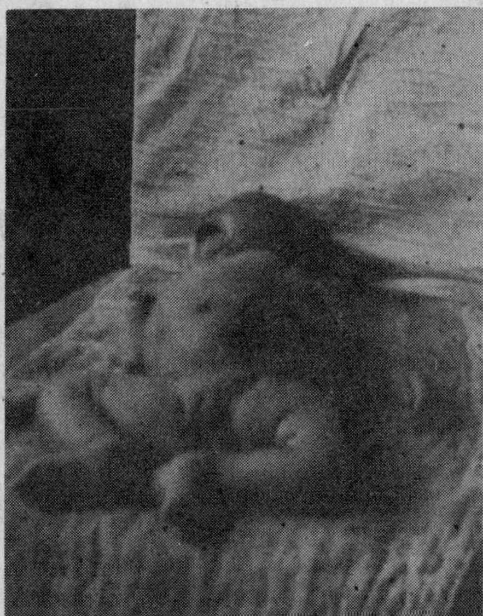

Fig.2.3 : Neonatal convulsion with carpo-pedal spasm

5. **Abnormal behaviour (CNS problems) :**

This week neonatal convulsions like facial twitchings, carpo-pedal spasm or even frank convulsion, jittery, apathy, poor feeding might take place due to deficiency of calcium and excess of phosphorus, due to feeding with cow's milk, pyridoxine deficiency and also from neonatal meningitis. The history of feeding and also presence of infections will help to differentiate the causes. The neonatal tetanus may present on the 7th day (Neonatal convulsion — see also in the chapter of Paediatric Emergency).

6. **Pallor :**

It might be due to perinatal hypoxia, hypoglycaemia, infection with septicaemia, shock, or adrenal cortical failure.

7. **Jaundice :**

The persistent jaundice for more than 2 weeks in the newborn period is termed as 'prolonged jaundice'. In some the intensity of jaundice gradually wanes off while in others the jaundice is prolonged for a couple of weeks more. In most of these conditions, the bilirubin rise is contributed by indirect reacting and direct fraction of bilirubin. To understand the pathogenesis of hyperbilirubinaemia both unconjugated and conjugated, one should follow the role of bilirubin metabolism, which is in transitional stage from the fetal stage, when the placenta was the principal route of elimination of the lipid soluble bilirubin, to the adult stage when the water-soluble conjugated form is excreted from the hepatic cell into the biliary system and then into the gastrointestinal tract.

The 'physiological jaundice' defined as jaundice observed during the 1st week of life in approximately 60% of full term infants and 80% of preterm infants. It is a clinically detectable jaundice becomes present after 30 hours of age, and the serum bilirubin rises to a maximum level of 6 mg/dl. on the 4th or 5th day of life, returning to normal by the 7th day. In prematurely born infants levels between 10 and 12 mg/dl. are commonly reached on the 7th to 10th day of life returning to normal on the fourteenth.

It is now considered likely that there is no single cause of physiological jaundice in the neonate but that it results from the complex interaction of factors which cause (i) increased bilirubin production, (ii) impaired hepatic uptake and excretion of bilirubin, (iii) enteric absorption of bilirubin. In the individual infant, all the factors influencing bilirubin metabolism cannot be rigorously investigated (Arias 1976).

1. Physiological jaundice exaggerated by (a) immaturity, asphyxia, acidosis, infection and excess drugs (Vit. K). (b) Rhesus and ABO isoimmunisation, (so called inspissated bile syndrome), (c) Breast milk jaundice, cretinism and galactosemia.
2. Obstructive jaundice due to neonatal hepatitis and biliary atresia,
3. Familial non-haemolytic jaundice, e.g. Crigler-Najjar, type I & II, Lucy Driscoll, Gilbert's disease and Dubin-johnson Syndrome.
4. Familial haemolytic jaundice, G 6 P D deficiency.

Pathogenesis :

To understand the pathophysiology of prolonged jaundice, one should follow the physiological bilirubin metabolism in the newborn period, the relative hyper-bilirubinaemia, its hepatocellular conjugation and also excretion in the biliary canaliculi.

The commonest form of jaundice in the newborn period is the result of functional immaturity mainly resulting in inadequate formation of glucuronyl transferase so that unconjugated bilirubin accumulates in the plasma known as physiological jaundice. It generally appears after 30 hrs, peak of bilirubin level reaches on the 4th or 5th day and disappears by 7th day. The bilirubin level usually does not exceed 10 mg./100 ml.

The bilirubin is the degradation product of haem and being potentially toxic (especially in the neonates) requires an efficient excretory pathway. The bilirubin being insoluble, is held in circulation by albumin binding when normally has a capacity upto 80 mgm. per 100 ml. The risk of toxic effects from elevated levels of bilirubin in the circulation hypoproteinaemia, displacement of bilirubin from its binding sites on albumin by competitive binding of drugs such as sulpha, acidosis, hyperosmolality due to intravenous alimentation, increased fatty acid concentration secondary to hypoglycaemia, starvation or hypothermia or by factors that increase the permeability of nerve cell membranes to free bilirubin or the susceptibility or brain cells to its toxicity and in the neonates where these conditions may exist there is therefore a real hazard of kernicterus. The signs and symptoms of kernicterus usually appear 2 to 5 days after birth in term infants and as late as the 7th day in premature babies, but hyperbilirubinaemia may led to the syndrome at any time during the neonatal period and may very rarely in later childhood.

The liver has a remarkable capacity to trap organic anions such as bilirubin but the mechanisms of dissociation from albumin and membrane transport into the cell is still not clear. On entering the cell it is bound by two recently discovered non-albumin proteins (Y and Z) whence it is transported to the site of conjugation in the smooth endoplasmic reticulum or microsomes. The conjugation predominantly over 90 percent involves transfer of glucuronic acid from uridine diphosphoglucuronic acid by UDPGA transferase to bilirubin. The bilirubin glucuronide is soluble in water and therefore in bile and its regurgitation back into plasma, as occurs in obstruction, means that urinary excretion can occur. It also tends to stain tissues more readily than unconjugated bilirubin. The delay in UDPGA transferase activity leads to jaundice of prematurity and accounts in part, though only partly, for the so called neonatal physiological jaundice. The suppression by material factors, in milk Steroid Pregnane-3, 20-diol and in serum due to transplacental passage of an inhibitory substance for the induction of hepatic enzymes for glucuronation of Lucy-Driscoll syndrome has been described as well as inhibition of drugs such as Novobiocin, Salicylates and long acting sulphonamides dissociate bilirubin from the albumin-bilirubin complex by competitive inhibition. Vit. K is an oxidant and increases haemolysis. It also blocks 'Y' protein (Cytoplasmic ligandin) necessary for bilirubin uptake by the cells. In the Crigler-Najjar Syndrome there is genetic total absence of the enzyme. An incomplete deficiency, partially correctable by enzyme induces such as phenobarbitone occurs in some cases of Gilbert's Syndrome but not in Crigler-Najjar Type I. Phenobarbitone both parentally given to the mother and postnatally to the neonate, has been shown to induce physiological jaundice by the same mechanism of enzyme induction. The excretion from the cell of conjugated bilirubin involves active transport, it needs some energy drive to transfer conjugated bile through the parenchymal cell membrane into the bile-duct system. Rarely this step may be genetically defective in the Dubin-Johnson and Rotor Syndrome and in Cretinism. It may also be suppressed by drugs, e.g., C-17-alkyl-substituted steroids and in addition, bilirubin has to compete with other substances such as cholecystographic media for the excretory pathway. The block to biliary flow, as may occur in atresia or hepatitis results in regurgitation of conjugated bilirubin, e.g. predominantly conjugated hyperbilirubinaemia.

The excretory process in the child or adult are very efficient. Even if bilirubin production is increased five fold, in the absence of hepatic disease, the serum bilirubin is maintained at levels of less than 1.2 mg./dl. virtually all of it in its unconjugated form. If bilirubin production is even more increased, as in severe haemolysis, there may be impaired hepatic bilirubin metabolism before conjugation can occur, producing an unconjugated hyperbilirubinaemia. Since only lipid soluble, water insoluble bilirubin is retained, the urine is not dark in colour containing no bilirubin. If disease processes cause hepatocellular injury or obstruction of the bile flow, a conjugated hyperbilirubinaemia the bile stained urine is the outcome. Since the causes, clinical features and management of these two types of jaundice are so different, it is most useful to classify the jaundice into these two categories-clinical features, investigations and diagnosis.

The diagnosis of prolonged jaundice is often delayed because failure to distinguish this form of jaundice from the much common form of neonatal physiological jaundice. As paediatricians we should take every opportunity to learn that jaundice in the newborn period with dark yellow or brown urine is not merely physiological beyond the first week in risk neonates and that it might turn to indicate a serious liver or biliary tract disease. Sometimes the diagnosis can rarely be made from clinical examination alone nor on the basis of results of standard lists of liver functions. The priority for investigations should be aimed to identify the causes and complications for which urgent treatment is required. And also to identify those newborns with haemolysis leading to unconjugated hyperbilirubinaemia and those conjugated hyperbilirubinaemia due to biliary atresia from neonatal hepatitis syndrome so that timely surgical corrections can be adopted in many cases of atresias.

The proper perinatal history and clinical examination of all the high risk pregnant mothers and neonates will help to evaluate the cause, the clinical features, investigations and timely intervention of neonatal jaundice. The erythroblastosis due to Rhesus or ABO incompatibility between the mother and fetus is an important cause of severe neonatal jaundice requiring exchange transfusion. The disease can be suspected prenatally by knowing the blood group of the mothers and estimating the titer of anti-D antibodies by indirect Coomb's test. The severity of the in-utero disease can be assessed by amniocentesis for bilirubin and optical density measurement. On the other hand maternal viral infection early in pregnancy, history of blood transfusion or infection leading on to hepatitis B infection in late pregnancy or genetic disease in the family or previous siblings will point to more common hepatocellular problem rather biliary tract obstruction in the neonates.

The appearance of clinical jaundice starting within 24 hours of birth will suggest Rhesus or ABO or very rare minor group incompatibilities. Again it may be due to intra-uterine, intrapartum infections due to toxoplasma, cytomegalovirus, Rubella syndrome. Haemolysis may be due to other enzymes may be due Crigler-Najjar or Lucy Driscoll or Homozygous alpha-thalassaemia. The jaundice starting between 30-72 hours after birth, the commonest causes are physiological jaundice and septicaemia. The jaundice starting after 72 hours of birth are infections due to bacteria also congenital syphilis, neonatal hepatitis and biliary atresia. There might be delayed jaundice due to breast milk feeding, galactosemia and cretinism and congenital hypertrophic pyloric stenosis.

The intensity of physiologic jaundice may be accentuated with the presence of liver immaturity in low birth weight infants, presence of asphyxia, acidosis, hypoglycaemia, use of drugs, associated haemolytic factors etc. The persistent or prolonged jaundice beyond second week of newborn life will suggest inspissated bile syndrome (which may follow hemolytic disease of the newborn) hepatitis, cytomegalic inclusion disease, syphilis, toxoplasma, famililial non-hemolytic icterus, biliary atresia, galactosaemia, cretinism and with parenteral alimentation.

The newborn's behaviour with the progress of jaundice should be noted to diagnose kernicterus. The clinical examinations also includes evidences of infection in umbilicus, skin or eyes, associated fever and splenic enlargement in septicaemia. Hepato-splenomegaly in haemolytic diseases, urine and stool colour-more deep in haemolysis, urine dark and stool chalky white in biliary atresia, waxing and waning in hepatitis syndrome. Ictometer scale reading is also helpful to assess the progress of clinical jaundice.

The laboratory investigations include –

Estimation of serum bilirubin, both direct and indirect, Coomb's test, haemoglobin level, blood groups Rhesus and ABO all from cord blood or afterwards from heel puncture and from peripheral veins. Routine blood examination with haematocrit values. Hbs, TC, DC, Blood film, platelet and reticulocyte count, fragility test, blood culture, Hb-electrophoresis, enzyme studies-G6PD and others. The urine for reducing agents, culture and virus studies. The liver function test, including liver biopsy and cholangiography. The special tests includes estimation of alpha-antitrypsin, alpha-fetoprotein, Rose Bengal excretion and scanning with radio-active iso-tope.

Management :

The diagnosis of prolonged jaundice in newborn period is more delayed due to presence of physiological jaundice at this age. The incidence in our hospital is approximately 1 in 500 of all categories of birth. Even physiological jaundice beyond first week should be taken due consideration and requires urgent investigation. The good antenatal care leading to the atraumatic delivery of a mature infant, also appropriate environment in the newborn period with adequate fluid and calories intake minimise aggravation of physiological jaundice.

The main objective of the treatment is to prevent elevation of serum bilirubin to toxic levels in order to avoid development of kernicterus. In this disorder, death or permanent neurological damage occurs following the deposition of unconjugated bilirubin in the brain. This is considered to occur when the serum concentration of unconjugated bilirubin exceeds the capacity of the serum protein to bind bilirubin. Thus bilirubin protein ratio appears to be a better index for identifying an infant at high risk to develop kernicterus. Bilirubin protein ratio of more than 3.5 is often associate with brain damage. In full term infants an unconjugated serum bilirubin concentration of greater than 20 mg./dl. is associated with a significant risk of kernicterus. It may occur, however, above critical level. In contrast, acidosis, hypoxia, hypoalbuminaemia, prematurity and the administration of drugs such as sulphonamides, a wide range of endogenous anions such as haematin, bile acids and fatty acids compete with bilirubin for albumin binding. Many methods have been proposed for determination of binding capacity of albumin for bilirubin.

As it is already mentioned prevention of hypoxia, administration of oxygen, treatment of acidosis and early feeding are necessary to prevent hyperbilirubinaemia. To stimulate the physiological metabolism of the bilirubin, phenobarbitone 5 mg./kg. daily could be used but it has got more of prophylactic value if given before the jaundice develops. Agar-agar given orally also stabilises the conjugated bilirubin in the intestine and prevents its hydrolysis to the unconjugated form and reabsorption into the blood stream.

The phototherapy as an alternate metabolic pathway for degradation resulting from photo-oxidation of bilirubin. Blue light is the most effective but the white or day light fluorescent tubes are also useful. Bilirubin absorbs light maximally at 450-460 mm wave length. Since phototherapy may require 12 to 24 hours to have a measurable effect, when identified the underlying cause of icterus should be treated e.g., antibiotics for septicaemia, physiologic factors that increases the risk of neurologic damage should also be treated e.g., correction of acidosis.

Exchange blood transfusion is most effective and reliable method to reduce bilirubin levels. It is indicated in the following situations. The jaundice of any etiology exchange transfusion is indicated when serum unconjugated bilirubin approaches 20 mg. per 100 ml. or bilirubin-protein ratio exceeds 3.5. In preterm and sick babies, it may be required even at lower serum bilirubin levels. If at any stage, early signs suggestive of kernicterus are manifested, immediate exchange transfusion should be done. However, a lusty term baby with a serum bilirubin of around 20 mg. per 100 ml. on the 5th or 6th day should not be hurriedly exchanged because improving hepatic maturity at this age is likely to clear off the bilirubin spontaneously. The rhesus haemolytic disease of the newborn exchange transfusion is required urgently soon after birth in the following situations :

(a) Maternal anti-D antibody titer of 1 : 64 or more in a baby with positive direct Coomb's Test in cord blood sample and a history of a severely affected previous sibling.
(b) Cord haemoglobin of 10 G. per 100 ml. or less and bilirubin of 5 mg. per 100 ml. or more.
(c) Serum unconjugated bilirubin of more than 10 mg. per 100 ml. within 24 hours or a level of 15 mg. per 100 ml. within 48 hours of age or if serum bilirubin is rising at a rate of 0.5 mg. per 100 ml. per hour or more.

Early exchange transfusion in these situations reduces the chances of later hyperbilirubinaemia and anaemia by removing antibodies and sensitised red blood cells. The administration of 25 percent solution of salt free albumin in a dose of 1 gm. of albumin per kg. half to one hour before the exchange is useful as it binds the bilirubin that has diffused into the interstitial tissues. Albumin transfusion is not necessary before each exchange. It should be avoided if there is evidence of congestive cardiac failure or severe anaemia.

The direct or conjugated hyperbilirubinaemia includes sepsis, intrauterine infections the after-effects of severe haemolytic disease, biliary atresia/neonatal hepatitis, choledocal cyst, cystic fibrosis, galactosaemia, alpha-l-anti-trypsin deficiency, tyrosinaemia, prolonged total parenteral nutrition, and hepatitis 'A' virus positive hepatitis. The management of sepsis, intrauterine infection and other specific causes are excluded one must consider biliary atresia and neonatal hepatitis. The diagnositc tests are Rose Bengal-I^{131} excretion, stool bile, peroxide haemolysine, serum glutamic oxaloacetic transaminase levels, serum glutamic pyruvic transminase levels, bilirubin levels, and percutaneous needle biopsy have been suggested. The direct exploratory laparotomy limited to liver biopsy and cholecystogram usually provide the definitive diagnosis. The surgical exploration has been shown to be safe and effective. The surgical correction of biliary atresia is rarely possible; however, it is effective when circumstanees are favourable.

Prognosis :

The prolonged jaundice should be considered a sign of gross risk for the infant with the degree of danger that it may represent dependent upon factors that affect primarily the underlying cause with production, metabolism, excretion and distribution of bilirubin after birth.

The genetic and ethnic factors may affect the severity of physiologic jaundice, may prolong jaundice in the neonatal period resulting in hyperbilirubinaemia of pathological nature both unconjugated and conjugated fraction of bilirubin. The mean peak serum unconjugated bilirubin concentrations in Chinese-Japannese, Korean and American Indian full term newborns are approximately double that of other populations. The incidence of kernicterus is increased in oriental neonates and in Greek infants from Lesbos and Rhodes independent of haemolysis from the increased incidence of Glucose-6-Phosphate dehydrogenase deficiency. The other factors that increase the rise of hyperbilirubinaemia mentioned before may result in severe or prolonged jaundice in these infants.

References :

Arles, I.M., Gartner, L.M., Cohen, M., Ben Ezzer, J. & Level, A.J. (1969) : Chronic non-haemolytic unconjugated hyperbilirubinaemia with glucuronyl transferase deficiency, American Journal of Medicine, 47, 395-409. Arles, I.M. (1976) : Extracellular and intercellular transport of bilirubin. In Liver Diseases, in infancy and childhood Ed. Berenberg, S.R. pp. 1-17 The Haque : Martlnus Nijin off.

Mowat. A.P. (1976) : Liver diseases in infancy and children.
In recent Advances in Gastroenterology Ed. Banchin, 1.A.D. Pp. 261-296
Edinburgh, Churchill Livingstone.

CHILD CARE – IMMUNIZATION.

The various immunization programmes launched in India from time to time include National Small pox Control Programmes (which has been abandoned after two years Survillence period was over in 1977 when there was not a single case of small pox was detected); National Tuberculosis Control Programme and recently expanded programme on immunization by Govt. of India in 1979. Since the International Year of the Child is over; it is important to know the immunisation status of the children of this vast country from different regions so that various need-based programmes may be launched and measures taken to improve the immunization status of the child population having low immunization status.

Eighty percent of all the children in the world live in the developing countries. In many rural areas, 25% of the children die before they reach their 5th birthday. In the developing world there are 80 million children born each year who require, but do not receive, protection. In rural as well as urban areas small pox vaccination has proved to be the most accepted vaccination. But now small pox is not a killer in India but the others the tuberculosis, tetanus, diptheria, whooping cough, poliomyelites, measles – these are important causes of mortality and morbidity in the pre-school children of 1-5 years. Moreover, due to rampant malnutrition in this vulnerable age group, they become easy prey of these infectious diseases which are easily preventable by proper immunization. In most of the studies, it has been shown beyond doubt, that the urban children are better protected than their counterpart of village children, though the fact remains that 80% of Indian population resides in rural areas. It has been further pointed out that the immunization status depends much upon the educational standard of the parents, especially the

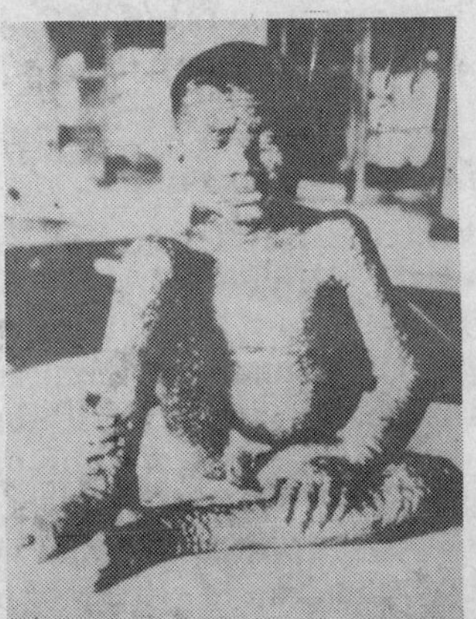

Fig.2.4 : A very rare case – small pox –

mother, and continuous health education has had a positive impact in improving the status of immunization in various regions. In addition to the above factor, the easy availability of vaccines also play a vital role. Besides in India door-to-door facility for these vaccines which is possible by primary health care delivery system, is still not available in 75,000 million villages scattered all over India. Here the people have a low educational standard and not health conscious. Moreover, their local customs and taboos, fear of complications, are a few of the positive hurdles — one encounters in the process of immunization. Immunization programme in India needs a complete re-evaluation through extended immunization programme launched in 1979 and stress should be laid on health education, primary health care, so that people will get care at their doorstep, they won't have to purchase their health like their essential commodities in their day to day life because most of the people still live below poverty level and finish their family income by purchasing food, clothes and shelter.

The slogan is 'small but healthy family' from all aspects — physically, mentally and socially. This can only be achieved by following proper child care, not only after the child is born but from the early date when the ovum is fertilized by the sperm. By and large, it is a team work of obstetrician, paediatrician, family doctor and the social worker, who will join hand in hand to share their individual responsibility to help the fertilized ovum to grow undisturbed as far as possible among the turmoils of unpredictable environmental influences in the pregnancy period, so that one day a healthy baby will be born and become an asset to the nation.

Preventive aspect in child care :

Measures adopted to protect the child from physical and psychological injury and those taken to prevent further deterioration of a child already a victim of disease, together contribute 'Preventive Paediatrics'. Illness in a child can be physical or organic and psychological but it is barely possible to dissociate these two. The physical well being is always modified by the psychological make up and psychological disturbances which nearly always accompany an ill child.

The aim of Preventive Paediatrics is to prevent as many of the above as possible. This can be achieved by —

(a) taking steps to recognise disease and disabilities before it is too late.-
(b) proper instructions in healthy habits, hygiene and sanitation,
(c) immunisation programme,
(d) prevention of deficiency diseases.
(e) prevention of accidents.

Immunisation programme :

Preventable diseases such as Tuberculosis, Diphtheria, Tetanus, Poliomyelitis and Measles are likely to remain a significant public Health problem in the near future. The establishment of an effective social and preventive health service is dependant upon the educational, economic and cultural development of the particular community. Health education and general education are inseparable. The provision of adequately trained personnel and of equipment sufficient to sustain the needs of a permanent preventive health programme, including mass immunisation, requires a sound national economy to support it, together with a national motivation to achieve and to maintain such a service. The ill effects of malnutrition on the outcome of infectious disease in childhood will continue until the results of health education have effectively improved the diets of preschool children and thus the physical standards of child health.

Immunisation may be active or passive. In active immunization antibodies are formed in the host by inoculating the vaccines. In passive immunisation the required antibodies are passively transferred to the patient. Artificial immunisation does not give absolute immunity and if the infection is severe, a child may still suffer from the disease, which may run a mild course.

Important physical illnesses caused by :

(a) Genetic disorders
(b) Infections –
Viral
Bacterial
Rickettsial
Spirochetal
(c) Infestations –
Protozoal
Helminths
By insects
(d) Birth defects
(e) Deficiency diseases
(f) Immunological disorders
(g) Neoplastic disorders
(h) Physical causes –
Accidents and injuries
Radiation hazards
Thermal injuries

(i) Chemical –
Poisonings.

B.C.G. Vaccination :

This vaccine, introduced by Calmette and Guerin, and named after them offers protection against Tuberculosis. Bovine attenuated tubercule bacilli are injected interdermaly.The body 'learns' to achieve sufficient resistance to fight turberculous infection in future. B.C.G. can and must be given to all those who have not suffered from tuberculous infection. Children already infected, as evidenced by a positive tuberculin test need not be given B.C.G. According to the present B.C.G. programme of the Government of India, B.C.G. is given to all children, who are not suspected to be suffering from tuberculosis, without preceding tuberculin test. This will help to increase the pace of B.C.G. immunization. B.C.G. immunization may be given soon after birth, as children are more easily available at this age and a prior tuberculin test is not required. Simultaneous B.C.G. and small pox vaccination has been carried out in the neonates with satisfactory results. B.C.G. vaccination should be avoided during an acute infection and physiological jaundice in the neonatal period.

The freeze dried vaccine is to be preferred as it is stable even at a temperature of 20°C. The liquid vaccine must be stored at a temperature of 2° – 4°C and should not be exposed to direct sunlight. Freeze dried vaccine has antigenic properties similar to those of liquid vaccine and these are maintained for 6 months at 20°C.

B.C.G. is administered intradermally over the left deltold region in upper arm. Subcutaneous injection may lead to complications, such as abscess formation. The usual dose is 0.75 mg. (0.05-0.1 mg.) of the moist weight of the organisms in 0.1 ml. A satisfactory injection should produce a wheal about 5 mm. in diameter. No dressing is required following the injection. Intradermal injection method has also been used for employing a dermojet injection. This method is rapid, painless and effective. Satisfactory reports have also appeared following oral administration of a highly attenuated B.C.G. vaccine. Following the intradermal injection, a papı e develops at the site of injection within 3 to 6 weeks. This gradually becomes large ‿uring the 2-3 weeks and later may or may not develop into a shallow ulcer, 5 to 10 mm. in diameter which completely heals after few weeks. At times, there may be a discharge of the contents from the ulcer in which case a dressing should be applied over the ulcer. The lesion usually subsides after 2 weeks leaving behing a tiny scar. This scar persists for several years and serves as an identification mark of past B.C.G. immunization. Moderate axillary gland enlargement may accompany the appearance of the ulcer. A successful B.C.G. vaccination leads to positive tuberculin conversion in 6-12 weeks and this is taken as an indication of development of immunity to tuberculosis. The level of protection conferred by this vaccine is usually 50-60 percent and may be as high as 80 percent. In the majority of cases adequate immunity persists for 5-10 years, after which a repeat immunization is necessary.

An Isoniazid-resistant B.C.G. has now been developed which is of some value in India where breast feeding is essential for the survival of newborn infants. By this means the baby of a mother with open tuberculosis may be protected with isoniazid (INH) and INH-resistant B.C.G. and breast feeding may be permitted. I.N.H. resistant B.C.G. given less immunity than the standard B.C.G. Even if INH-resistant B.C.G. is not available, the newborn should be protected with INH until the mother stops coughing out acid fast bacilli and then B.C.G. should be given to the baby. The mother should receive full anti-tuberculous treatment, the baby being isolated from her for the first 48 hours to allow the protective blood level of INH to be reached. There after, feeding at the breast is permitted, INH being continued until Mantoux conversion has occurred.

B.C.G. as a diagnostic Test :

In a tuberculin test survey it has been noted that due to negative reaction above 40% of children with active disease and also high drop out rate, tuberculin test could not be read in many cases. Hence a procedure of doing B.C.G. vaccination after the prior TT in a mass immunisation has been considered futile and impracticable. It is under these circumstances that many workers have recommended direct B.C.G. vaccination in B.C.G. vaccination without prior TT. The main objectives of the various workers in recommending direct B.C.G. was to cover as much population as possible particularly in mass immunization.

However, it was emphasized by some of these workers that B.C.G. could be used as a test to detect tuberculous infection and disease. The B.C.G. in proved cases of tuberculosis are found that direct B.C.G. did not produce any adverse reaction. Moreover, it will show accelerated reaction in active tuberculosis where the TT was negative. So B.C.G. can be used as a diagnostic test.

Complications :

Serious complications of B.C.G. are rare and are mostly due to the wrong selection of cases.

1. Recurrent ulceration and discharging of the contents at the site of injection of several months (to be left alone).

2. Undue enlargement and liquefaction of the regional lymph modes. This requires radical excision of the glands but no antitubercular treatment. Some physicians aspirate the local abscess and give a short term isoniazid therapy.

3. Abscess and sinus formation due to break down of axillary lymph nodes (drainage of abscess and scraping of the sinus with antitubercular treatment).

4. Occasional development of lupus vulgaris at the site of injection (to be treated with anti-T.B. drugs).

5. Keloid formation at the site of injection (can be surgically removed).

6. Very rarely generalized lesions following B.C.G. vaccination have also been described (this requires anti-T.B. treatment).

In general terms it can be said that local lesions produced by the freeze dried vaccine are much smaller than those produced by liquid vaccine and hence whenever available one should prefer the freeze-dried vaccine.

SMALL POX IMMUNIZATION

The first vaccination against small pox was carried out by Edward Jenner in 1978 in St. George Hospital, U.K, although the same was practised in India as arm to arm inoculation long before this date. Small pox immunization has been responsible for saving more lives and preventing more disfigurement than all other immunizations. Universal and repeated vaccination is the only sure method for prevention of small pox.

There are three types of small pox vaccines available for routine immunization —

(a) Fluid type — containing vaccine virus in glycerinated calf lymph.

(b) Freeze-dried vaccine — It is much more potent than the fluid type and maintains its potency for several months at room temperature even in tropical countries and hence this is the vaccine of choice for our country. From 1967 onwards, this type of vaccine is being manufactured and used in our country.

(c) Highly attenuated vaccine (Kempe's vaccine) — for use in children with eczema, other allergic reactions and in cases of hypogammaglobulinaemia — this is at present not available in India. But after 1977, The Govt. of India has stopped supply of this Vaccine.

The optimal age for small pox vaccination in our country is between one and three months but, it could be given in the latter half of the first week of life, before the child leaves the maternity hospital, simultaneously with B.C.G. The rate of 'non-take' are comparatively more in the newborn period than between one to three months. In case of an unsuccessful take, vaccination should be repeated every 1-3 months till the child shows a definite positive take. Negative take does not mean natural immunity against small pox as the disease is known to occur in persons who had unsuccessful small pox vaccination repeatedly. Following a successful take, the child should be reimmunized every 3 years to maintain the immune status. Primary immunization is compulsory and every child is required to receive it by the age of 6 months, but there is no compulsion for repeat immunization. This rule is not in vogue now. Postvaccinal encephalitis is commoner in older child.

The sites of primary vaccination are (1) right upper arm over the lower part of the deltoid, (2) leg vaccination over the calf, (3) thigh, upper lateral aspect of thigh, (4) and sole — the hollow of the sole. Any of the above sites is satisfactory for primary immunization. Anterior surface of the forearm is preferred for revaccination. The selected area should be washed with soap and water before the vaccine is applied.

Spirit or alcohol should not be used as it sterilises the vaccine. Ether or acetone may be used following washing with soap and water but should evaporate completely before the vaccine is applied. The following techniques have been used for inoculation :-

(a) Scratch method — which is the one in vogue in our country,
(b) Multiple — puncture method,
(c) Intradermal injection (undesirable),
(d) Jet injection.

The best (preferred) is the scarification technique. Only one insertion is enough due to high potency of Russian freeze dried vaccine now available in India because two insertions may increase the chances of complications. More insertions do not guarantee greater immunity.

Observation of results :

A successful primary reaction would pass through the stages of papule, vesicle, pustule and crust formation. The papule appears on the fourth or fifth day, the vesicle on 6th or 7th day and the pustule on 8th to 10th day. The pustule starts drying up from the 12th day leaving a crust which sheds by the end of the 3rd week. An accelerated reaction occurs in persons previously immunized when the whole process is rapid and may complete within a week.

Complications are uncommon :

They are more frequent after primary vaccination in older children and adults.

1. Secondary infections —

   (a) Abscess, (b) Osteomyelitis, (c) Tetanus.

2. Abnormal viral distribution —

   (a) Because of auto-inoculation secondary vaccinia infection may occur at ectopic sites on the skin.

   (b) Eczema vaccinatum. Eczematous skin gets infected with vaccinia. Mortality rate is high.

3. Abnormal host response —

   (a) Generalised vaccinia,

   (b) Vaccinia gangrenosa — a prolonged progressive infection with viraemia. This is usually fatal if not treated with hyperimmune vaccinial gammaglobulin, but is fortunately very rare.

4. Skin eruptions — allergic reactions are frequent.
5. Post-vaccinal Encephalitis —

This is a rare but serious complication and carries a high mortality. This usually occurs 11-14 days after primary vaccination especially in older children.

Contraindications to vaccination :

1. Pregnancy in women — especially in the first trimester of pregnancy.
2. Children with allergic or other chronic skin diseases as eczema.
3. Children on corticosteroid therapy.
4. Hypogammaglobulinaemia.
5. Child who have recently suffered from any infectious diseases.

Passive immunrzation against small pox is carried out by means of specific hyperimmunoglobulins prepared from the serum of recently vaccinated donors or from convalescent serum. This could be used for household contacts of small pox who have never been vaccinated or vaccinated long back. Hyperimmune vaccinial gammaglobulin is life saving in vaccinia gangrenosa.

Alternately Methisazone (n-acetyl isalin-thiosemicarbazone) may be used. Recently immunisation against small pox is not compulsory and it is a choice of the parents.

Triple vaccination (Diphtheria, Pertussis, Tetanus) :

It offers protection against Diphtheria, Pertussis (Whooping Cough) and Tetanus. It differs from B.C.G. and small pox vaccines in that it requires three doses at intervals of 4-6 weeks before adequate immunity is built up, whereas one dose of B.C.G. and cow-pox vaccine is adequate. It is preferable to start in the fourth month as that 3 injections are completed by the end of sixth month. Booster injection is given after one year of primary immunization and second booster at the age of 4-5 years. It is better to avoid the pertussis vaccine from the tripple vaccine for the second booster. Post-vaccinal encephalopathy due to pertussis vaccine in the triple antigen has been reported rarely.

Diphtheria Prophylaxis :

The maximum incidence of diphtheria is in the age froup, 1-5 years, although it is seen in older children and even in adults. All children below the age of 10 years should be immunized against diphtheria. Injections of diphtheria toxoid to children upto the age of 5 years is not likely to give rise to any significant general reactions.

When used alone, the recommended dose for primary immunization is 2 injections of 1 ml. at an internal of 4-12 weeks. A third dose is given within 6-12 months of the second dose. Following the full immunization booster doses are required every 5 years. If a child so immunized comes in contact with a case of diphtheria a booster dose of 0.5 ml. is sufficient in most instances. ADS for passive immunization of such children is seldom required and should generally be avoided. Non-immunized contacts, however, should be given a dose of 3,000-5,000 units of ADS.

Complications :

Directly attributable to diphtheria immunization are uncommon.

This can be minimised by the following precautions :

1. The antigens containing mineral carrier should be given deep into the muscle.
2. Cautious immunization of children above the age of 10 years and those with an allergic diathesis.
3. During periods with high prevalence of poliomyelitis in the community, poliomyelitis immunization should take precedence over diphtheria immunization.

Pertussis Immunization :

The inherited immunity against pertussis is of little importance and hence every child needs to be protected against whooping cough infection. The usual course of active immunization consists of three doses of 1 ml. of plain vaccine containing 20,000 million organisms per ml. given at intervals of 4-6 weeks by the subcutaneous or intramuscular route, starting at the age of 2-3 months. Booster doses are given at the age of 18 months and 4 years respectively. Subsequent booster doses are to be avoided as the vaccine causes more severe complications when administered to children above the age of 5 years.

Reactions to pertussis vaccine :

Local reactions like redness, swelling, pain and tenderness and general reactions like fretfulness and a moderate rise in temperature, is to be expected in about 50 per -cent of the children. These reactions tend to be more severe in older children. It may precipitate convulsions in a child with a convulsive tendency, in which cases further doses of the vaccine should be given, to such children, with the strictest precaution and under close medical supervision. Rarely pertussis immunization may lead to encephalopathy, anaphylaxis and even death. Pertussis vaccine should not be given in a child with history of convulsions.

Tetanus Prophylaxis :

Tetanus is very prevalent in India, and carries a high mortality. The administration of anti-tetanus serum which is of equine origin, as a prophylactic measure in case of injuries is undesirable, may be dangerous and at times may end fatally. It carries risk of sensitizing the individual to further injections of horse serum. Cases are on record of patients developing tetanus, even after seroprophylaxis. The best way of protection against tetanus is by active immunization. Tetanus toxoid available now-a-days, causes practically no unpleasant reactions.

Immunization against tetanus consists of 3 injections of 1 c.c. each, of aluminium absorbed toxoid. The first two injections are given at interval of 4-6 weeks, whereas the 3rd dose is given 6-12 months after the second injection. A high degree of immunity is conferred following the third dose which can be maintained throughout life by administering a dose every 5-10 years and also in case of a tetanus prone injury. It may be re-emphasized that in case of a major tetanus prone injury A.T.S. may have to be given in addition to the toxoid. The perons who have not been immunized properly should be protected by human tetanus immuno globulin (TIG). It does not produce serum sickness.

The best way to treat fresh tetanus-prone injuries in previously non-immunized persons is by carrying out thorough surgical debridement of the wound, followed by administration of antibiotics for seven days.

If required, human tetanus anti-toxin should be preferred in the prevention of tetanus, as unlike antitoxin of equine origin, homologous antitoxin does not cause sensitization. The dose of TIG is 3,000 — 6,000 units, given intramuscularly (IM).

Since there is no natural immunity against tetanus, immunity may be induced in the mother, by actively immunizing her while she is pregnant. This is done by administering to her, two injections of the absorbed toxoid, at 6 weekly intervals, commencing from the 4th month of pregnancy. A 3rd dose is given 2-4 weeks before the expected date of delivery. This regimen produces a high degree of immunity in the mother, and in the newborn child. This will be effective in reducing the incidence of tetanus neonatorum. Mild reactions like fever, local swelling, erythema and lymphadenopathy may occur in a small number of cases, severe reactions are unknown.

Poliomyelitis immunization :

In our country, poliomyelitis is essentially a disease of infancy and childhood. The emphasis should be on the immunization of all infants during their first 6-9 months of life.

Types of vaccine :

Two types of vaccine are available for immunization against poliomyelitis (1) Salk's inactivated vaccine, developed in 1952-53, (2) Sabin's live attenuated vaccine, developed by 1955. In India, a modern polio virus vaccine production centre for the manufacture of live attenuated vaccine has been set up in Coonoor. By 1960 attenuated polio virus vaccine prepared from the Sabin's strain got universal recognition, and because of its ease of administration this vaccine has now practically replaced the inactivated vaccine all over the world. WHO report (1966) shows oral polio virus vaccine is the safest live antigens in use and hence it can be safely used in all susceptible persons. There are 3 types of polio virus — (1) Brunhilde, (2) Lansing, (3) Leon.

Polio virus vaccines provide protection against paralytic strains of poliomyelitis virus. Each type of attenuated live virus multiplies in the intestinal tract, produces localized gut resistance to virus of the same type and also stimulates the production of type specific humoral antibodies. The protection offered by the development of localised resistance in the intestinal tract to virus growth is independent of specific circulating antibodies.

A polyvalent oral vaccine effective against all the three types is being used for routine immunization in our country. The immunization may be carried out simultaneously with triple antigen from the age of 4 months by administering the vaccine in 3 doses at 4-6 weeks interval, in a dose of half to one ml. (the dose of the vaccine depends on the concentration of the antigen). The schedule for booster doses for polio vaccine is not well established. Some physicians give a booster dose after 12-18 months and after 3 years. Booster doses are probably necessary in our country as primary vaccine might not have established due to interference of the other enteroviruses in the intestinal tract with establishment of polio vaccine virus. As the alimentary tract is comparatively free of enteroviruses during winter, this is the ideal season for oral immunization. Sabin vaccine should be given to the entire vulnerable population in the community during an epidemic of poliomyelitis without any untoward effect. It helps in curtailing the spread of the epidemic quickly. The same does not hold true for the Salk vaccine. Breast feeds should be avoided for 2 hours before and after a dose of oral vaccine as the antibodies against polio in breast milk may interfere with its antigenic effect. Polio vaccine can not be freeze dried and liquid vaccine has to be used which has a short life and needs to be stored at low temperature.

Inactivated poliomyelitis vaccine should be stored at 2° - 5°C, at which temperature it remains potent for about 12 months. Live attenuated poliomyelitis vaccine retains its potency for at least two years when stores at minus 20°C. At 4°C, the potency is retained for 6 months, whereas at 18° - 20°C, the potency is retained for not more than 7 days. Polyvalent polio vaccine should be given even to those children who have suffered from active polio as they may develop immunity from infection, for only one type of the virus. Vaccination in these cases could be started a month after the acute attack.

Poliomyelities vaccine should be avoided in (a) acutely ill patients, (b) patients on high dosages of corticosteroids and during (c) first trimester of pregnancy.

Salk vaccine is given i.m., in three doses, 1 ml. at sixth month, seventh month and a third injection after six months. This interval from the first injection and the time interval between the injections is chosen after large field trials, because of the very satisfactory antibody production response. A booster dose needs to be given every two years.

There are few dangerous complications of polio immunization if the vaccine is reliable and cases for immunization are not selected properly. A case with fever, respiratory infection or gastroenteritis should not be vaccinated until completely symptom free. It is not possible to protect other children by administering this vaccine if a child in the family is suffering from poliomyelitis. Gammaglobulin should be used for family contacts under five years old. Older siblings and parents do not usually need gammaglobulin or active immunisation as by five years most children develop a sufficient titer of antibodies.

Measles Vaccine :

This recent addition to immunization programme is still under trial in the United States, U.K. It is now available in India. Measles has high morbidity and mortality, bacterial complications are frequent and encephalopathies following measles are not rare. Pre-existing disease like tuberculosis worsen the prognosis. Measles should therefore be prevented with the use of this vaccine. It is included in the EPI programme in India.

Active immunization is now available. Killed vaccine should not be used. Live attenuated vaccines require a single injection only but is more liable to cause reactions, particularly fever and rashes, but occasionally convulsions which are usually 'febrile'. The risk of convulsions after live vaccine is much less than with a natural attack of measles.

Vaccination is carried out at 9-12 months of age; infants younger than this may fail to respond owing to neutralization of the virus by maternal antibody. It is wise not to vaccinate infants with a history of convulsion. It is also contraindicated if the child is receiving drugs such as steroids, which would affect the antibody response.

Pregnant women should not be vaccinated since, on theoretical grounds, there is a risk that the virus could damage the foetus as is known to occur with vaccinia. Recently vaccinated children are not infectious to others. There are different opinions regarding immunization against Cholera and Enteric fevers. Better hygiene and sanitations, will reduce the need of immunization.

In passive immunization methods the use of gamma globulin deserves mention. It is an established fact that the various antibodies are present in the gamma globulin fraction of human plasma. The proper amounts of antibodies introduced in the human system are expected to prevent or at least to minimise the severity of the disease. Human gamma globulins as prepared from placental blood appear to offer such a promise and have been tried for prevention and attenuation of diseases like measles, infective hepatitis, poliomyelitis, German measles, chicken pox, mumps etc. An I.M. injection of gamma globulin in the dose of 0.04 to 0.05 ml./kg. body weight to contacts of such cases is recommended. There is no contraindication or complication with its use.

The following schedule is recommended by the Government of India

Immunization Schedule

3–9 months	Triple antigen (DPJ)	: 3 doses at monthly interval
	Polio	: 3 doses
	BCG	: 1 dose
9–12 months	Measles	: 1 dose
1½–2 years	DPT	: 1st booster
	Polio	: 1st booster (4th dose)
School entry (5 years)	DT	: 2nd booster
	Polio	: 2nd booster (5th dose)

10 years	Typhoid	: 2 doses at monthly interval
Pregnant women	TT	: 2 doses at monthly interval

The aim should be to complete the immunization as soon as possible and certainly within the first year. Unfortunately the EPI coverage is still low. The coverage for 1982 was — DPT (3 doses) 35%, Polio (3 doses) 11%, BCG 14% and TT (2 doses) 25%. Every effort must be made to improve the situation and mothers and young children should be immunized wherever they are.

Bibliography

Udani, P.M. : Tuberculin Test in Pediatric Practice.

Preventive Paediatrics — A seminar on extended immunization programme and various others immunisation held in Delhi in 1980.

Ghosh Shanti — The Feeding and Care of infants and young children — *New revised edition — VHAI.*

CHAPTER – THREE

FEEDING PROBLEMS OF NEWBORNS AND INFANTS

Nutrition is the basis of child health the world over and a knowledge of its essential is necessary for all physicians, most of all for pediatricians, as it is, during the early years that health and growth, depend most on our adequate and properly balanced nutrient intake (Jelliffe, 1974).

Modern scientific nutritional knowledge gives approximate guidance concerning the needs of the growing infant and young child for calories, protein, fat, minerals and vitamins. Moreover, recent work indicates that the situation is more complicated than previously thought in relation to the reliability of such estimates, to the interaction of nutrients present, and to the presence of previously unsuspected ill-understood components particularly in human milk (e.g. nucleotides, polyamines and linoleic fatty acids).

BREAST FEEDING

The advantages of breast feeding are numerous although perhaps more evident in India where the mother's inclination and ability to breast feed may be the principal factors which determine whether the infant will survive the first year of life. This is due to the relative freedom from gastrointestinal infections enjoyed by breast-fed infants. The factors which contribute to this freedom from infection include :

1. Lack of contamination from domestic receptacles.
2. The presence of anti-bacterial agents in breast milk, such as lactoferrin and the bifidus factor which inhibits the growth of infecting organisms.
3. The secretion of immunoglobulins notably IgA, lysozyme in human milk which interact with intestinal mucosa of the infant gut.
4. The induction of appropriate conditions in the infant gut lumen which enhance its colonization by non-pathogenic bacteria. In addition large numbers of live cell present, particularly active phagocytic macrophages.

Breast feeding is a skill which needs to be taught. Ideally, instruction should take place in the antenatal clinic and should include a practical demonstration by a nursing mother and advice concerning breast hygiene. Gentle manipulation of the nipples using an emollient cream is often adviced during the last three months of pregnancy but the value of this procedure remains to be established.

The infant should first be put to the breast within a few hours of birth but sucking should initially be restricted to a few minutes to avoid damage to the nipple epithelium. By the end of the first week the milk supply should be regulated to the infant's demand. The bulk of the milk from each breast is obtained during the first few minutes of feeding so there is little advantage in keeping the infant at either breast for more than 10-15 minutes. Only thing to be reckoned that 'hind' milk contains more fat than 'Fore' milk. Both breasts should be given at each feed. The conditions in which feeding takes place are important since anxiety or disturbances diminish the flow of milk. The mother and infant should be comfortably positioned in calm and quiet surroundings, conditions which are not always readily obtained in hospital. The volume of milk secreted increases progressively with the demands of the growing infant. Thus after 3 to 4 months a secretion of 800 ml. of breast milk per day would not be unusual. Such a volume will provide 560 calories together with 10 g. of protein and 240 mg. of calicum. It is, therefore, important that the additional nutritional burden for the mother is adequately met by corresponding supplementation for her diet.

There are few contraindications to breast feeding such as maternal tuberculosis, acute infections in the mother as temporary and chronic conditions such as heart disease, chronic nephritis, each case should be evaluated on its merits. Although in most cases the supply of breast milk matches the infant's demands this is not always immediately achieved.

Test Feeding :

When an inadequate supply of milk is suspected, it should be confirmed by test weighing the infant before and after each feed to provide a measure of the milk ingested over a 24 hour period, since the flow of milk vary throughout the day.

Aerophagia :

Infants who are inadequately feed tend to swallow air during and between feeds. They might suffer from 'air colic', weight gain is impaired and such infants are initially constipated but later on may have small, greenish, often frequent 'hunger stools'.

Lactation Failure :

The causes are in the mother and also in the baby. Maternal causes may be local such as inverted or depressed nipples and general causes including anxiety, fatigue and malnutrition. The causes in the infant low birth preterm and small for date babies underlying disorders for example nasal obstruction, structural anomalies of the palate or incoordination of swallowing and respiration.

ARTIFICIAL FEEDING

The mother who is unable or unwilling to feed from the breasts and also those mothers who just after delivery cannot provide breast milk supply, an additional source of nourishment for the infants must be provided. This is normally an animal milk such as cow, goat, buffallo and ass's milk in various parts of India or common milk available as 'Tin Food' in powder forms, which is offered after each breast feed as 'complementary' feeds in distinction from total replacement of a breast feed, known as 'supplementary' feeds. The volume and nature of the complementary and supplementary feeds to be offered should be determined by experience but the

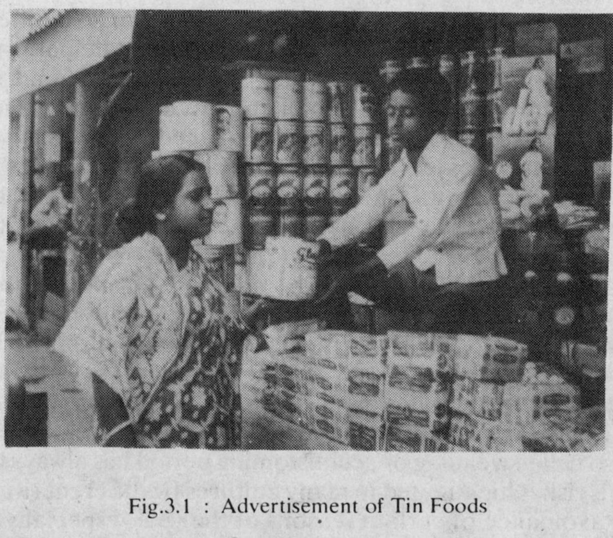

Fig.3.1 : Advertisement of Tin Foods

differences between expected and measured intake on 'test weighing' may be taken as a guide.

Cow's milk, most usually, is employed as artificial feed, either fresh or on one of its processed, tinned forms, is very different from human milk in particular contains about two to three times the content of protein (especially relatively indigestible casein), the same amount of fat, but bigger molecular size and about half as much milk sugar (lactose) as is found in breast milk. The cow's milk has to be boiled, both to kill harmful bacteria and also the heat makes the protein and fat more digestible. Unless from a reliable source, fresh liquid cow's milk is often a rather uncertain dangerous fluid, as, in many places it is likely to be contaminated, diluted and adulterated.

The dried or powdered milk is made in India by different firms as full cream, three-fourth and half cream, according to their content of fat. Powdered milk has the advantage of being compact, light in weight and hence easily transportable. It is also sterile untill the tin is opened, when it soon becomes contaminated.

Full strength cow's milk can be approximately reconstituted by adding one rounded teaspoonful (with a volume of about 5-6 ml.) of full cream powdered milk to 1 ounce of boiled water. This method is very approximate, as the compactness of different brands of dried milk and size of spoon both vary, but has to be as simple as possible. The modification of fresh cow's milk for babies under 3 months can be carried out by (i) diluting with water (2 parts of boiled milk : one part of boiled water), (ii) adding sugar (1 level teaspoonful of household sugar to each feeding). Boiled undiluted cow's milk, with sugar added, can be given after the age of 3 months. Even there are controversies about dilution of Cow's milk seeing 3 months of age. Full cream powdered milk can be used at the strength of 1 rounded teaspoonful to 1 fluid ounce of boiled water, and evaporated milk can be diluted 1:1 with boiled water. Always sugar should not be added to both. Many other animal milks are customarily used in different parts of India, and can be employed in much the same way as has been suggested for fresh liquid cow's milk. Even buffallo's milk which has a much higher fat content (9%), can be diluted and reinforced with sugar in the same manner. As a rough guide, young infants in the first 6 months of life need approximately 150 ml./kg. of body weight (2.5 fluid ounce/lb.) per day of modified cow's milk, prepared from fresh cow's or powdered milk. It is then possible to calculate the daily amount of milk needed by knowing the baby's weight. Number and timing of feedings as in breast feeding on demands, the baby should be allowed to develop his own schedule of feeding and sleeping. However, usually this will settle into an approximate pattern of about three hourly feeding upto three months and then four hourly feedings. For artificial feedings, the feeding bottles, cup and spoon etc. are used. One should be careful to advise the mothers regarding the sterilisation of feeding utensils so that bacterial contamination could be avoided. The vitamins and artificial feeding, addition of Vit.C be added to the diets from 1 month of age either in the form of fruit juice or as ascorbic acid tablets (30 mg. each day). An addition of extra Vitamin 'D' is not required in our tropical environment but in premature or low birth weight infants extra dose of Vit.D — 400 — 800 I.U. daily should be added and also the babies should be adequately exposed to sun rays. Those who are fed with skimmed milk formula, Vit. A must be added to the diets. Artifically fed babies in our country should be introduced to a wider diets earlier than breast fed infants. They are already at risk of developing weaning diarrhoea as a result of artificial feeding and usually will be receiving less milk than desirable, so that extra calories, protein and other nutrients are needed. The so called weaning or accoustoming period has always been recognised as dangerous. This risk is highlighted in many cultures by different rituals to propitiate the Gods, by the avoidance of certain seasons of the year, especially the hot seasons and also by classical time periods when weaning was to be started and finished. The deferral is made on the plea that this is only 'milk teeth' were so termed, because in many cultures the weaning process was often concerned when the first tooth appear and completed when the last teeth had erupted. Plainly one has to supply the young child's nutrient requirements to enable him to grow, to be healthy and from a negative point of view, to avoid developing malnutrition, especially protein energy malnutrition. It is well to recall that during this transitional period there are found different sources of food during the weaning period. The first of this is the weaning diet itself, the exogenous foods the child is taking. Secondly, in many cases, breast milk should be a component in the weaning diet over a period of taking off as the other exogenous foods take over. Thirdly, the weaning diet is also directly related to the stores the child has achieved in the uterus. Lastly, as a fourth source of nutrients, there is the irradiation of the skin as far as Vitamin D is concerned. In India home made weaning foods of cheapter variety from the family diet is the ideal weaning food. One type of areal to be added to start with e.g. milk with sugar. Also DGLV (Darkgreen leafy vegetables) to be added with the weaning foods to supply Vit.A.

Calories have been under appreciated for a long time, Proteins have been the main concern and must continue to be an important consideration. But calories have tended to be disregarded. In many surveys it has been shown that calories are more significantly inadequate than proteins though of course both are totally interrelated in young children. The question in many weaning diets, especially in some parts of the world, is much related to calories, and often to the question of compact calories. In some parts of the world the staple food such as plantain is used, which is especially high in water, high in glucose, and low in calories therefore lacking in compact source of calories which is very important. The oil seeds, sugar, honey, the combination of cereal and pulses, the fish and butter may be mentioned as examples. The protein content of the weaning diet is obviously important, and it is quite plain that for economic reasons and for reasons of food avilability in most parts of the world, most children will not get most of their protein from animal sources alone, but from blends of vegetables foods plus small amount of available animal protein.

Most communities have by age-long experiment come to use foods in mixtures, so that their nutrients complement one another. In fact, an important generalisation in relation to human diets is that the wider the range of foods included and the greater the variety, the less the likelihood of nutritional deficiency.

References :

Jelliffe, D.B. (1969) : I. Pediat. 14, 808.

Morley, D. (1973) : Paediatric Priorities in Developing Countries. London, Butterworths.

CHAPTER – FOUR

GROWTH AND DEVELOPMENT

Developmental paediatrics is concerned with both growth and development – physiological and pathological. It is concerned with normal fetal development, with perinatal physiology and with the normal growth and development of children – physical intellectual, emotional and social. It is concerned with the prevention of

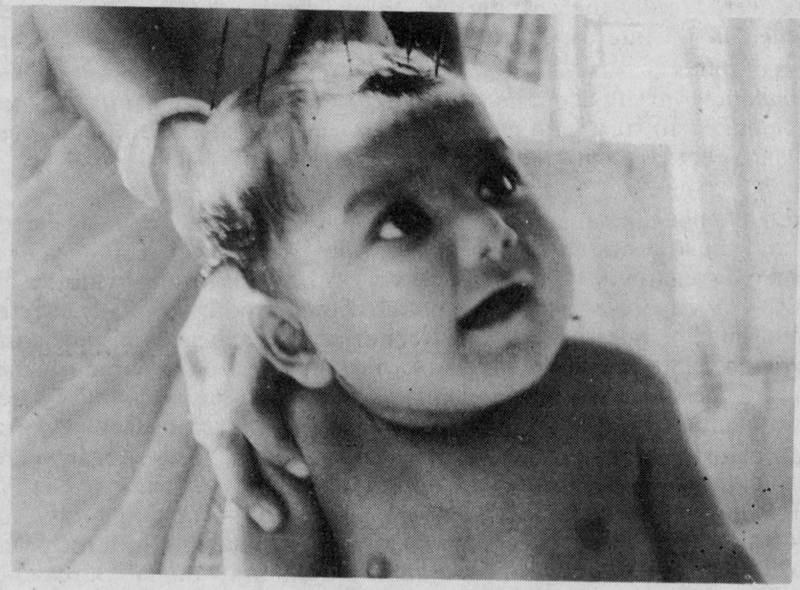

Fig.4.1 : A smiling infant at 9 months

optimum health and the early detection of handicap, its total assessment and the methods by which it may be minimised. However, upto recently the principal foci of attention have been : the newborn (first 30 days), the infant (0-1 year), the pre-school (1-5 years), the school child (5-12 or 15 years) and the adolescent. Normal puberty and adolescence may occur over a variable period of time between 11 and 16 years and is 1-2 years earlier in girls. It will be noted that the titles for these categories can only be applied literally if formal schooling is customary, and in some cultures, children are graded according to their physiological development or their ability to do certain tasks such as 'able to walk' capable of herding cows'.

Normal development can be described as a unified development of intelligence, emotional maturation, adoption to society and increasing physical size and powers. Whilst intake intelligence is considered to be genetically determined, performance is modified by emotional difficulties, environment, physical defects and illnesses. For example, deprivation of maternal affection in the early years may have permanent effects upon personality; the child may be inadequate at making close personal relationships and may have lost the ability to sustain long-term ambitions or to keep to permanent employment in adult life. Lack of stimulus and of the normal experiences of childhood may result in apparent retardation of development. Physical defects such as deafness may impair speech development and lead to poor school performance. Allowance must also be made for any prolonged illness, which may cause temporary retardation of progress.

It is easier to assess growth (increase in size) accurately. Assessment of development (maturation), is difficult. Though there may be individual variations, patterns of growth and development in general are predictable.

Growth :

(a) Birth weight : 2.8 — 3.0 kg. 10% loss after birth, birth weight regained by 10th day. Average daily weight gain — 25 gms. (1st three months), 15 gms. during the remainder of first year. Birth weight is doubled by 5 months and trebled by one year.

Growth :

(a) Birth weight : 2.8 — 3.0 kg. 10% loss after birth, birth weight regained by 10th day. Average daily weight gain — 25 gms. (1st three months), 15 gms. during the remainder of first year. Birth weight is doubled by 5 months and trebled by one year.
Quadruple by two years and then 2.5 — 3 kg. per year of age upto the age of 12 years.

(b) **Length/Height :**

At birth	...	20 inches (50 cm.)
at 6 months	...	26 inches (65 cm.)
at 1 year	...	30 inches (75 cm.)
at 4 years	...	40 inches (100 cm.)

and then 2 inches (4.5 cm.) per year of age upto the age of 12 years.

(c) Head and chest circumference and midarm circumference.

	Head circumference (Cms)	Chest circumference (Cms)	Midarm circumference (Cms)
At Birth	35.0	33.0	12.0
At 6 months	42.0	39.0	12.2
At 1 year	45.0	45.0	12.6
At 2 years	48.0	49.0	13.0
At 3 years	49.0	50.0	23.6
At 5 years	50.0	50.8	14.2
At 9 years	50.3	57.3	16.3
At 12 years	51.3	62.9	17.4

Abnormal Growth :

In traditional tropical communities, the abnormal weight curves seen are due to a variable combinations of the following :-

Malnutrition :

In the first 4-6 months of life the breast milk is usually abundant and more than adequate as a source of protein and calories, while body stores of minerals and vitamins are sufficient for the baby's immediate needs. As a result, weight is gained as fast as if not faster than western babies — so much so that they may often have to some extent, made good the often relatively low birth weight.

Indeed, a few solely breast fed babies to remain in fair nutritional condition, although often anaemic, for even longer. Usually, however, after about 4-6 months of age, the infant's increasing calorie and protein needs cannot be met by even an optimal flow of breast milk, together with the starchy carbohydrate weaning foods usually given. The slowing in weight gain so produced becomes even more marked between the ages of 1 to 3 years, unless adequate food, especially protein, becomes available in significant quantity of milk being obtained by prolonged breast feeding is cut off as a result of the child being weaned, due to the development of a subsequent pregnancy or for other reasons. In some tropical countries, it is correct to say that most individuals reach their nutritional life peak at 6 months of age. (ii) Besides malnutrition, infection as Malaria, infestation by intestinal parasites, maternal deprivation and also various other infections resulting from the poor hygiène associated with 'filth and overcrowding diseases' — including gastroenteritis, coryza, bronchitis, scabies and boils is undoubtedly important, especially as for most tropical children these may occur in an almost uninterrupted flow and produce cumulative effects.

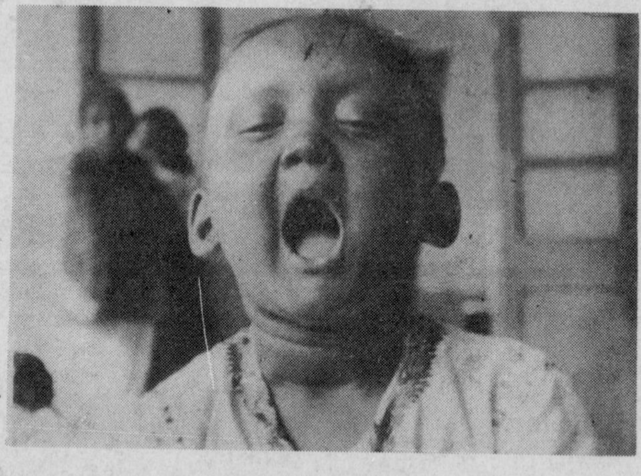

Fig.4.2 : Ectodermal dysplasia

Development :

The general developmentof the infant and young child is directly related to the maturation and progressive myelinization of the central nervous system, but is modified to some extent by the facilities available for practice, the individual child's personality, and by the influence of the cultural group into which he has been born.

All workers in this field stress the great range of normal variation in a child's general development, although the sequence is usually the same. The following approximate average figures may be quoted based on western children growing up in Europe or America, using the cephalo caudal sequence :

(i) appearance of social smile at 6 weeks of age.

(ii) holds head up (when sits up) at 3 months.

(iii) sits supported at 6 months,

(iv) sits unsupported at 9 months,

(v) stands holding on at 10 months,

(vi) stands unsupported at 12 months,

(vii) walks alone at 15 months.

As far as can be judged it seems likely that the rate of a child's development may be influenced by the cultural surroundings in which he finds himself, whether, for example, this is dominated by the over riding importance of competitive success or not. Each area will have to define its own variation from the general pattern.

References :

Arnhold, R. (1969) : J. trop. Pediat. 15, 243.

Illingworth, R.S. (1975) : The development of the infant and young child. Edinburgh Churchill Livingstone.

Singh & Dhatta : Pediatric, Residents Handbook, February. 1980.

PROBLEMS RELATED TO GROWTH

Obesity :

The over weight child presents a different problem and is less frequently the cause of parental anxiety. Numerous causes of obesity have been recognised, including hypothyroidism, and the Cushing, Prader-Willi and Laurence-Moon-Biedel Syndrome, although these are all relatively rare. Genetic predisposition has been suspected in many cases but in clinical practice it is difficult to distinguish from obesity due to environmental factors.

Over nutrition leading to obesity is common in the developed countries. In the developing countries like India it is already common in the more privileged sections and is becoming a problem amongst the less affluent social groups. Although the exact relationship of obesity to health and disease cannot be clearly defined, there is agreement that in adult life over weight is associated with increased mortality rates, and that there is an association between obesity and ischaemic heart disease, hypertension and diabetes mellitus. Obesity also causes disability and reduces the quality of life by reducing physical fitness, work capacity and respiratory function by exacerbating osteoarthritis, by increasing liability to post operative complications and poor obstetric performance, and by causing emotional and social disability, especially in women. Because about one-third of adult obesity originates in childhood or adolescence and obesity in children tends to persist into adult life, prevention during childhood is of major importance.

Strictly defined obesity is a condition in which the whole adipose mass (adipose organ) is enlarged out of proportion to other body tissues. This definition is, however, of limited practical value because of the difficulty of assessing the size of the adipose organ. Thus obesity is usually defined in terms of relative body weight or of skin fold thickness. For several purposes estimation of the thickness of subcutaneous fat by measurement of skin fold thickness has been used both alone and in conjunction with weight for height indices. The skin fold thickness must be determined on standard sites, for examples over the tricep muscle, by means of calipers. The measurement of body weight in relation to height at given age is a useful index and an arbitary value of 20% above the predicted value has been used to define the upper acceptable limit of body weight. Inspection is of particular value in recognising children in whom an unusual degree of muscular development results in above average weight for height.

A child may have a low height for the age because he is thin or because he is stunted due to past malnutrition or a combination of both. The best way to identify these children is to compare their weights with the table or 'the thinness chart' by save the Children Fund showing the grades of malnutrition in different colours. It makes easy for a health worker to use the weight-to-height (age independant anthropometry) method for assessing growth and the nutritional status and also see whether or not the weight is in the normal range (i.e. above 80 percent) for a child of similar height.

The increased storage of fat in obesity is due to an energy intake in the form of food in excess of the individual's requirements including in the case of infants and children, requirements for growth. Many factors can disturb energy balance and they differ in their importance not only between individuals at different times. Furthermore, the etiology of obesity is complicated by the development of certain vicious circles. To give two examples physical inactivity may cause obesity which then further restricts activity, emotional disturbance may cause over eating and the resulting obesity then worsens the emotional upset. Energy is consumed as food. The composition of the food, the periodicity with which it is eaten, and the absolute amount of energy derived from it are all relevant to the etiology of obesity. The attribution of infant obesity in early cereal feeding and the possible determination of adult obesity in early life, may, therefore, have been over-emphasized. By contrast, children presenting with obesity, usually after the age of seven years, are likely to become obese adults.

The management of the obese child is a prolonged affair and not so much rewarding. The aim should be reduced food-intake and increase exercise. Although initial success may be there but chance of relapse is always a tiring affair if the child and more so the parents do not cooperate. For children of school age, a providing 800-1000 Kcal/daily is given but a further reduction to 600-800 Kcal/daily may be necessary if the previous calories fail. The diet should contain an increased proportion of protein in relation to fat and carbohydrate. Appetite suppressants are not normally used to treat an obese child.

Reference

FOMON, G.J (1974) : Infant Nutrition, 2nd ed.
Philadelphia, Saunders.

DWARFISM

The dwarfism may be defined as failure of skeletal growth with no alteration in sexual growth and maturity. If hypogonadism subsequently persists beyond puberty in association with dwarfism, the term infantilism is applied. Pure dwarfism as opposed to infantilism is rarely of endocrine origin and may be an ethnic or familial characteristic without evidence of disease. Dwarfism may be associated with a low birth weight despite a full gestational period.

If the height is below 3rd percentile, the growth may be consisdered as stunted or dwarfism. Common causes of dwarfism are summarised below :-

Causes of dwarfism :

1. Constitutional.
2. Nutritional dwarfism.
3. Chronic visceral disease.
   (a) **Chronic infections :**
   Tuberculosis, malaria, kala-azar, syphilis, empyema, chronic urinary tract infections.
   (b) **Birth defects :**
   Congenital heart disease, anomalies of urinary tract and nervous system.
   (c) **Metabolic disorders :**
   Chronic renal disease due to tubular malabsorption syndrome, diabetes insipidus, glycogen storage disease, Vit. D resistant disease and diabetes mellitus.

(d) **Miscellaneous :**

Subdural hematoma, cirrhosis of liver, severe asthama, bronchiectasis and uraemia.

(f) Chromosomal disorders, Turner's syndrome, Mongolism.

4. Bone disorders.

Inherited skeletal disorders, such as achondroplasisa, dyschondroplasia and oesteogenesis imperfecta, give rise to gross stunting of stature. Acquired skeletal disease, such as the various forms of rickets and spinal caries giving rise to spinal deformity are important causes.

5. Endocrine disorders.

Hypopituitarism (HGH deficiency), Hypothyroidism, hypogonadism, precocious puberty and pseudohypo-parathyroidism.

6. Miscellaneous causes.

(a) Genetic short stature (Familial).

(b) Low birth weight dwarfism (Primordial or intrauterine growth retardation).

(c) Emotional deprivation dwarfism syndrome.

(d) Use of anabolic steroids for a long time, prolonged use of corticosteroids — leads to earlier growth spurt and epiphyseal fusion and arrests further growth.

Nutritional dwarfism :

Protein-calorie malnutrition causes wasting of the muscles and poor weight gain. The child becomes less active and conserves energy, growth in height is slowed. Long standing malnutrition, starting early in life, is the commonest cause of stunting. As weight and height are affected concurrently, the child looks smaller for his age.

These children with nutritional dwarfism may not look apparently wasted and therefore the diagnosis may be missed if adequate history is not obtained.

Hypothyroidism :

This condition may be present from birth or acquired subsequently, in the former case — it is termed cretinism.

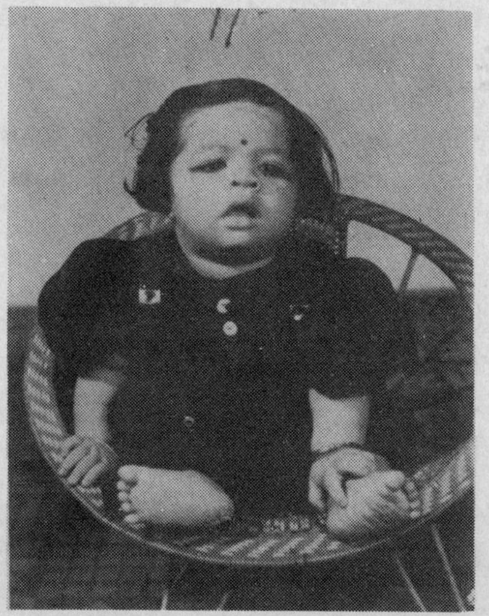

Fig.4.3 : Cretin at 8 months

The thyroid gland develops as an epithelial proliferation in the floor of the pharyngeal gut. Thyroid glands have two types of secretory cells, viz., the follicular cells and the parafollicular cells. The former secretes thyroxin and the latter secretes calcitonin. Secretion of thyroxin is regulated by the thyroid stimulating hormone (TSH) of the anterior pituitary. The latter released under the influence of thyrotropic releasing factor (TRF) from the hypothalamus. The thyroid function starts during the fetal life. The fetus depends on its own thyroid for maintenance of normal growth and development. At birth, the serum T4 level of the fetus is slightly less than that of the mother, but may rise to 10-15/ug./dl. within a week of birth. The level declines by the age of 4 months. The weight of the thyroid gland at birth is 1 gm. and it increase to 35 gm. in adults. During puberty, there is a physiological enlargement of the thyroid gland leading to goiter.

Test for thyroid function :

1. Protein bound iodine (Normal 4-8/µg/100 ml.) includes T4, T3 and the thyroglobulins.
2. Thyroxin or T4 (Normal 4-11/µg/100/ ml.).
3. Tri-i-odothyronine levels T3 by radio-immuno-assay (RIA) (Normal 100-250/ng 100 ml).
4. TSH level (Normal upto to 10/iu/ml.).
5. 131 uptake (Normal 15-40% at 24 hours).

Causes of hypothyroidism :

Congenital :

1. Agenesis or dysgenesis of the thyroid gland.
2. Familial goitrogenous cretinism.
   - (i) Iodide trapping defect.
   - (ii) Iodide organification defect.
   - (a) Complete absence of peroxidase.
   - (b) Failure to bind thyroidal appoperoxidase by the prosthtic hematin group.
   - (c) Pendred syndrome-goiter and nerve deafness.
   - (iii) Coupling defect.
   - (iv) Deiodinase defect.
   - (v) Defects of thyroglobulin synthesis.
3. Endemic cretinism due to iodine deficiency in the maternal diet.
4. Administration of drugs to the mother during pregnancy, e.g., iodides in cough syrups and antithyroid drugs.

Acquired :

1. Primary hypothyroidism.
2. Hashimoto's thyroiditis due to auto-immunisation.
3. Thyroidectomy.
4. Ingestion of drugs, e.g., PAS and antithyroid agents.
5. Panhypopituitarism —
   - (a) Hypothalamic lesions deficiency or TRF from hypothalamus.
   - (b) Damage to the pituitary, deficiency of TSH.

Clinical features :

The cretin is pale and has a yellow tinged, rough, dry skin. An umbilical hernia is present in 50% of cases. The hair is straight, dry and sparse, the cry is hoarse and low pitched. The tongue is enlarged and protrudes, because it is too large for the mouth. The child is slow in all his movements, the smile comes and goes slowly and the mentality is greatly retarded. He is very backward in learning to raise his head, get up, crawl and walk. The temperature is subnormal, the hands and feet being cold, and the pulse slow. Growth is slow. A radiograph of the wrist will show delay in the appearance of the carpal centres.

Dysgenesis of the epiphyses of the humerus femur, and tibia is of diagnostic importance, the epiphysis being formed by multiple foci of calcification. The teeth are late in appearing and when they do, tend to be carious. No such simple laboratory investigation besides specific clinical changes will help to diagnose the condition early. Only serum cholesterol is found to be raised above 300 mg. per 100 ml. and ECG reveals a low voltage tracing. The diagnosis is confirmed by measuring the circulating thyroid hormone thyroxin (T4) and Triiodothyronin (T3) in the peripheral blood. Determination of circulating thyrotrophic hormone (TSH) will show increased values in cases associated with primary thyroid defect and decreased or absent values in cases with a pituitary disorder.

The prognosis depends largely on how early and how efficiently the child is treated. There are, however, a few cases in which there is mental retardation despites very early therapy.

Treatment must be started immediately the diagnosis is made and continued for the rest of the patient's life. L-Thyroxine sodium is the preparation of choice and for an infant a few months old the dose should be 0.05 mg. daily. This is slowly increased, week by week until the greatest dose is reached which the infant can tolerate without diarrhoea, loss of weight, tachycardia or hyperactivity. The dose varies with the age of the child and with the individual patient. A child of one year may tolerate 0.1 — 0.15 mg. daily and a child of five years 0.1 — 0.2 mg. but there is wide variation. The patient improves with relief of constipation, warm hands and feet instead of cold, hairs again becomes dark and curly, the excess of subcutaneous fat disappears, the skin becomes soft and that yellow tinge with pallor disappears, becoming pink. The treatment should be guarded by repeated measurement of height to ensure that skeletal growth is maintained.

Undeveloped child :

The deviations from expected rates of weight gain are common causes of presentation in paediatric practice. Parental anxiety is usually associated with complaints of diminished appetite and failure to 'put on flesh' and attempts to induce the child to increase his dietary intake are invariably accompanied by domestic friction. In fact, most allegedly thin children are extremely healthy and have weights which lie within the normal range for their age. In each case a careful dietary history should be taken and the child examined clinically to exclude underlying organic disease. Ideally, serial determinations of height and weight should be made and the growth velocity determined. These will allow repeated opportunities for contact with the parents and appropriate reassurance.

The nutritional requirement is defined as the least amount of nutrient that will promote and optimal state of health.

The failure to thrive is defined as a rate of gain in length and/or weight less than the value corresponding to two standard deviations below the mean during an interval of at least 56 days for infants less than 3 months of age and during an interval of at least 3 months for older infants. The advisable intake of nutrients refers to the amount of various nutrients recommended for the individual. It is presumed that requirement of nearly all normal individuals of the stated age under nearly all variations of living conditions will be satisfied by intake twice the average requirements. The protein quality depends on its ability to supply essential aminoacid in sufficient amounts to fulfil all the requirements for maintenance and growth. The essential aminoacids are those that cannot be synthesised by the animal body from the materials readily available at a speed commensurate with the demands for the normal growth. For the human infant these are arginine, leucine, isoleucine, lysine, methonine, phenylalanine, threonine, tryptophane, valine and histidine.

In the first four months of life, at least 6.5 percent of the calories in the diet must be provided by protein of high biological value. It is, however, advisable to provide about 9 to 10% of the calories metabolised, from protein of good quality. This approximates to about 1.6 to 2 gm/kg. as nutritional requirement or about 2.5 gm. to 3 gm/kg/day as advisable intake. After the age of 4 months, the growth rate slows down and lesser quantities of protein may be adequate. Thus the requirement may vary from 1.2 to 1.6 gm/kg/day about 1.6 to 2.5 gm/kg/day may be the desirable intake. In older children the needs may be slightly lower.

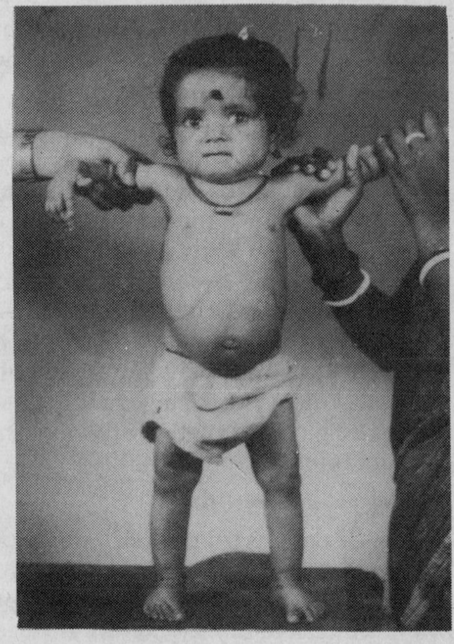

Fig.4.5 : Malnutrition with congenital Typhilitis diagnosed at 9m. of age

The children below 5 years constitute over 15% of the population in India. A majority of them are from poor rural communities. Children of the preschool age group are not only the most vital but from the nutritional standpoint, the most vulnerable segment of our population. Some of the worst ravages of malnutrition are seen in this age group. About 40% of the total deaths in the country take place in children below 5 years as against 4% in the developed countries. Though there has been a steady decline in the infant mortality rate in India over the last 20 years (on an average varies from 70 to 120 per thousand), the preschool child mortality has more or less remained stationary. (The mortality between 1-4 years is about 45/1000, described by C.Gopalan in 1972). In India the incidence of severe PEM in preschool children is 1-2% and that of mild to moderate malnutrition nearly 80%. As there are at present 90-100 million pre-school children in India, the number of malnutrition children there is simply staggering. Such rapid turnover of the population in this unproductive period is a serious economic wastage and acts as a disincentive to our family planning programme.

The programme.

The protein calorie malnutrition and Vitamin-A deficiency are the major nutritional problems among pre-school children. Anaemia due to iron deficiency is also widely prevalent. In addition, manifestations of Vitamin B-complex deficiency and nutritional rickets are frequently seen among children.

PROTEIN-CALORIE MALNUTRITION IN CHILDREN — PAST, PRESENT AND FUTURE

Introduction :

India had the dubious distinction of being among the countries, with the highest of infant mortality. (The infant mortality rate of the urban section is 77.5 and that of the rural sector is 114.8 per 1,000 live births) As it is an important index of health status of the community, it reflects the dismal failure of health planning in our country inspite of tremendous investment of resources. Even in 1986 the problem of malnutrition and undernutrition confronting children and infants poses another serious difficulty for the health of the people of our country, while many children die, many others survive only to carry with them the prolonged effects of malnutrition to their adult life. This may result in permanent detorioration of physical and mental health. We must bear in mind that maximal rate of growth of the human brain takes place at an early age, this rate slows down rapidly and becomes minimal after the age of 6 years when the brain has reached 90% of its ultimate volume. Therefore it is easy to imagine the importance of the first years of life, a period during which the greatest number of cases of the protein-calorie malnutrition to be found[3].

Astiology :

Malnutrition is mainly due to (a) poverty, (b) ignorance. Malnutrition of pre-school children (1-5 years) constitutes one of the major public health problem in India. Children of 0-5 years of age constitute 15% of the population while it accounts 44% of total deaths. Malnutrition is one of the most important cause of death. This hazard is more prevalent among poor children in the slum areas of urban community. The epidemiologic basis for the development of this condition is (i) maternal malnutrition, (ii) inadequate nutrient intake due to poverty, (iii) faulty feeding programme arising from ignorance, defective dietary habits, superstition, food prejudices and belief, (iv) infections and infestations, (v) unhygienic environmental condition and (vi) lack of consciousness of health care. All these factors precipitate malnutrition of different degrees resulting in retardation of growth and skeletal maturation.

Classification :

Grading of protein caloric malnutrition is necessary for formulating therapy individual patient and defining provision for combating malnutrition. Gomez et al defined 76 to 85% of normal weight as first degree malnutrition between 61 and 75% as second degree malnutrition and less than 60% as third degree malnutrition. A better and simple alternative is to express the planes of malnutrition in categories. More than 90% of the mean weight for age of the reference standard is normal nutrition. In first degree malnutrition, weight falls between 81 and 90% in second degree between 71 and 80%, in third degree between 61 and 70% and in the fourth degree, it is below 60% of the reference standard. Children with weight less than 60% of the reference standard are listed as marasmus, when oedema is also present these are defined as Marasmic Kwashiorkor. If the weight is between 60 and 80% of the reference weight, they are classified as under weight or pre-Kwashiorkor. Oedematous and skin changes in this weight range are graded as Kwashiorkor.

Clinical story :

Epidemiological evolution of these malnutrition cases were the same. As long as the child was completely breast fed, he remained well. When the breast milk failed completely or partially, mothers added starchy foods like sagoo, barley etc. or become the victim of 'Tin Foods' without the proper knowledge of dilution and

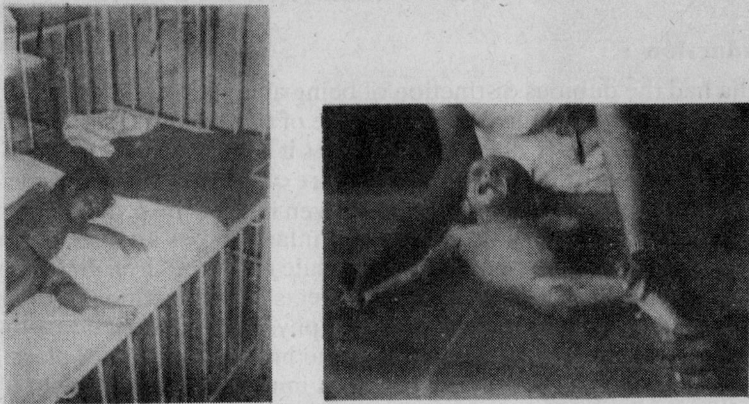

Fig.4.6(a), 4.6(b) : Marasmus — Marasmic Kwashiorkor

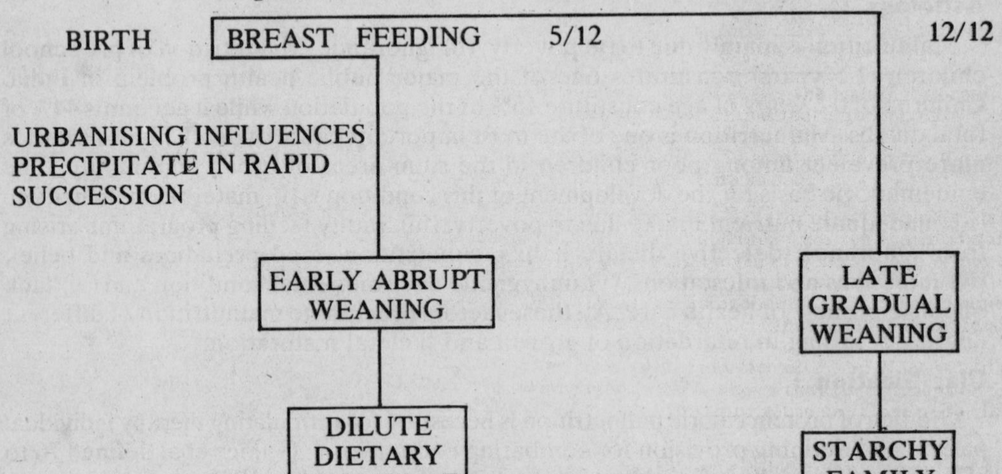

Flow chart showing — Paths leading from early weaning to nutritional marasmus and from protracted breast feeding to kwashiorkor (By courtesy of Dr. D.S. Meharen and the editor of the Lancet).

calorie requirements and introduces infection, resulting in diarrhoea. The usual belief was that the milk should not be tolerated by diarrhoeic children and mother stopped milk, sometimes even she stopped her own breast milk, thinking that it did not suit her child. She (the mother) and even the doctors would never believe that carbohydrates could give rise to diarrhoea while child was having diarrhoea and the diet was restricted only to those carbohydrates and no protein and suffer from more of infection like measles and whooping cough which might tigger off the nutritional balance, resulting in hypoprotinaemia. In a few months time oedema sets in and also other signs of Kwashiorkor develop. Not only that the children were getting very much restricted calories which ultimately result in marasmus..

(Paths leading from early weaning to nutritional marasmus and from protracted breast feeding to kwashiorkor (By courtesy of Dr. D.S. Meharen and the editor of the Lancet).

A subclinical or very early state of protein deficiency in children, known as 'Prekwashiorkor' in which a failure in growth, a reduction in the serum albumin and increased liability to diarrhoea and respiratory infections, are the salient clinical features. This type of malnutrition is extremely common in regions where the fully developed syndrome is found.

In the middle of the spectrum, between kwashiorkor and marasmus there is marasmic kwashiorkor in which children have the clinical features of both the disorders.

Role of infection and infestation :

The role of infection and infestation in protein-caloric malnutrition is an important one and is receiving increasing attention. It is, however, difficult to disentangle the effects of malnutrition and infection. 375 cases of protein caloric malnutrition in children admitted to the Department of Child Health of Calcutta National Medical College Hospital during the period from January 1956 to december 1961 were studied. Each patient was studied clinically with special reference to history of infections. Each and every child was admitted in the hospital and observed for various periods, ranging from one week to two months. Their progress was studied from day to day and in most of them routine blood, urine, stool, chest x-ray, tuberculin test and relevant blood biochemistry and liver histological studies were done.

In many cases diarrhoea was associated with some of the above mentioned infections with some respiratory infections, pyelitis etc. as a presenting feature.

A history of diarrhoea at the onset of illness was obtained in 66.8% of cases. Thirty-two percent of the children had diarrhoea while in the hospital. In one-third of them the dirrhoea subsided with dietetic correction alone. The diarrhoea thus appeared to be non-specific and attributable to irregularities in diet in already malnourished children. In two-thirds of the cases, on the other hand, diarrhoea was associated with fever and toxemia. Chemo-therapeutics or antibiotics has to be used to obtain clinical response in these cases, suggesting besides malnutrition, presence of an infective agent. A number of children (55%) had febrile episodes at the onset of illness — it was due to respiratory infections (non-tuberculous) in (56%) ear infections in 4.0%, skin infections in 3.6%, urinary tract infections (E.Coli) in 12%. In a few of these cases, however, no cause could be ascertained but antibiotics such as penicillin with or without streptomycin injection controlled the fever. Tuberculosis of the lung was found in 21 cases on routine chest x-ray examination and was confirmed by tuberculin test. Though of doubtful value as a diagnostic test in malnutrition. It was more common in marasmic group (in 15 cases). It will be seen that in marasmus and marasmic kwashiorkor group

Fig. 6 (Table 1)

Showing the nature of infective condition in various clinical types of malnutrition.

Infective Conditions	Classical kwashiorkor	Pre-kwashiorkor	Nutrition marasmus	Marasmic kwashiorkor
N0. of Clases	48	33	198	96
1. Tuberculosis	2	4	15	—
2. Respiratory infection (Non-specific)	8	11	90	26
3. Ear infections	4	4	5	3
4. Pyelitis	8	10	15	12
5. Skin infections	2	4	5	3
6. Poliomyelitis (after effect)	—	—	1	—
7. Congenital syphilis	—	—	1	—
8. Enteric fever	—	—	5	—
9. Diarrhoea —	9	11	130	50
(a) Infection and infestation	7	10	16	14
(b) Non-infective	8	2	115	5

out of 294 cases, only 58 cases were without any obvious infection in kwashiorkor and pre-kwashiorkor group as many as 24 cases were suffering from some type of infection. These figures show that in our country, infection plays a major role either in initiating or keeping up a condition of malnutrition. The merit of this observation is obvious. In those cases who had no infection, we could build up our therapeutic programme on dietetic measure alone, but in those cases where infections were supervened, without the control of infection, none of them were cured; of these tuberculosis demanded special mention, as in many of these cases (21 cases) we found associated tuberculous infection.

Prevention :

The prevention of protein caloric malnutrition should be an action of education. Poverty is not the single chief cause of this pathology which in most cases is essentially due to the lack of knowledge. This lack of knowledge is not peculiar to the less privileged classes but in the most primitive as well as the most sophisticated groups, whether we come across a belief, a taboo or an outdated opinion, these phenomena have a common denominator; ignorance of an adequate diet,an existence of detrimental habits and customs. It is rash to generalize about child care, because customs vary from place to place. It is wise to interfere with established customs as little as possible and then only when they are harmful .

The historyof malnutrition will no doubt evolute rapidly in the years to come, the urbanisation phenomenon known in our country will change the picture. The children affected by malnutrition will be younger and younger since the mothers tend to reduce breast feeding (working mothers, a fashionable trend or snobbery, victim of wide publicity of tin-foods) and because the diet of the city children differs from that of rural children. We must bear in mind that there are two kinds of people, the urban and the rural population, there are also those who are not rural any more for they have become as refugee or settled in the out-skirts of the city due to deterioration of economic life and are neither urban. They have almost no way to cultivate or breed; they do not have a fixed salary, they are not integrated in the urban economy or in the urban way of life, they are inhabitants in the slum areas, road sides, pavements and under high way bridges. Among these people protein caloric malnutrition are particularly frequent, upto now various studies carried out bore mainly on problems of nutrition in city areas, in some provinces particularly in West Bengal rural exodus has become quite important and the deficiencies in urban and pre-urban areas should soon be considered in order to be able to formulate prevention programmes adopted to the various situations, before these diseases become too important to be dealt with.

Management :

Emergency management of initial problems were diarrhoea-dehydration and infection which were dealt with by giving fluid and electrolytes and appropriate chemotherapy or antibiotics. It is essential that one should make every effort to detect any signs of infection, however, trivial even severe infections may provoke little rise of temperature.

Survival of the malnourished children with diarrhoea is limited by calorie deficit to a greater extent than by water and electrolyte deficit. Reparative calories can be given by slow drip through an indwelling nasogastric tube while electrolyte and water are given parenterally. Initial parenteral therapy is designed to improve the circulation and to expand extracellular volume. The repair solutions are — (i) half strength Ringer lactate with 5% dextrose, (ii) 5% dextrose with 0.45 gm. % of sodium chloride, (iii) and half strength Darrow's with lactate and 5% dextrose, if urine output is good. Rate of administration and quantity of fluid should be reduced from recommended levels if oedema is present, to avoïd pulmonary oedema. Blood should be given if the patient is in shock, severely ill, or anaemic. Potassium salts can be given early if urine output is good. Controlled trials suggest that survival can be improved by the intramuscular injection of 1.0 to 1.5 ml. of a 40 percent solution of magnesium sulphate (4.0 mEq. per ml.) every 12 hours for 1-3 days. Clinical and electrographic improvement may be more rapid with magnesium therapy and seizures occuring during recovery from diarrhoea complicating severe malnutrition may respond to magnesium.

The principles of the dietary treatment were to offer in a digestible form diet rich in protein and calories. These categories of diet were tried during the study period and one given in tabulated form (Fig.7 - Table 2).

Fig.7 : Table-2

Showing the ingredients, modifications, calories and daily cost of three categories of diet used. (cost in 1979)

Type	Ingredients	Modification	Calories	Cost (approxi)
P_A	Milk 24-32 oz. (Protein 2.5%, fat 4%, carbohydrate 4%)	Can be modified by diluting, skimming and addition of extra sugar. Modified by addition of lactic acid or with addition of extra casine, protein milk can be prepared from it.	480-640 or by modification it can be increased up to 1000 calories.	Re.0.63 to Re.0.84 and by modification Rs.1.05
P_B	Milk same as above with 1 egg or 1 sandesh, 1 orange or banana (ripe), soft rice (50-100 g.), fish (25 g,), vegetable (50g.), and dahi (10-20g.)	Here also milk can be modified as mentioned above and solid foods varied from 50-100g. normally and it can be increased or decreased accordingly.	990-1100 calories or by modification it can be increased up to 1500 calorises.	Rs.1.93 and by modification Rs.2.25
P_C Breakfast	Milk 8 oz. to 18 oz., 1 egg or 1 sandesh, 1 orange or 1 banana (ripe)	Here also milk can be modified as mentioned above and solid foods varied from 50-100 g. normally and it can be increased or decreased accordingly.	1500 to 1800 calories or by modification it can be increased up to 2000 calories	Re.2.25 and by modification Rs.2.55
Lunch	Soft rice fish, vegetables, dahi 50-100 g.			
Dinner	Soft rice or bread, fish or meat 50-100 g.			

This diet is suitable for the age of 6 months to 3 years and in cases where oral feeding started gradually after intravenous fluids, this diet might have to be given in stages, so that the children can digest easily. Infections must be treated concomittantly[6] with the dietary therapy, whereas treatment of parasite infestation, if not severe; may be postponed until recovery is underway for a few weeks. Owing to loss of oedema, weight loss may occur even when oedema was not previously obvious, and will reflect in apparent oedema or unusual distribution of water within body fluid compartments. During recovery, serum and intestinal enzymes return to normal and intestinal absorption of fat and protein improves.

First few months the infant thrives on breast milk and even if there is shortage of breast milk some supplementation with cow's milk is usually attempted. The decline in the production of breast milk varies much from one mother to another, if lactation is poor, after 6 months, marasmus may be seen after this age if no other food or milk is offered. In the treatment of these cases, these who have received too little of cow's milk mixture should have the feeds first increased in amount until all the fluid requirements are met with and the infant will take no more, in quantity and then the strength (quality) should be increased slowly until the calorie requirements are met. If diarrhoea is severe with dehydration, the first step is to correct electrolyte disturbance, especially that of potassium and to overcome dehydration. Subsequently dietary treatment is to be cautiously instituted, judging every case individually, subject to the general principles mentioned above.

Comments and conclusion :

In conclusion, it is probable that in future protein-calorie malnutrition will become of increasing clinical importance in our country as a consequence of a continuing decline in breast feeding and the urbanisation of the uneducated families, socially insecure and living in poor, insanitary houses or even in pavements or roadsides with insufficient money to buy adequate supplements of milk or milk substitutes. On the contrary, recently our National Government is aware of the fact of immense importance of balanced nutrition in the age group of 1-5 years among the poor children in the slum areas of urban community. The comprehensive nutritional programme has been organised to look after the nutritional need through, 'under five clinics', supplement of extra protein to pre-school children (1-5 years) through Balwadi Services and anganwads services or integrated child development scheme (ICDS) and establishment of mobile paediatric services, during the seventh five year plan period and also various rural economic and agricultural development programmes.

References

1. Ghai, O.P. — Editorial, Indian Paediatrics, 10 : 1, 1973.
2. Stein, Hermand, D. — Planning for the Needs of Children in developing countries — Report of a Round Table Conference, Published by United Nations Children's Fund, italy, 1964, P.51.
3. Raimbault, A.M. — Prevention of Malnutrition — Children in the Tropics, 81, 21, 1972.
4. Datta Banik, N.D., Nayar, Sushila, Krishna, R. and Lila Raj — A study of epidemiologic basis of malnutrition in pre-school children in Slum Areas in Delhi, 10,19, 1973.
5. Gomez, F., Ramos Galvan, R., Cravioto, J. and Frank, S. — Malnutrition in infancy and childhood with special reference to Kwashiorkor in Advance Paediatric, Vol.VII, Lewine S.Z., ed. P.131, Chicago, Year Book Publishers, 1955.
6. Chakraborty, Bijon — J. Indian M.A., 60, 129, 1972.
7. Paterson's Sick Children — A Text Book of Paediatrics, ninth edition, 1971. Diseases of Children in the Tropics and Developing Countries, Child Care and Nutrition, P.661.

CHAPTER – FIVE

MALNUTRITION AND DEFICIENCY DISORDERS

In order to have balanced nutrition, the child should have a diet to cover his needs in terms of growth and output of energy. The due consideration should, therefore, be given to the proximate principles of diet containing protein, fat and carbohydrate content of the diet and to the needs for vitamins and minerals.

The vitamins are naturally occuring substances present in normal food stuffs in small amounts which are required for normal metabolism and health. The deficiency states are most commonly encountered in the developing countries like India and may arise in association with malnutrition specially Vitamin A or as a result of the improper preparation and selection of the diets. The fat soluble vitamins (A, E, D and K) deficiency may thus arise in infants with steatorrhoea. The water soluble vitamins are (B and C) deficient in tropical countries mainly due to intestinal trouble and more of starchy and carbohydrate content of diets. In some cases the requirements for vitamins are related to the composition of the diet as mentioned earlier, another example increased protein intake requires additional Vitamin B_6 and diet rich in poly unsaturated fatty acids require extra amount of Vit. E. The distinction should be made which allows for substantial margin of safety. The excessive provision of some vitamins, notably A and D, may result in toxicity.

The xerophthalmia due to Vit. A deficiency presents a sinister prognosis, with malnutrition, the mortality had twice as high compared with those without. The difference was ascribed to a lesser resistance to infection. The incidence is highest in South India, West Bengal, where upto 70% of malnourished children may have eye lesions and where the bulk of corneal blindness (BCM — Blinding Corneal malnutrition) might be attributed to it. The only way for a doctor to prevent its consequences is to look for xerophthalmia in every case of child with malnutrition. In the first year of life the retinal (1 mg. of retinol = 3,300 Iu performed Vit. A) status of a child is still in constant evolution. It is influenced by the liver storage at birth, which from a well-fed mother may be about 5-7 mg. Afterwards, it often depends on the Vitamin A content of breast milk alone. Accepting an average milk yield of 850 ml/day this should give a total of 0.4 mg. retinol per day during the first 6 months. But sometimes the total quantity of breast milk and its Vitamin A level may both be low. After weaning, in many infants, Vit. A activity become only from the intake of Vit. A precursors especially β carotene which again may be low or subject to defects in conversion and absorption hampered due to associated worms infestation. Even without any improvement in their poverty, these children still need not go blind and die. In the green tropics carotene is around them on all sides. But leafy vegetables are often withheld from their diets. Besides xerophthalmia, the other eye changes are progressive night blindness, xerosis of various degrees. Bitot's spots, keratomalacia in young infants. Although other epithelia are involved, the principal changes are in the skin-follicular keratosis (toad skin) involving the thighs and outer aspects of the upper arms, plasma Vitamin A level fall below (20/ μ u/100 ml.). The normal requirement for Vitamin A is of the order of 10/ μ u/kg/day (30 IU) in infancy. But daily intakes of the order of 2000 IU for infants and 3000-4000 IU for older children are recommended. The therapeutic dose requires larger doses so that blindness and keratomalacia require 6-10 injections intramuscular 100,000 IU to 300,000 IU, chronic poisoning or toxicity is characterised by hepatic and splenic enlargement, headache, joint pains, muscle weakness, coarse and sparse hairs, bleeding episodes and periosteitis. The diagnosis is confirmed by high level of plasma Vit.A.

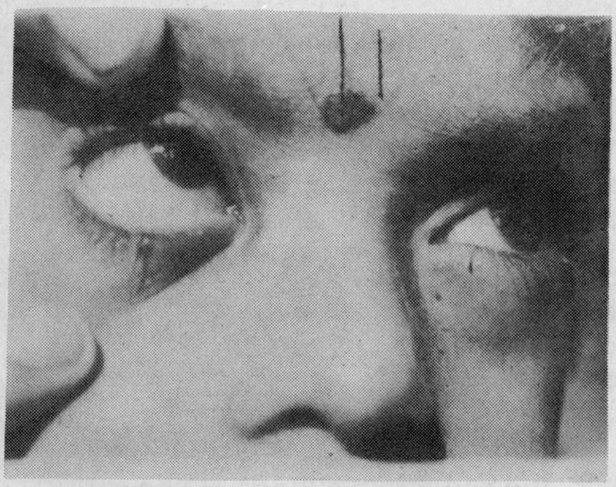

Fig.5.1 : Xerosis Bitot's spots. (XIB)

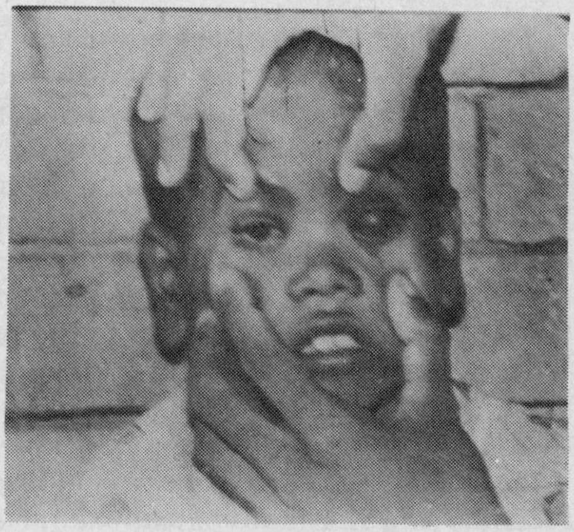

Fig.5.2 : BCM — (Blinding Corneal Malnutrition due to Vit. A deficiency).

Vitamin B :

Vitamin B_1 (Thiamine) deficiency leads to infantile beriberi — is a disease of the first year of life, but is most commonly found between the ages of 2-3 months. Almost all infants who suffer from beriberi are breast fed and diets of their mothers are usually deficient in thiamine. The nursing mother gives a history of numbness and weakness, particularly of lower limbs, the baby develops early signs of cardiac failure, also presents with aphonia. The treatment is with parenteral injection of thiamine hydrochloride, 50-100 mg. immediately and followed by a maintenance dose of 5-10 mg. daily. The mother should be treated similarly and breast feeding should be continued.

Nicotinic Acid :

B_2 fraction known as Niacin and other B_2 as riboflavin. The deficiency is mainly but not exclusively associated with communities in which maize forms the main source of carbohydrate and leads to a condition known as pellagra. Clinically, the deficiencies are maintained as dementia, diarrhoea and dermatitis and also with painful red and swollen tongue. The vitamin is also deficient in those patients who are with long term isoniazid therapy.

Vitamin B_6 or Pyridoxin :

However, pyridoxin dependant convulsions have been described in new born infants fed with a B_6 deficient milk formula and pyridoxin responsive hypochromic anaemia has been reported. The deficiency is also noticed in these patients who are having isoniazid therapy for tuberculosis.

Folic acid and Vit. B_{12} deficiencies :

Causes megaloblastic anaemias. Folic acid deficiencies may complicate malabsorption syndrome and arise as a complication of therapeutic use of folic acid antagonists for example, methotrexate and also in case of anti-convulsive drugs — phenytoin in epilepsy. Increased requirement in prematurity and haemolytic anaemias are also noticed. B_{12} deficiency may arise as a result of inadequate diet as in vegetarians or as a consequence of malabsorption due to lack of intrinsic factor, small bowel disease or infestation with fish tape worms.

Vitamin C :

The deficiency states are now relatively rare and in Indian sub-continent it is more rare in infants because breast milk contains ascorbic acid, due to mothers habituated in taking citrous fruits and green vegetables and thereby the children get vitamin C from breast milk. Though it might be seen associated with rickets in malnutrition states, typically it occurs between the ages of 9 months and 1½ years of age, and may be precipitated after an acute infection. The infant ceases to grow and widespread capillary bleeding occurs particularly beneath the periosteum near the growing ends of the long bones and in relation to the teeth. In the initial stage, the presentation is excessive crying during handling the baby and they prefer to be kept in frog position. The urine examination reveals evidences of bleeding and the radiological examination reveals characteristic changes.. The treatment is with ascorbic acid 300-500 mg. daily. The normal requirement of ascorbic acid in childhood is 15-30 mg./day.

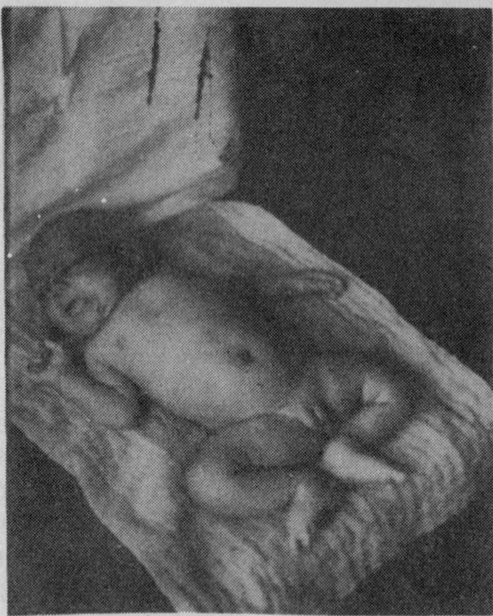

Fig.5.3 : Frog position : Scurvy

Rickets :

Rickets is a disease of bones in infants and children, the development of which required the simultaneous lack of dietary Vitamin D., calcium, phosphorus and sunlight. The rickets is highly prevalent in many tropical countries even inspite of sunning, which should more than ensure the small amount of endogenous cholecalciferol synthesis sufficient to protect against rickets. A poor and more of starchy diet, often rich in phytate, gastrointestinal infections and infestations with varying degrees of malabsorption and absence of Vitamin D supplements and excessively protective clothing due to strong traditional beliefs are important contributory factors.

The richest sources of Vitamin D in the human diet are from the oils derived from the livers of several species of fish and to a lesser extent from the dairy products. After absorption the vitamin undergoes 25-hydroxylation in the liver and the product is in turn further hydroxylated in the kidney to give the active form 1,25 dihydroxycholecalciferol. This substance facilitates calcium absorption from the intestine by stimulating the synthesis of a specific calcium binding protein. It is also thought to enhance the renal tubular reabsorption of phosphate. In excess, the vitamin will cause the reabsorption of bone with liberation of calcium.

The signs of Vitamin D deficiency may also arise as a result of an inherited defect in the 25-hydroxycholecalciferol-hydroxylase, or as a complication of treatment with anti-convulsants drugs. In Vitamin D deficiency there is failure of calcium deposition at the epiphysis and replacement of the line of calcification with osteoid tissue.

The peak prevalence is observed during the second six months of the first year and usually does not appear much before the third month and is seldom encountered after the third year. The child is usually pale and fretful, excessive sweating over the head, flabby with toneless muscles. There is often a coincidental iron deficiency anaemia. The abdomen is distended due to hypotonia and fermentive diarrhoea and they often suffer from respiratory infections.

The earliest bone change called 'craniotabes' can usually be observed over the occipito-parietal bones. The other bone sign include the enlargement of the lower end of the long bones and costochondral junctions of the ribs known as rickety-rosary, the lower ends of tibia and fibula. If the disease continues into the second year of life, closure of the fontanelle and the primary dentitions are delayed. The formation of new subperiosteal bone produces frontal and parietal bossing giving the head a square or boxed appearance. The forceful sucking of the softened ribs on inspirations during respiratory infections produces bilateral depressions on the chest along the attachment of the sternum up to the midaxillary line (Harrison's Sulcus). This deformity in turn gives the sternum undue prominence producing the so called 'Pigeon shaped', appearance. Sitting and crawling result in kyphosis of the spine while standing causes scoliosis. When the child begins to walk, deformities of the legs are 'knock-knees' or 'bow legs' add to the clinical picture. The fracture of the extremities occur easily and due to deformity of pelvic bones — in future difficulties may lead to obstructed labour in later life. In the presence of active rickets serum phosphorus is generally lowered, calcium normal or slightly lowered and alkaline phosphatase increased. The radiological examination of long bones, preferably the radius and ulna shows characteristic loss of definition of the metaphysical line with flaring and cupping of the ends as well as generalized osteoporosis. The treatment is with Vitamin D_2 125/μg. (5000 IU) per day will produce demonstrable radiological and biochemical improvement within a few weeks. The normal recommended intake of Vitamin D is given as 10 μg. daily thereafter. The excessive intake of Vitamin D may cause signs of toxicity.

Vitamin E :

The deficiency has been best recognised in premature babies, in whom haemolytic anaemia may occur at 6-10 weeks of age. The prophylactic administration of 5-10 mg. of Vitamin E daily to premature infants has been advocated. The normal intake of Vitamin E help in absorption of polyunsaturated fatty acid content in the diet. It also helps in reducing oedma in premature babies in the newborn period.

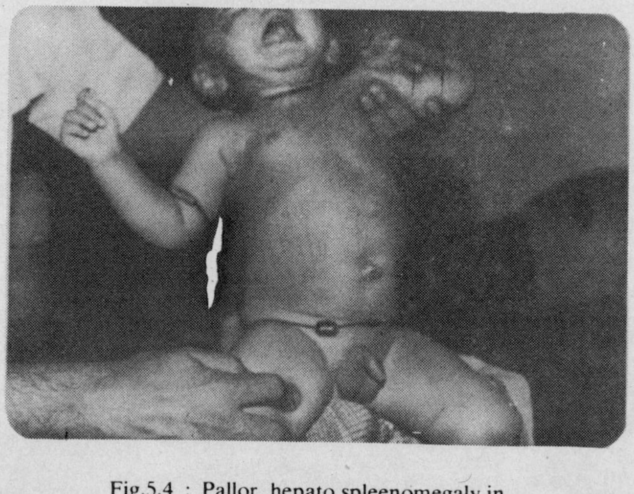

Fig.5.4 : Pallor, hepato spleenomegaly in Anaemia (Nutritional)

Anaemia :

This is mainly due to iron deficiency but folic acid and Vitamin B_{12} deficiency also may play a part. The child looks pale, his conjunctiva, lips, tongue and nail bases are pale. The nails may become flat or spoon shaped. The anaemia may, be due to lack of iron in the diet, lack of absorption from the gut, or hookworm infestation. It may also be seen in infancy under the age of 6 months as a result of inadequate iron stores in the liver because of anaemia in the mother. The ferrous sulphate is as good as any other more expensive salt. One tablet of 200 mg. containing 50 .ng. of elemental iron is enough for a child upto 5 years. Because of widespread an emia, it is better to give iron as a prophylactic, 10 mg. of elemental iron in the first year and 20 mg. after that. The tablets issued by Government containing 20 mg. elemental iron and 0.5 mg. folic acid are very convenient, and 1 tablet a day is a good prophylactic as well as treatment for milder anaemia. Anaemia is very common in pregnant women. It is recommended that a pregnant woman should be given 60 mg. of elemental iron and 0.5 mg. of folic acid a day during the last 100 days of her pregnancy. The foods, rich in iron like meats and green vegetables, should, if possible, be added to the diet. The possibility of fortifying some articles of food with iron has engaged the attention of nutrition research workers for sometime. It may be practicable to fortify common salt with iron in the not-too-distant future.

Iodine; Zinc and Fluoride :

These are micronutrients, essential component for thyroxine — thyroid hormone, body growth and also acrodermatitis enteropathica — related to Zinc deficiency, fluorine is needed for teeth. The colostrum of brest milk has high concentration of zinc. The deficiency of iodine in water and food is common in the population in mountaineous region and leads to goitre. It has been studied that children of these mothers, might develop mental retardation due to constant inadequacy of iodine in the mother. This is of epidemological importance and as a therapy these mothers can take iodised salts to replenish their iodine deficiency.

Bibliography

McLaren, D.S., & Burnow, D. (1976) : Paediatric Nutrition, Edinburgh and London, Chuchill Livingstone.

CHAPTER – SIX

DIARRHOEAL DISEASES IN YOUNG CHILDREN.

The diarrhoeal diseases specially acute diarrhoeic diseases in small children are one of the major medico-social scourge in most of the developing countries. It is the dominant cause of the excessive morbidity and mortality in the young populations of under developed and developing communities. It is closely related to the socio-economic and cultural conditions which prevail upon these people a suboptimal nutritional status, unhygienic environment and limited health care facilities available. The fact that the seasonal peaks of summer diarrhoea observed many years ago in Europe and North America have vanished, points to climate as only an incidental factor. The diarrhoea in small children wrecks the worst havoc in the lower economic state, where poverty goes hand in hand with ignorance, over crowding, poor hygiene and a limited food supply, inadequately safeguard and often unclean. Diarrhoea may be defined as increased frequency of stools which may be watery or may contain blood or mucus.

Etiology :

The causes of diarrhoea cannot always be identified. According to WHO, however, major advances have been made by well equipped laboratories, and it is now possible to assert that 'the recognition of the role of new viruses and bacteria makes it possible to identify aetiological agents in more than 80% of diarrhoeas; this is a reversal of the situation present of few years ago when 80% of the cases remain undiagnosed.

A. The main causes of acute diarrhoea;

1. Viruses and bacteria;

Enterotoxigenic Escherechia coli produces a dysenteric syndrome similar to that of cholera.

The Rota viruses, recently discovered, are the most usual cause of diarrhoea in age group of 6 to 24 months.

The cholera Vibrio

Shiegella.

Salmonella.

2. **Parasites :**

Amoebiasis (Entamaeba histolytica)

Lamblia — giardia — only the most frequent agents of diarrhoea.

3. **Miscellaneous or parenteral causes :**

Since diarrhoea is only a symptom, it may be the indication of a non-intestinal infectious ailment — secondary to infection elsewhere in the body — Oto-rhino-laryngological, urinary, meningeal or pulmonary infections. Quite often it accompanies episodes of malaria and measles. For a three months to three years old these pathogenic agents constitute continual aggression during a most vulnerable time of life when growth is rapid and with immature immunological responses and particularly the malnourished non-breast fed young infant with a history of low birth weight, abrupt weaning provide the most fertile ground for invasion.

Other elements are :

The role of the feeding bottles.

A poorly washed, poorly sterilized bottle is an excellent culture media; the plastic bottle is indeed even more dangerous since it cannot be boiled. The presence of flies on a poorly cleaned nipple further multiplies the risks.

The practice of repeated purgatives inflicted upon the child so that he or she will have regular bowel movement, irritates the lower intestinal tract and causes diarrhoea.

4. **Mal-nutrition and diarrhoea :**

It makes infants more susceptible to viral and bacterial intestinal pathogens and renders their effect more ravaging. The regeneration and maturation of intestinal mucosal cells is slower in infants specially associated with malnutrition and so is the production of the locally protective secretory immunoglobulin 'A', an important barrier to invasion of the mucosal cells.

B. **The main causes of chronic diarrhoea :**

1. Malabsorptive disorders.
   Acquired disaccharidase deficiency.
   Tropical sprue (rare causes).
   Cystic fibrosis of the pancreas.
   Gluten induced enteropathy.
   A- β lipoprotinaemia.
   Protein loosing enteropathy.
2. **Metabolic and endocrine disorders :**
   Hyperthyroidism.
   Addison's disease.
   Juvenile diabetes.
   Hypoparathyroidism.
   Chronic renal disease.
3. **Local intestinal disorders :**
   Intestional tuberculosis.
   Regional enteritis.
   Ulcerative colitis.
   After surgical resection of bowel.

The alimentary tract dysfunction is not an entity, but represents the reaction of the bowel to a wide spectrum of conditions of varied aetiologies.

Diarrhoea means increased frequency of stools which may be water or may contain blood or mucus. Management of acute diarrhoea with dehydration in children depends upon the correction of physiological disturbances. This is to try to combat dehydration by proper replacement of fluids and electrolytes. In the next phase, therapy should be aimed at to reduce the number of loose motions and vomiting and thereby lessening the dehydration and toxaemia by proper use of antibiotics and chemotherapeutic drugs. Although biochemical studies are useful for proper evaluations of fluid therapy, one must also be conversant with managing such cases on clinical assessment without the help of laboratory aids, since majority of diarrhoea cases will not be able to get the help of biochemical investigations in remote villages and more so in the non-teaching hospitals. Acute diarrhoea in infancy and early childhood is still a major cause of morbidity and mortality. Most of the deaths are due to dehydration and so the survival depends more on the correction of physiological disturbances than immediate removal of the cause. Modern biochemical concept has changed the rationale of fluid therapy in children.

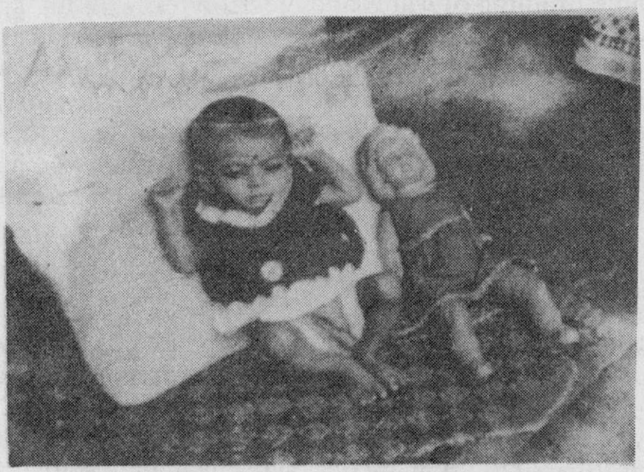

Fig.6.1(a) : Lactose intolerance diarrhoea — at 3 months

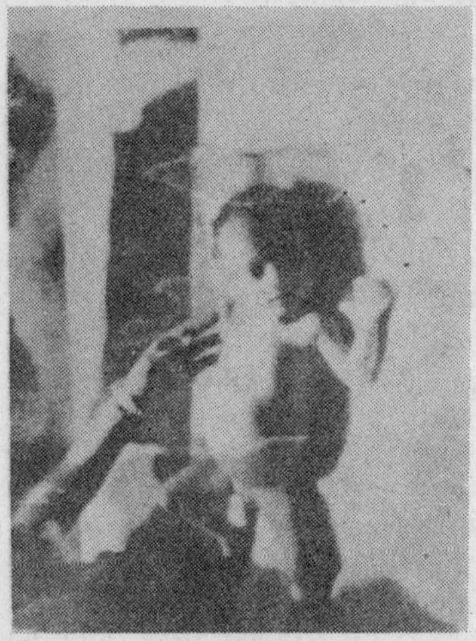

Fig.6.1(b) : Lactose intolerance diarrhoea — at 6 months.

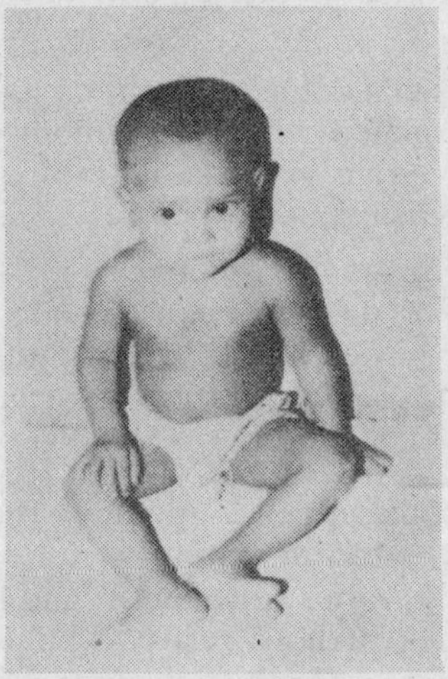

Fig.6.1(c) : Lactose intolerance Diarrhoea — at 9 months.

Prophylaxis :

Acute diarrhoea is largely confined to artificially fed babies and is a disease associated with poor hygiene and dirty methods of feed preparation. Moreover in a breast fed baby the colon is mainly populated by *Bacillus acidophillus* whereas in a baby fed on cow's milk it is mainly populated by *Escherichia coli,* thereby increasing the chance of infection with a pathogenic *Esch. coli* (Jolly, 1968). In poor and uneducated communities every possible step should be taken to pursuade the mothers to continue breast feeding at least for 3-6 months. During management of diarrhoea cases in hospitals, a strict barrier nursing should be imposed. No one with bowel disorders should be allowed to nurse or handle the feedings in the neonatal nurseries.

The cholera vibrio, or Koch's Vibrio, named after the man who discovered it in 1884, includes two pathogenic species :

Vibrio cholerae, the classical agent of cholera.

Vibro El tor, producing clinical forms, which may be minor or in apparent infections least, infection to case ratio — 90% of cases. Cholera is an intestinal toxic infections producing a veritable draining of water and electrolytes, with massive extra cellular then overall dehydration. Vaccination against cholera has been justifiably criticised. Vaccinal immunity is insufficient and only protects 50% of those who receive one injection and 60% of those who are given two injections, for three to six months theoretically. The possibility of reducing the number of cases of cholera by 50% during an epidemic is far from negligible, however, physicians who have been obliged to fight an Indian epidemic claim that mass vaccination puts an end to an epidemic assault.

Management :

Assessment of dehydration —

(a) Clinical assessment as mild, moderate and severe are characterised by depression of the fontanelle and eye balls, dryness of tongue, lips,mucous membranes, loss of tissue turgor-of the skin and scanty or no urine. Moreover, in severe dehydration the child appears very ill; systolic blood pressure below 80 mm. of Hg., cold and clammy extremities with mottling of the skin are noticed. The mental state may vary from one of the lethargy to coma. The pulse rate and volume are dependant upon factors other than the state of hydration and must be interpreted in the light of the child's general condition.

(b) This clinical assessment as mild, moderate and severe dehydration could be easily correlated with loss of body weight, and determination of plasma specific gravity by using graded dilutions of copper sulphate solution, known as Philip's method (Krishnan et al, 1974).

If specific gravity is between 1024 and 1028 in mild degree of dehydration, where loss body weight is between 2.5 and 5 percent, in moderate degree of dehydration, the lose of body weight is 5 to 10% and specific gravity will be between 1028 and 1030 while in severe dehydration associated with shock, the loss of body weight is more than 10 percent and the specific gravity is more than 1030.

(c) In some institutions, where the biochemical investigations could be done, the assessment of dehydration is done by estimation of serum sodium where serum sodium level varies between 135 and 140 mEq./1. the dehydration is known as isotonic; most of the diarrhoea cases develop this type of dehydration. Where sodium level is below 130 mEq./1., the dehydration is known as hypotonic, this type of dehydration is present in cholera where sodium is above 150 m Eq./l., the dehydration as known as hypertonic dehydration. Where there will be more loss of fluids as in the hot dampy atmosphere after profuse perspiration. Practical assessment of prognostically risk cases should be done as early as possible because even with the best of facilities available in management of acute cases, the death rate is still high, almost from 10 to 15 percent, so that one should spare no time to detect an early case before it takes an adverse turn and to prevent development of a serious picture. Clinical examination of the child and at least a microscopic examination of a specimen of stool should be insisted upon before suggesting the line of treatment. A mere history from the parents cannot be relied upon for a correct diagnosis. It is a better practice to enquire as to the number, quality and quantity of stools so that replacement therapy can be balanced. In infective diarrhoea the colour of the stools are greenish, offensive, with fishy odour in *Esch. coli* and *Shigella* infection, rice watery in cholera, mucoid in amoebic dysentery and mucopurulent with blood and less faecal material in bacilliary dysentery. Besides frequency and physical character of stools, one should note presence of vomiting, output of urine, hyperpyrexia, convulsion, presence of acidotic breathing and air hunger and also associated malnutrition in a patient of acute diarrhoea, for evaluation of the nature of therapy and ultimate prognosis of the case.

Nature of therapy —

In mild, moderate and in severe cases, where there is no vomiting, oral route is preferred for replacement therapy. Even if vomiting occurred oral fluids may be withheld for several hours and then started in teaspoonful amounts with gradual increments. But in severe dehydration with shock and moderate dehydration with vomiting, intravenous replacement should be the ideal route.

Type of fluid according to state of dehydration —

In our country most of the cases of acute diarrhoeas will develop isotonic (70 percent) or hypotonic (20 percent) dehydration and a few will develop hypertonic (10 percent) dehydration.

Due to presence of malnutrition in more than 70 percent of cases (Khatua, 1974) in our country, the type of dehydration is modified with addition of acidosis in 62 percent (Krishnan et al, loc. cit) in almost all the degrees of dehydration and so marked hypokalaemia in almost 42.3 percent (Krishnan et al, loc. cit) of cases. In isotonic dehydration, the fluid of choice is 5 percent dextrose with 0.45 g. percent sodium chloride and half strength Ringer lactate with 5 percent dextrose. The solution of 'glucose saline' can be made by the mother by adding three teaspoonful of sugar and a pinch of salt to every two tea cups of boiled water for oral use. In hypotonic dehydration, the fluid of choice is moderately hypertonic fluid with 5 percent dextrose with 0.9 g. percent sodium chloride and full strength Ringer lactate. In hypertonic dehydration, the fluid of choice is 4.3 percent dextrose with 0.18 g. percent sodium chloride. As for oral hydration, there are some 'salt packets' (oral Rehydration Salts — ORS) which are marketed under different names; and when these packets are mixed with requisite amount of water, it will supply proper electrolytes. As for example WHO packet contains sodium chloride — 3.5 gm., sodium bicarbonate 2.5 g., potassium chloride — 1.5 g., and glucose powder — 25 g. and 1000 ml. of water to be mixed with it.

Amount to be replaced —

The therapy during the initial phase should be aimed to correct the shock and restore the circulatory volume, so it needs rapid replacement; 20-30 ml./kg./hourly up to 4-6 hours should be given preferably with isotonic fluid. The maintenance fluids are needed during the subsequent hours, the amount being 120 ml./kg. in 24 hours or if possible oral replacement. During intravenous therapy, one should keep watch on developing pulmonary oedema, hyperpyrexia, convulsion, signs of water intoxication and circulatory overload. These are the hazards due to rapid infusion, contaminated fluids with infection, and hypo-or hypertonic fluid infusion.

Associated vomiting, hyperpyrexia and convulsion —

If vomiting is present, it might prevent oral replacement, so one should go for intravenous replacement and oral fluids may be withheld for several hours and then started in teaspoonful amounts with gradual increments. No drug is beneficial to combat vomiting. Only stomach wash with normal saline or sodium bicarbonate will help.

Hyperpyrexia may be a side effect of infusion or sometimes it is present due to toxaemia or due to dehydration itself not corrected after infusion of small amount of calculated fluids. Convulsion in acute diarrhoeas might be due to hypertonic dehydration or with more sodium retention or due to hyponatraemia and water intoxication. The new concept is the relative hypomagnesaemia associated with malnutrition in diarrhoea cases. Low serum magnesium produces hyperirritability and convulsions (Krishnan et al, loc. cit).

Acidosis is a common feature in acute diarrhoea cases with dehydration; 62 percent of the diarrhoeal children had moderate to severe acidosis (Krishnan et al, loc. cit.). Our children with their inherent low resistance and in the presence of malnutrition, may withstand the degree of acidosis seen in relation to fluid loss and dehydration. Thus sodium bicarbonate 7.5 percent or 1/6th molar lactate — 4 ml./kg. will increase the plasma bicarbonate level by 1 mEq. In case of malnutrition with liver damage, better fluid is sodium bicarbonate than sodium lactate. The incidence and severity of acidosis are not similar in the well nourished and malnourished children. Sodium bicarbonate needs to be used with caution in malnourished children as the sodium infused may rapidly expand the extracellular compartment producing cardiac failure. Also in presence of hyperkalaemia, rapid rise in blood pH may precipitate tetany. Sodium bicarbonate should be given in small amounts attempting 2-3 mEq. correction and preferably after initial correction of hypokalaemia.

Hypokalaemia (Potassium below 3.5 mEq./1.) was always encountered in acute diarrhoea with malnutrition. In 42.3 percent (Krishnan et al, loc. cit.) of the cases studied varying degree of hypokalaemia was observed. Inspite of such marked potassium deficits, potassium cannot be fully replenished on the first day itself since any excess beyond 40 mEq./1. of potassium in the infused fluid will have toxic effects. Potassium depletion appears to play an important role in disturbances of renal function, water and sodium balance and cellular function. In oral replacement of potassium, 3 mEq./kg./day should be aimed at and more so in malnutrition with diarrhoea. It is also important to realise that potassium correction ought to be achieved in 72-96 hours time. Oral replacement of potassium is much safer than intravenous replacement. Oral replacement should be as potassium chloride 0.5 g. as tablet or one teaspoonful of syrup at 4-6 hourly interval, if renal function is satisfactory as indicated by good urinary output. It is better than intravenous replacement and not more than 40 mEq./1. of infused fluid should be used.

When to start oral therapy —

After 24-36 hours of intravenous infusion, when the signs of dehydration have been corrected, number of stools and vomiting have diminished, and there is no sign of toxaemia only then one should start oral replacement. It should be very gradual and the choice of fluid should be the same as the patient was having as the last intravenous fluid. Hypertonic glucose solution orally might lead to increased hyperosmolarity in the stomach and thereby draw in more fluid and again loose motions. So a better oral replacement fluid will be an electrolyte solution such as WHO fluid or half strength Darrow's or Ringer lactate solution. Milk feeds should be gradually introduced with modification. For example milk should be diluted, boiled, skimmed off the fat and if necessary acidification and addition of extra sugar, so that the diarrhoeic children may get required amount of calories and at the same time digest the milk properly. One should take at least 7 days for going back to normal diet. The breast fed baby will be put on breast again as soon as the dehydration has been corrected by replacement fluids. In the newborns with acute diarrhoea, the fluid of choice is 4.3 percent dextrose with 0.18 g. percent sodium chloride because of sodium retention is more if hypertonic fluid is used. The amount should be calculated as 90 ml./kg./day as intravenous replacement with the help of scalp vein needle. Subcutaneous replacement with the help of hyalase in some cases as preliminary replacement before transferring the case to hospital, is sometimes advocated in remote village where there are no trained personnel for intravenous replacement. But chance of infection by the secondary invaders through the subcutaneous route is more, so it is better to make simultaneous use of parenteral antibiotics such as pencillin and with an oral antibiotic such as neomycin.

Antibiotics and Chemotherapeutics –

In the introduction it has been mentioned that in acute diarrhoeas, the first aim is to treat dehydration and secondly to treat the loose motions because if loose motions continue, then there will be more dehydration and fluid electrolyte imbalance. So, the use of antidiarrhoeal agents comes afterwards to combat the bacterial infection or in some cases infestation by parasites and worms. It was recognised that the prescription of antibiotics was useless in most cases of diarrhoea, and be reserved for cases of severe Enterotoxigenic coli, Shigellosis and Cholera. Various drugs are used, among them, the drug of choice for Esch, coli, is neomycin sulphate (25-30 mg./kg. body weight) orally in 24 hours. For shigella, the drug to start with sulphaguanidine (240 to 480 mg./kg. body weight) orally for Ent. histolytica and Giardia intestinals the drug of choice is di-iodohydroxyquinoline, chloroquine phosphate and furazolidin (6 mg./kg. body weight in divided doses), metronidazole (20 mg./kg. body weight in divided doses), for 7-10 days duration. For various worms specially round worms, piperazine, is given as a single dose (60 to 80 mg./kg. body weight) at bed time.

Convalescent treatment –

During the phase of recovery a quick but speedy return to balanced nutrition should be made to prevent a malnutrition state developing with prolonged starvation with hypocaloric diet because the stools are not yet perfect, is a common mistake for restricting calories leading to marasmus after an attack of acute diarrhoea.

References

Joly, H. : Diseases of Children 2nd., 1968, Blackwell, London, pp. 18-28.

Khatua, S.P. : Indian Med. J. 68 : 9, 1974.

Krishnan, B.R. Senthana, Deendaysis, K. and Raju V.V. : Indian
Pediat., 11 : 345, 1974.

Villod, M.T., Raithault, A.M., Guerin : Children in the Tropics.
A seminar on diarrhoeic diseases, ICC/W.H.O., June, 1979.

CONSTIPATION IN CHILDREN

Definition :

It is a condition of passage of very hard stool with pain and straining during defaecation. Constipation is usually a chronic affair but acute constipation may result from acute intestinal obstruction.

Causes :

1. Dietetic defects :
   Underfeeding or starvation.
   Insufficient intake of water.
   High protein content of the diet.
2. Gastrointestinal causes :
   Faulty training.
   Emotional upsets.
   Pyloric stenosis.
   Fissure in ano.
   Congenital anal stenosis.
   Hirschsprung's disease.
3. Other causes :
   Cretinism.
   Juvenile myxoedema.
   Drugs e.g., opiates.

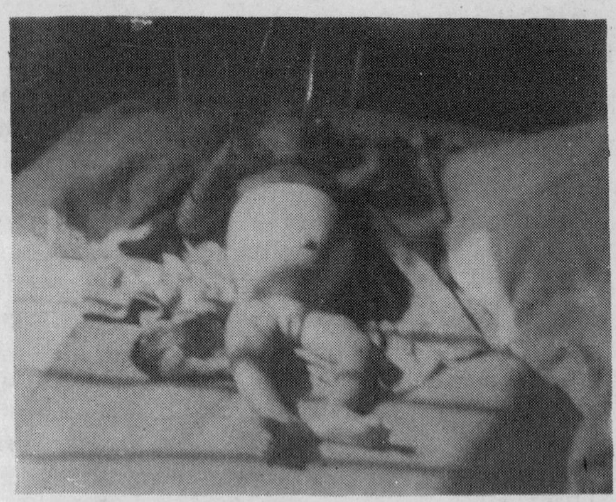

Fig.6.2 : Abdominal distension — Hirschprung's disease.

Diagnosis :

Usually in all constipated children rectum is very much dilated and contains hard faeces. Accumulated faeces in the rectum may cause irritation leading to false diarrhoea.

Treatment :

The underlying cause should be diagnosed properly and treated as far as practicable. The diet should contain cellulose, bread, fruits and vegetable. Fluid should be given adequately. Senna preparations are better tolerated and may be given.

References

Hinton, J.M. and Lannard-Jones, J.E. (1968) : Constipation — Definition and Classification. Post Grad. Med. J., 44 : 720.

CHAPTER – SEVEN

RESPIRATORY DISEASE OF INFANTS AND CHILDREN

ACUTE BRONCHIOLITIS :

Acute bronchiolitis is a disease of early infancy caused by infection with a respiratory virus which leads to inflammatory reaction. Confined to the walls of bronchioles and the peribronchial tissues, the alveoli being spared. The plugging of the bronchioles by inflammatory exudate gives rise to obstruction of the lower respiratory tracts which is responsible for the characteristic clinical findings.

The respiratory synctial virus (RSV) is the main pathogen. Most cases occur between the ages of 6 weeks and 10 months, the typical clinical picture is never seen in the newborn period and becomes increasingly rare after 1 year of age. The recent evidence from New Castle strongly suggests that breast feeding affords some protection against RSV infection. Williams has found an association between bronchiolitis in infancy and asthma in later childhood.

The condition usually starts with coryza, but is followed by a rapidly developing severe illness. The degree of fever is moderate. There is distressing dry cough, increasing dyspnoea and tachypnoea with an expiratory grunt,marked intercostal and suprasternal retraction occur with each inspiration. There is restlessness and disturbed sleep. There is minimal stridor. In severe cases there is cyanosis which can often be relieved by removal of tenacious mucoid secretion blocking the mouth, nose and oropharynx. The physical signs are scattered inspiratory crepitations, but wheezy rhonchi are also common. The lungs are hyperresonant on percussion on account of acute emphysema. The illness has a significant mortality but one which can be greatly reduced by modern treatment in skilled hands. If it is not complicated then improvement starts within one week.

The diagnosis is made on clinical examination and is easy in epidemic periods. The X-ray shows increased lung markings, but no frank consolidation unless the condition has progressed to patchy pneumonia. The segmental collapse from the occlusion of a bronchus may occur. An attack of asthma may be suspected in a mild case and the distinction may not be easy. The possibility of a foreign body in a bonchus or cystic fibrosis must be remembered. The management is urgent and great vigilance is required in the nursing of these patients. The infant should be nursed in a semi-upright position. The oxygen should be given in sufficient concentration to overcome restlessness and cyanosis. The oxygen and humidity are of accepted value, and are satisfactorily provided only in a tent with a mechanical humidifier. The maintenance of hydration is essential. While the infant is unable to suck, the feeds may be given by a fine nasal polyvinyl feeding tube. Occasionally, parenteral fluids may be given. To induce sleep choral hydrate 5-10 mg. or phenobarbitone 15 mg. twice daily are helpful. In severe cases with generalized toxaemia, here is a need for digoxin in view of the possibility of cardiac failure. It should be introduced cautiously, the full digitalizing dose being given over a 48 hour period. The antibiotics are not indicated unless a secondary bacterial infection is suspected. If there are signs of circulatory collapse then steroids should be given hydrocortisone acetate in doses of 25-50 mg. even six hourly by I.V. or I.M. is appropriate for a child of 6 months to 1 year of age. After 48 hours the dose should be gradually tapered and omitted after 5-7 days time. The respiratory acidosis may occur and need correction by alkali. The obstruction by secretions of the main bronchi and trachea require frequent suction. The postnasal drainage and suction at the back of the pharynx which also stimulates the cough reflex, are essential to clear the airway. After recovery from the acute state, there may be localized segmental collapse which is resolved less rapidly and which can become the site of secondary bacterial infection.

THE PNEUMONIAS

The pneumonias are defined as an acute inflammatory process involving the alveolar walls and spaces of the lung parenchyma. Infants and children of all ages are affected and a wide range of bacteria and respiratory viruses may be responsible. The older classification of acute chest infections in children into bronchitis, bronchiolitis, bronchopneumonia and lobar pneumonia needs revision. The true pneumonia, either localized to one area of the lung or more widespread has its own clinical picture.

To elaborate some points on aetiology, some further light has been thrown by a small comprehensive study of actue non-tuberculous lower respiratory infections in children under 4 years of age in Calcutta, Hughes et al, 1966, found evidence of a virus infection in 44% of children studied, H. influenzae was recovered from one quarter to one-third of cases by percutaneous lung aspirations. The same workers cultured Mycoplasma pneumoniae from the nasopharygeal secretions of a child with pneumonitis, moreover, emphasis has been given on the role of respiratory viruses and mycoplasma in the causation of pneumonia in a representative Indian urban population. Nevertheless, it seems likely that the relative importance of viruses and bacteria in the causation of pneumonia will be different in tropical and temperate climates, still playing a rather larger role in the former than is now the case in the west. The pneumococci, H. influenzae and staphylococcus aureas, are the bacteria most often involved. The recurrent attacks of pneumonia suggest an underlying abnormality such as tracheo-oesophageal fistula, cystic fibrosis, malnutrition with primary tuberculosis, or immune deficiency state. Before the age of two years classical pneumococcal lobar pneumonia is rare. Staphylococcal pneumonia is commonest in this age group. In a newborn infant aspiration of infected liquor amnii, in cases of premature rupture of the membranes, is the usual cause. The infection is often by **E. Coli.** In pneumonia developing some days after birth the usual pathogens are staphylococci and pneumococci. The humid environment of an incubator favours the growth of pseudomonas organisms.

The pneumonia in an infant may supervene on an upper respiratory infection or may begin abruptly without evidence of upper respiratory tract involvement. The infant is likely to appear seriously ill with fever, cough, tachypnoea, dyspnoea, with grunting expiration, active alae nasi and intercostal and lower costal recession and with abnormal moist sounds in the lungs. There may be fine crepitations in one or more zones or there may be evidence of consolidation with diminished air entry impaired percussion note and bronchial or tubular breath sounds. The cyanosis may be present. This clinical picture is very clear cut and the diagnosis is not likely to be in doubt. However, in neonates, or in malnourished or otherwise debilated infants, the signs may be very much less definite, with no clear pointer to the respiratory tract as the site of infections. The staphylococcal pneumonia the onset is sudden and within hours of onset, the infant is running high fever and seriously ill with localized signs of consolidation appearing early. If the diagnosis is not made promptly and appropriate antibiotic therapy started, pneumatococeles are likely to develop with the risk of emphysema, pneumothorax or pyopneumothorax. A tension pneumothorax with rapidly progressive shift of the mediastinum and cardio respiratory collapse is not an uncommon complication. The chest X-ray is of great assistance and there is a great contrast between the physical signs and the X-ray picture. Generally, it will show whether the distribution is scattered and patchy or whether confined to one or more lobes. The tension cysts which are so characteristic of staphylococcal pneumonias may be seen in X-ray, but tension cysts also occur in pneumococcal pneumonia.

The laboratory findings also support the evidences of infection due to bacteria or viruses. The increase total count with increase of polymorphs suggest bacterial infection and leucopenia with relative lymphocytosis favour the diagnosis of viral aetiology.

The confirmation of the diagnosis of virus pneumonia is obtained from samples of serum taken at the onset and again after a two week interval in this way active infection with adenovirus, coxsackie, ECHO virus, psittacosis, Ornithrosis and Q Fever may be identified. The direct virus isolation can be obtained from nose and throat washings.

It is a known fact that most of pneumonias in children are due to viruses, all cases should be treated as though of bacterial in origin. The radiological appearance of consolidation caused by the alveolar exudate of a bacterial infection and the interstitial pneumonia of a virus infection cannot be distinguished, and all causes must, therefore, receive antibiotics. In the less seriously ill cases treatment may be started with penicillin, co-trimoxazole, or sulphadiazine. A single injection of a massive does of penicillin is an effective simple form of therapy useful for out-patient treatment where large numbers of children are involved where as in severe infections, the combination of cloxacillin and ampicillin is a logical first line of treatment, cloxacillin for a possible penicillin resistant staphylococcus and ampicillin for H. influenzae, both being effective against the commoner pneumococci and streptococci. The treatment should be started parenterally in high dosage and changed to the oral route after 48 to 72 hours if there is a good therapeutic response. Chloramphenicol by mouth is a reasonable alternative in case of ampicillin in H. Influenzae infection. Oxygen should be administered in severe cases with cyanosis, and fluids and alkalis to be infused in case of dehydration with respiratory acidosis respectively. Digoxin should be given in a dosage to achieve rapid digitalization if there is any suspicion of cardiac failure. Where pneumonia is complicated with PCM or other nutritional deficiency, this should be corrected as rapidly as possible. Associated anaemia may need blood transfusion where signs suggest pleural fluid or pneumothorax, the diagnosis should be established by immediate pleural aspiration and the appropriate treatment instituted. The septicaemia with metastatic pyaemic abscesses or meningitis is now rarely seen, except in staphylococcal infections. The prognosis depends on several factors but probably the most important is the age of the child. The children with malnutrition, cerebral palsy and primary muscular diseases are associated with bad prognosis.

WHEEZY CHILD.

The wheeze or bronchospasm in a child, is an evidence of bronchial obstruction, specially of lower respiratory bronchi. It may be caused by extrinsic pressure from a mediastinal mass (cyst, neoplasm or lymph nodes, by involvement of the bronchial wall in an inflammatory process, laryngotracheo bronchitis or in association with a contiguous tuberculous lymphadenitis), or by aspiration of material such as blood, or secretions formed in the course of a respiratory tract infection or of a foreign body. Also the combination of respiratory infection and pulmonary congestion which can occur in young children with congenital heart disease which includes a significant left to right cardiac shunt in VSD, ASD and patent ductus. The likelihood that wheezing in a child is due to migratory parasites such as Ascaria lumbricodies (Loffler's syndrome), Toxocara canies (Viseral larva migrans) or filaria pp. (tropical eosinophilia) is of course very much greater than bronchial asthma of allergic origin and should be excluded by eosinophil counts, chest radiographs and appropriate parasitological investigations. In true asthma the range of antigens involved will certainly differ from usually responsible in western children.

However, in true asthma, in more than half the cases there is a family history of asthma, hay fever, eczema or urticaria. This suggests a marked tendency for asthma to be inherited or at least a constitutional tendency to this type of reaction under stress.

The various factors may precipitate an attack of asthma. Among the commonest are (a) infections, specially of nasopharynx, (b) hypersensitivity to inhalants and (c) Psychogenic; there is no doubt that excitement and nervousness without other influences can initiate attacks. The bronchospasm or wheeze is due to (a) spasm of the bronchial muscles, (b) swelling of the lining mucous membrane of the smallest bronchioles by plugs of mucous.

The child may be put to bed with what appears to be a slight cold, with or without a temperature, but wakes during the night, much distressed, coughing and wheezing and unable to get his breath. His difficult breathing worries him and he looks anxious and may complain of a 'tight chest'. The attack may be over in a few hours or cease on waking in the morning; on the other hand, if accompanied by a fever, it may continue for some days and manifest some degree of true bronchitis. In other situations such as exposure to a known precipitating allergen such as dog or horse hair or pollens may rapidly precipitate an attack. In some children bronchospasm appears to be induced by exertion.

In some children, where it is prolonged for some years, the chest might be deformed and is of barrel shaped. The percussion is hyper-resonant due to accompanying emphysema. On auscultation expiration is markedly prolonged and expiratory rhonchi are heard. These are high pitched and sibilant. The excursion of the chest is small and the air entry extremely poor. In every case, other pulmonary disease must be carefully excluded as wheeze or bronchospasm may be simulated by such condition as tuberculosis or tropical eosinophilia and in a young child, inhalation of a foreign body into a bronchus. An X-ray of the chest and a tuberculin test are of value as a routine. The repeated attack of 'bronchitis' for no apparent cause in a child should always suggest asthma. The blood count may show an eosinophilia of from 4 to 10%. Asthma should also be suspected if the child has a previous history of well marked eczema or urticaria. The family history may be suggestive. Primary obstruction is reflected in impaired FEV% values compared with normal standards for age and sex.

A large number of methods of treatment advocated indicate that all have limitations. During severe attack the child should be put to bed, clothes put on but not overclad, with plenty of fresh air. During mild attack every effort should be taken to cut it short as soon as possible and then allow the child to return rapidly to normal activities.

In the fully developed attack the most useful routine measure is subcutaneous injection of 1/1,000 solution of adrenaline 0.3-0.5 ml. This may require to be repeated at half hourly interval to maintain relief from bronchospasm. If adrenaline fails to provide relief, aminophylline 125-250 mg. may be injected I.V. diluted with 5-10 ml. of water over a period of 10 minutes. This drug can cause syncope but the risk can be avoided if given slowly. Aminophylline can be given as rectal suppository, 50-100 mg. for children between one to five years, 100-200 mg. for older children. The acute attacks of asthma can frequently be aborted if treated at the first sign of tightness of the chest with oral ephidrine hydrochloride ½ gr. 6-8 hourly interval. Alternatively, isoprenaline sulphate may be used, either as 10 mg. in tablet form sublingually or as a 1% solution which is spread into the pharynx from an all glass nebulizer during forced inspiration, this is only practicable in older children.

Recently introduced, salbutamol which is a sympathomimetic drug with a selective beta-2 stimulatory effect is an effective safe bronchodilator. This may be used in a dose of 0.15 mg./kg. body weight upto four times a day by mouth. In severe attacks, salbutamol inhaled by means of a nebulizer can be dramatically effective. Recently, salbutamol is available in injection form.

Status asthmaticus is an emergency. If it has not responded to the treatment outlined above, the use of corticosteroids on a short term basis can be life saving. In dire emergency hydrocortisone I.M. in six hourly doses of 50-1000 mg. for 24 hours, to be followed by an oral steroid for another five to six days. Where there are antigens involved, the management concerned with the exclusion of or reduction of sensitivity to selected antigens by hyposensitization technique, may be relevant but the recently introduced protective regimens based on the regular inhalation of disodium cromoglycate or of a topical steroid like beclomethazone dipropionate would certainly be effective.

The deep breathing exercises supervised by attained physiotherapist and preferably in a class with other children are of undoubted value in chronic asthmatics. As long term management in some asthmatics where there is possibility of psychological problems, the family physician with his knowledge of the home background, is in a position to help the poor child and judge the nature of the affliction in its home background. Specific psychotherapy is rarely of benefit, but common sense advice should be given for instance — releasing child from over- protection by mother. The long term use of corticosteroids in some resistant cases might be used but among the side effects of corticosteroids such as slowing of growth, obesity, osteoporosis, peptic ulcers, steroid diabetes and acne-hirsutisms render the decision to institute such treatment a difficult problem. Better steroid is ACTH during the growth period, which has got less side effects and moreover steroid addiction and slowing of growth is less marked.

References

Hughes, J.R. and Sinha D.P. (1966) : Indian Pediat., 3, 52.

Chakraborty, B.K. : Archives of Child Health, Vol. 10, No. 1.

Pp. 16-18, 1968

Hutchinson, J. : Paediatric Problems, 3rd edition, 1978.

Lloyd Kukes, London.

CHAPTER – EIGHT

TUBERCULOSIS.

The prevalence of tuberculous infection is an yard-stick of the national health, community status and moreover the nutrition and environmental hygiene of a nation. More of clinical tuberculosis in children points to prevalence of open cases of tuberculosis in the adult population. The specific prevention through BCG, though controversial after WHO Organisation study in Madras and use of prophylactic antituberculoùs drugs are effective where these agents are correctly used as part of a national programme to reduce childhood tuberculosis from its position as a common happening to a rarity. The infection is usually through droplet infection and the primary site of infection is in the lung. The incubation period is 6-8 weeks until sensitivity and immunity develops. The primary complex that is the parenchymatous focus, the involvement of the regional gland, the involvement of the lymphatics, with it the development of hypersensitivity and immunity. It takes 6-12 weeks time. During this process of development the organisms may escape into the blood stream. The primary complex may develop commonly in lungs, intestines, lymph glands, any other viscera, except brain. The tuberculin test is a measure of hypersensitivity. The clinical story of a tuberculous infection is, therefore, a balance between the immune response and the acquired sensitivity. Associated malnutrition reduce the immune response and favour rapid spread of the disease from its initial site. The fate of primary complex may follow (a) extension of the primary focus known as progressive primary complex, (b) Caseation and rupture of a gland with involvement of the lung parenchyma leading on to blockage of bronchus segmental or endobronchial tuberculosis, (c) dissemination into blood pulmonary arteries, miliary tuberculosis and veins, disseminated tuberculosis including tuberculous meningitis, bone tuberculosis, visceral tuberculosis, involvement of kidney, liver etc. Any of these may occur at the same time, and the risks of all are greater in young children, decreasing gradually with age until puberty, when the risk increases again.

A child who has apparently overcomed a primary infection is not free from risk of tuberculosis where his own resistance is low, or when he is expected to a large infecting dose of organisms, reinfection may occur. It may also happen that the apparently healed primary lesion 'lights up' e.g., if corticosteroids are being administered. Reinfection differs in that the immune response is more rapid, dissemination is less likely, and so the disease is usually localised to one organ.

The miliary tuberculosis and tuberculous meningitis are most often seen about three months after the primary infection has been established. The caseation of lymph nodes is more likely to occur within the first year after infection. The blood spread is most likely in the first few weeks after primary infection, but bone lesions do not often appear until three or more years later. Renal and epididymal lesions are uncommon in childhood and are more often seen at puberty. 15-20% of children infected in the first year of life develop tuberculous meningitis or miliary spread within two years compared with only 4% of all children infected under the age of 5 years (Miller et al, 1963).

The prevalence of tuberculosis in children in India below the age of 14 years has been reported as 27%. The annual incidence of new cases is 1.0% (Raj Narain, 1963). Studies by Raja and other show that 40% of the child population below 14 years and 25% of those below 6 years are infected with tubercle bacillus. as evidenced by positive tuberculin test.

The diagnosis of tuberculosis (Chakraborty et al, 1978) in children possesses a problem. History of sickness is invariably vague, family history or history of contact is lacking in many patients. The clinical signs are ambiguous, radiological evidences may be inconclusive and bacteriological determinations are invariably negative. However, primary tuberculosis with various forms and progressive complications can be completely cured with adequate early treatment.

The tuberculosis may involve practically any organ or tissue of the body. Symptoms of any tuberculous lesion may be varied and may simulate many other diagnosis of the majority of chronic infections and acute ones, the possibility of tuberculosis must be considered.

Intrathoracic tuberculous infection accounts for at least 90% of recognised tuberculous diseases in children. Parenchymal and lymph node involvement always occur but the foci are not always apparent on clinical or roentogenographic examination. The extent of the infection in the pulmonary parenchyma or in the lymph nodes is largely responsible for the various clinical patterns. Among the various intrathoracic types primary complex (9.8%) bronchopneumonic types (3.0%) pleural effusion (4.5%) mostly in elderly children, collapse, consolidation in segmental tuberculosis (4.5%), bilateral infiltration through bronchi or local pulmonary vessels 1.5% and acute milliary tuberculosis were classified both on clinical and roentgenographic examination. Udani et al (1976) observed intrathoracic tuberculosis was most common 41% in their series, the mortality was low as 4.4%. The acute miliary tuberculosis is fourth 3.9%, its mortality was on an average 41.3% which is very high as most of the cases were brought late for treatment. Chakraborty et al, 1978 presented acute miliary tuberculosis as 6.1% and 2 cases with thrombocytopenia with massive bleeding episodes and one with anaemia resistant to usual haematinic therapy respectively. Mortality was nil though this is a very small series and the age incidence in all cases were above 3 years. The acute miliary tuberculosis is a blood borne infection characterised by multiple tubercle formations. It is more frequent below 1 year of age than in older children. Practically all organs of the body may be involved. The tubercle bacilli became lodged in the small capillaries involved the parenchyma and a tubercle is developed. If the life is sufficiently prolonged then these tubercles may be generalised in the lung parenchyma and show radiological appearance after 6-12 weeks known as 'snow storm' appearance.

The clinical picture is usually those of general infection with toxaemia, fever, enlargement of spleen with ambiguous signs in the chest. May be associated in 60% of cases with central nervous system involvement as tuberculous meningitis. Here the choroidal tubercles in the eyes though rare may be an associated findings and may be detected by opthalmoscopic examination. Death usually occurs within four to six weeks in untreated cases but recovery is possible in the majority of cases if treatment is instituted sufficiently early.

Among the extra thoracic type of tuberculosis (58.3%) the CNS tuberculosis is 35.6%, bone tuberculosis 3.1%, abdominal tuberculosis 9.0%, tuberculous kidney 0.08%, cervical lymphadenopathy 3.7% and only tuberculin positive of more than 10 mm. induration 6.1% were observed by Chakraborty et al, 1978. The mortality in CNS tuberculosis, among tuberculous patients was 80.8% and 9.2% among the total deaths.

Abdominal tuberculosis :

This includes tuberculous ulceration of the bowel, tuberculosis of abdominal lymph nodes (tabes mesenterica) and both the ascitic and plastic forms of tuberculous peritonitis. It is usual to find two or more of them at the same time, in fact they develop one from the other and all will have been present to some extent in most cases. The abdominal tuberculosis is usually due to a primary focus in the bowel, spreading to the mesenteric glands or peritoneum, sometimes, especially in the much older child, there is a previous pulmonary lesion which has secondarily infected the bowel, In our country this is the cause because abdominal tuberculosis in our country mostly due to human tubercle bacillus. Moreover, our cattle population is not much infected with Bovine tubercle bacillus and so the infected milk is not the source, which was once common is western countries.

Abdominal pain and perhaps fever and also irregular bowels with alternate loose motions and constipation are the commonest symptoms. In a few cases there is a history of colicky pain and diarrhoea sometimes mucus and a little blood are noted. The clinical picture resembles that of sprue syndrome or amoebic or bacillary dysenteries on account of the passage of pale, loose and offensive stools, possibly due to interference with the absorption of fats. On palpation in tabes mesenterica, the enlarged mesenteric glands may be felt, in some cases radiologically calcified glands may be demonstrated. More than 75% of abdominal tuberculosis in our country are associated with clubbing of the fingers and toes possibly due to malabsorption. In ascitic forms, fullness of the abdomen, doughy feel and sometimes mass of enlarged glands and rolled up omentum may be felt on deep palpation. The child is pale, wasted and languid. In the plastic form of peritonitis, the abdomen feels more doughy. Very often associated with toxaemia and feature of sub-acute intestinal obstruction.

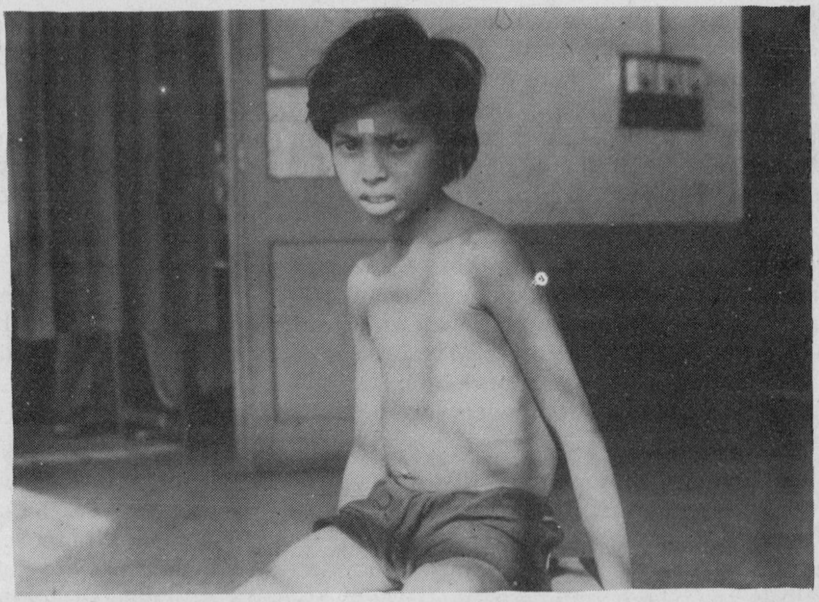

C N S Tuberculosis :

Among the CNS tuberculosis, the tuberculous meningitis is the commonest. It is again common under 5 years of age, those who are not immunized with BCG at birth. The disease develops as a complication of tuberculosis elsewhere in the body usually following within a few months of the primary infection. The tubercle bacilli are thought to reach the meninges from caseous foci in the brain due to blood borne spread from the primary complex or other distant tuberculous lesions such as lymph glands, abdomen and bones, generalized miliary tuberculosis is found in about 60% of cases. Generally, from an adult tuberculous person as a close contact in the family, the child is affected and the bacilli responsible here is human type. Although the clinical picture is variable, the untreated disease usually shows three ill defined stages, each lasting about one week. The onset is generally insiduous, a previously active, normal child losing his vigour, weak sometimes vomiting without loose motions, drowsy, may complain of headache and often severe irritability. Such changes in a child's behaviour should always be taken seriously. In the second stage the temperature rises and signs of raised intracranial pressure, and sometimes of meningeal irritation, become more obvious. Vomiting, drowsiness and irritability increase. The curled up attitude, dislike of bright light on the eyes, periodic high pitched cry, teeth grinding or frank convulsion may result. The neck rigidity, the kernig signs and opisthotonic attitude may develop suggesting more of meningial irritation. In the eyes ocular palsies, squints and nystagmus may be seen occasionally at this stage or later, there is 'papilloedema and choroidal tubercles' may be seen by ophthalmoscopic examination. With the third stage the child sinks into stupor and finally coma; with fixed and dilated pupils, irregular respiration, widespread paralysis, hyperpyrexia and sometimes generalized convulsions and deliberate rigidity preceding terminal death. The diagnosis depends on examination of the CSF. This is almost always under raised pressure and either clear or faintly turbid with a ground glass appearance and on standing there is formation of 'Cob-web' coagulum. The cells are increased to 300/cmm. mainly lymphocytes, though occasionally polymorphs may present in early stage. The protein content is increased and the sugar reduced (but not like pyogenic meningitis). The combination of a moderate mainly lymphocytic pleocytosis and a low sugar content is diagnostic of tuberculous meningitis. The acid and alcohol fast bacilli can usually be seen in the centrifuged deposit of CSF stained by the Ziehl-Neelsen method or by flourescent microscopy. The culture of CSF should prove positive and guineapig inoculation tests are often helpful, but both these methods required several weeks befor their results are available.

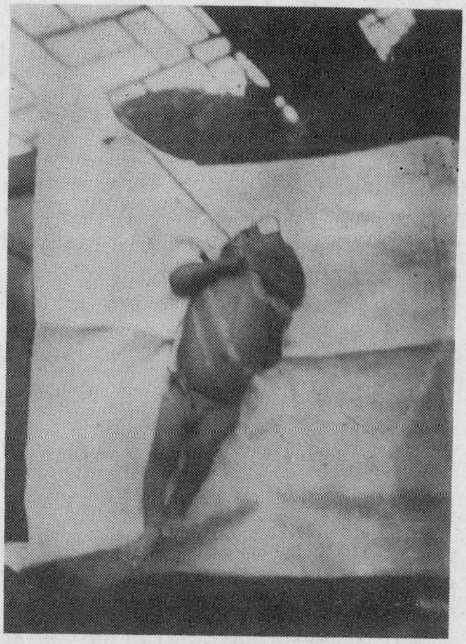

Fig.8.2 : A nine month old baby with T.B. meningitis and opisthotonic attitude.

INTERPRETATION OF THE TUBERCULIN TEST AND BCG VACCINE AS A TEST IN THE DIAGNOSIS OF TUBERCULOSIS

The object of performing skin test with tuberculin is to find out the hypersensitivity with tuberculous infection. The most widely used test is the Mantoux Test in which a low dose of 1 TU or 1 in 10,000 dilution of old tuberculin or 2TU of PPD of RT23 is given intradermally by means of tight syringe, on the anterior aspect of the left forearm, using 0.1 ml. of a standard dilution to raise a wheal about 6-8 mm. in diameter. The test is read 72 hours later and the size of the induration is recorded in mm. An induration of 10 mm. or more is generally accepted as positive. A negative reaction excludes tuberculosis in the great majority of well-nourished children. Tuberculin deteriorates fairly quickly in warm climates. The freshness of the solution and the technique of testing should, therefore, be checked at intervals. If these are satisfactory, the tuberculin test will only be negative in the presence of active tuberculosis when it is administered during the incubation period or if the body's allergic response is depressed by malnutrition, miliary or meningial tuberculosis, treatment with corticosteroids or recent infectious diseases, e.g., measles or whooping cough.

In the recent years, the experience of findings negative tuberculin test in proved cases of tuberculosis has led to the use of BCG vaccination as a test reagent. In a non-tuberculous child, often BCG is given there is no reaction for two or three weeks. Then a papule slowly forms with induration, which develops into a pustular stage in 6 to 8 weeks, while a scar is formed at the site of BCG vaccination in three months. In some children, instead of a scar, there is nodule. In a child with tuberculous infection BCG is followed by the formation of a papule with induration within 24 to 48 hours, a pustule by 5 to 7 days, and a scab by 10 to 12 days. This acceleration of the whole BCG does not produce any adverse, reaction — local, focal or general, even if frank tuberculous cases. Direct BCG is a more sensitive and reliable test than tuberculin test and is of great advantage in developing countries not only in the diagnosis, but also immunization (Udani et al, 1971), control programme.

Chemoprophylaxis :

(1) Extensive trials have demonstrated that the daily administration of isoniazide to children who have a high probability of exposure to tuberculosis significantly reduces the incidence of new tuberculous infections. In addition, it is recommended that all tuberculin positive children upto 4 years of age, all older children who have known to have become tuberculin positive within recent months and all positive reactors who are or have been in recent contact with open tuberculosis irrespective of the time of acquisition of their tuberculin sensitivity, should receive INAH in doses of 10-12 mg./kg.a day for about a year, whether or not they have a demonstrable lesion. Udani et at (1970) mentioned isoniazide and thiacetazone and/or ethambutol to sputum positive population where 76% of the total tuberculosis cases exists. This chemotherapy is meant to make these infections cases into non-infectious one, so that they are no more a danger to the society, particularly children. However, if chemotherapy is only provided to sputum positive cases most of the children who have primary tuberculous infection, post-primary complications in the lungs, disseminated tuberculosis, abdominal tuberculosis and CNS tuberculosis will not be covered by National Tuberculosis Control Programme. It is possible that the available resources do not permit the programme to cover the diseases in children. However, it should be pointed out that tuberculosis is the fourth cause of death in children in the hospitals: the other from the top are gastroenteritis,

respiratory infections, malnutrition respectively. Nearly 75% of tuberculosis deaths are caused by CNS tuberculosis, while many who are saved as permanent liabilities to the family and community. Hence some cover of the primary tuberculosis and its complications by chemoprophylaxis should be included in the National Tuberculosis Control Programme. BCG immunization, though WHO study in Madras, demonstrated that pulmonary tuberculosis could not be prevented, yet BCG can prevent CNS and bone tuberculosis in children. Moreover, it will go long way to prevent dangerous complications of primary tuberculosis and even reduce the incidence of adolescent and adult tuberculosis in future. The most useful drugs in the treatment of tuberculosis are 'isoniazide, streptomycin and PAS, other agents include rifampicin (most potent anti-tuberculous drug), cycloserine and possibly pyrazinamide, ethionamide and ethambutol. Clinical experience with these drugs is limited in children. At the moment their usefulness is largely limited to patients infected with tubercle bacilli resistant to isoniazide and streptomycin.

(2) Direct BCG vaccination to new borns, children and also to adolescent under 20 will produce definite though incomplete protection against tuberculosis. The practice of administering BCG vaccine to children who live in areas with high tuberculous mortality rates to thos who are ultimately exposed to adults with inactive or 'arrested' tuberculosis is less frequently recommended than previously, since equal or greater protection is afforded by the daily administration of isoniazide as chemoprophylactic agents.

Protective value of BCG :

Udani et al pointed out that the present contribution is from a study of large material of ours as well as various workers in the country. It was found that the BCG provides partial protection against tuberculous disease. This may result into modified clinical picture particularly of neurotuberculosis when brain and meninges are involved by tubercle bacilli. BCG will be least effective particularly when children of younger age group come in contact with infectious tuberculous adults. They will get the tuberculous disease inspite of BCG vaccination but the incidence and severity are less compared to non-vaccinated children. In the autopsy material it was found that the incidence and severity are less compared to non-vaccinated children. In the autopsy material it was found that the incidence of serious tuberculous disease responsible for the death of the child was 2-3 times higher in non-vaccinated compared to vaccinated children. Though miliary tuberculosis and meningitis can occur in BCG vaccinated children the incidence of these serious complications is lower in vaccinated than in non-vaccinated children. Studies of ours as well as studies of other workers emphasize that inspite of BCG vaccination serious tuberculous disease can occur even in vaccinated children, particularly those who have come in contact with open infectious cases. Various morbidity and mortality and autopsy studies of ours and others in children and experimental studies have revealed that BCG vaccination cannot protect children or animals against entry of tuberculous infection but is certainly useful in preventing the spread and thus outcome of tuberculous infection because of the inmates provided by the BCG. However, this protective value is adversely affected when the child gets massive or repeated doses of tubercle bacilli from an infectious adult and in children who have severe PEM, and are victims of recurrent inter current infections and communicable diseases like measles.

Realizing that BCG vaccination has some value in modifying the manifestation of serious disease and reducing the incidence of serious tuberculous disease, it should be confirmed in the vulnerable childhood population as they should not be deprived of the possible benefit of BCG vaccination. However, it is essential to carry out a large control trial in the Pediatric population with a research methodology which should take into consideration practical situations in day to day life. Such a trial of BCG vaccination to evaluate its protective value in children is an urgent necessity.

STANDARD TREATMENT SUMMARY (FROM NATIONAL TUBERCULOSIS CONTROL PROGRAMME IN INDIA WITH MINOR MODIFICATIONS) :

Initial daily treatment (8 weeks) :

The success of treatment is, however, dependent on two important conditions, namely (1) the combined drug regime and dosage must be strictly followed, and (2) the treatment must be taken in full dosage, long after an apparent clinical remission of the illness which is usually quickly achieved. Full co-operation of the patient is essential for this purpose.

Dosage Schedule :

Streptomycin 20-40 mg./kg. (maximum of 0.5 g. under 5 years of age and 0.75 g. in older children upto 10 years of age), 'Thiacetazone + INAH' (150 mg. TB_1 + 300 mg. INAH, combined tablet) : Under 12 kg. — ¼ tab. + 50 mg. INAH; 12 to 30 kg. — ½ tab. + 100 mg. INAH; 30 kg. and above — 1 tab. (and no extra INAH). For developing countries like India the WHO expert committee on tuberculosis recommends a regimen of twice weekly streptomycin and high dosage of isoniazide for 12 months. Although rifampicin with isoniazide gives better results it involves higher cost of treatment. Streptomycin 20-40 mg./kg. (maximum of 0.5 g. under 5 years of age and 0.75 g. in older children upto 10 years of age) INAH 15 mg./kg. The factors which govern the choice of these drugs are efficacy, cost, toxicity and acceptability.

The toxicity is a less problem in children than in adults. Isoniazide is less likely to cause toxic effects which present as peripheral neuritis or pellegra, and which respond to pyridoxine and nicotinic acid. Streptomycin may cause eighth nerve damage, but this is more frequent in older adults. PAS and TB_1(thiacetazone) have both caused agranulocytosis. There is marked variation in the incidence of thiacetazone side effects from country to country and an assessment of side effects should be made before thiacetazone, rifampicin and ethambutol is released for general use. Hypersensitivity reactions of fever, pain in injection site, skin rash, loose motions and vomiting, jaundices may occur with any of the drugs, and necessitate withdrawal of all, treating with one at a time to identiry the cause. Severe reactions of the Steven-Johnson type and hepatitis as chronic active hepatitis are described after INAH and Rifampicin and may require treatment with corticosteroids.

References

Miller, F.J.W., Seal R.M.S., and Taylor, M.D. (1963) : Tuberculosis in children, Lodon, Churchill.

Raj Narain : Tuberculosis Prevalence Survey in Tumken district in "The Indian Journal of Tuberculosis — 10 : 85, 1962.

P.M. Udani, Usha, S. Bhat (nec Parekh), S.K. Bhave, S.C. Ezuthachan and

V.V. Shethy : Problem of tuberculosis in children in India —

Epidemiology, Morbidity, Mortality and Control Programme — XI, 1,

12 December 1976, India Paediatrics.

Chakraborty, Bijon, Chakraborty (nec Maitra), Sumitra : Primary Tuberculosis in Childhood, Indian Medical Journal, November 1978.

CHAPTER – NINE

CARDIOVASCULAR DISEASES

Congenital Heart Disease :

At birth a little under 1% of all infants have a cardiac defect. The incidence is seen approximately 6 to 8 per 1000 live births (Shankar, 1981). Little is known of the aetiology of congenital heart disease. It is recognised to be very common in infants with Down's syndrome, Turner Syndrome and to be frequent when the mother has had rubella or taken certain drugs specially cortisone during the first trimester of pregnancy. A familial predisposition is common in those who give history of congenital heart conditions common in siblings though less well recognised in the simultaneously present in the parents and their offsprings. So, congenital heart disease is of multifactorial aetiology pertaining to gene abnormalities with some environmental factors such as nutrition, drugs or infections in the mother specially in the earlier part of antenatal period. Among various congenital heart diseases there are eight commonest varities ventricular septal defect (VSD), patent ducts arteriosus (PDA), aortic stenosis, pulmonary stenosis, coarctation of the aorta the tetralogy of Fallot and transposition of the great arteries, all of which are amenable to surgical correction, Certain specific defects exhibit a definite sex preponderance such as atrial septal defect and patent ducts arteriosus are frequent in females, and aortic valvular stenosis, coarctation of the aorta, tetralogy of Fallot, and transposition of great arteries are noted more frequently in males.

The congenital heart diseases may be classified on the basis of presence or absence of cyanosis and may be further subdivided on the basis of the pulmonary blood flow.

1. **Acyanotic heart disease :**

(a) Normal pulmonary flood flow : Malposition of the cardia, Coarctation of the aorta, aortic stenosis, endomyocardial disease, malformation of the aortic arch and malformation of the mitral valve.

(b) Increased pulmonary blood flow : Atrial septal defect, ventricular septal defect, patent ductus arteriosus, aorta pulmonary septal defect, and endocardial cushion defects.

2. **Cyanotic heart disease :**

(a) Normal or decreased pulmonary blood flow : Tetralogy of Fallot, Tricuspid atresia, pulmonary atresia, severe pulmonary stenosis, Ebstein's anomaly and Eisenmenger's syndrome.

(b) Increased pulmonary blood flow : Complete transposition of the great vessels, total anomalous pulmonary venous return, tricuspid atresia with transposition, hypoplastic left ventricular syndrome, truncus arteriosus.

Dextrocardia, laevocardia and asplenia :

There can be abnormalities in the position of the cardia, with heart lying either in the right side of the chest with its apex formed by the left ventricle and directed to the right (dextrocardia) or in the midline (mesocardia). The heart may be located normally in the left side of the chest with its apex directed to the left but with abnormal position of the viscera (isolated laevocardia). In dextrocardia the viscera may be in their normal (isolated dextrocardia) of completely reversed position (mirror image dextrocardia situs inversus totalis) further situation occurs when there is absence of spleen and a midline liver. The abnormalities found include single ventricle.

transposition, pulmonary atresia, and anomalous pulmonary venous drainage, often occuring simultaneously. Surgery is, therefore, only rarely possible.

Tetralogy of Fallot :

After the first year of life, Fallot's tetralogy is the commonest cause of cyanotic congenital heart disease, but quite often patients are not cyanosed during the early months after birth. Fallot described four features of this condition. The two essential ones are ventricular septal defect and pulmonary stenosis — valvular or infundibular. The third is over-riding of the aorta over the ventricular septum, is not a constant feature. The fourth one right ventricular hypertrophy is simply a result of the pulmonary stenosis. In 25% of cases of Fallot, there is associated right sided aortic arch.

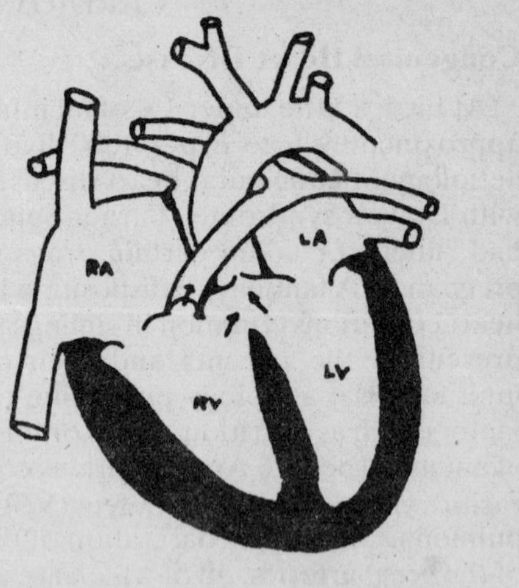

Fig.9.1: Pulmonary Stenosis with Patent Inter-ventricular Septum (Fallot's tetralogy)

The children those who are cyanosed at birth with severe obstruction to the right ventricular outflow tract, marked degree of right ventricular hypertrophy results. There is a right to left shunt and the magnitude of the flow depends on the extent of obstruction to the pulmonary blood flow. Severe obstruction is associated with decrease in pulmonary blood flow resulting in a shunting of a large volume of unsaturated blood into left ventricle and aorta. It results in hypoxic state, central cyanosis and polycythaemia. The general growth is retarded. The children exhibit dyspnoea on exertion. The central cyanosis becomes increased by exertion and emotional stress. There is development of clubbing of the fingers and toes. The children assume squatting posture while resting after exertion. Periodically they exhibit hypoxic spells and it is precipitated by infection and emotion. The cyanosis and tachycardia are increased with crying. The spell may last for a variable time and it may be associated with syncope and convulsion. Examination reveals normal cardiac size. Apex is difficult to palpate and there is tapping impulse of right ventricle in the left parasternal region.

The most characteristic sign is a loud systolic ejection murmur in the pulmonary area due to pulmonary stenosis. There is no murmur associated with the VSD since it is large and has equal pressure on either side. The murmur becomes much quieter and may disappear during cyanotic attacks where there is little blood flowing through the obstruction. The second heart sound is sometimes loud, but this is due to the aorta being more anterior than usual, the pulmonary element being inaudible.

The chest radiogram shows a boot shaped cardia with its apex, being elevated, should not be confused with boot shaped heart of left ventricular hypertrophy where there is a large smoothly rounded prominence at apex. Here the apex is upturned due to outward displacement of the small left ventricle by the enlarged right ventricle. Proper terminology will be 'Coeur en sabot' likened as to be shape of a dog nose or sabot. There is hypertrophy of right ventricle. The aortic shadow is increased and there is absence of pulmonary artery curve. The pulmonary blood flow is decreased. The aortic arch may be right sided in some cases. The E.C.G. shows right axis deviation and right ventricular hypertrophy. Echocardiogram shows lack of echoes between the ventricular septum and anterior aortic wall. During cardiac catheterisation, catheter enters the left ventricular aorta from right ventricle and its entry into pulmonary artery is difficult. Angiocardiogram reveals opacification of aortic arch and left ventricle, following injection of the dye into the right ventricle. The congestive cardiac failure is unusual. There is likelihood of development of subacute infective endocarditis, paradoxical embolism and cerebral abscess. The condition is associated with polycythaemia and iron deficiency anaemia. Most of the children will require operative correction of the defects at some stage. The defect is closed with a patch and the obstruction is relieved. The age of election of surgery for those not severely disabled is about five to seven years but earlier palliative operations are required if the symptoms are severe. The operation is aimed to increase the pulmonary blood flow by connecting the pulmonary artery with systemic artery, i.e., one or other subclavian artery or direct anastomosis with aorta and pulmonary artery. The cyanotic spells have to be treated with oxygen and the patient has to be placed in knee-chest position. The sedation with Morphine 0.1 – 0.2 mg./kg. I.M. is given. The dehydration has to be corrected with intravenous fluids and metabolic acidosis with sodium bicarbonate. The beta adrenergic blockers such as propranolol, which reduces the speed of contraction of the infundibular muscle and allows more blood to pass into the lungs is used. The infections are to be controlled with antibiotics. The polycythaemia may require phlebotomy to reduce the hematocrit level. The anaemia should be corrected with iron replacement.

Ventricular Septal Defect :

The ventricular septal defect is one of the commonest forms of congenital heart disease. Its incidence in the population at birth is about three per 1000. It can be an isolated defect or it can exist in association with other anomalies such as tetralogy of Fallot, pulmonary stenosis, coarctation of the aorta, transposition of great arteries, truncus arteriosus and tricuspid atresia. The ventricular septum is formed from three portions, the major part from the apex of the primitive ventricle and the minor parts from the endocardial cushion in the atrioventricular canal and from the conotruncal septum which separates the primitive truncus into aorta and pulmonary artery. A defect in the ventricular septum may occur where these fail to join up most commonly due to a failure of the conotruncal septum to join the main ventricular septum (Roger's disease) so that the commonest place for a ventricular septal defect is just below the aortic valve. Generally the defects are of variable size and may be single or multiple the functional disturbances depends on the size of the defect, volume of pulmonary blood flow, degree of pulmonary vascular resistance and presence or absence of pulmonary stenosis. The condition can be distinguished into four categories. The haemodynamic is not dependent on the site of the defect. When the defect is small (less than 0.5 cm. diameter), there is a left-to-right pressure gradient allowing the blood flow from the left ventricle. There is no elevation of pressure of right ventricular or pulmonary artery. The pulmonary vasculature accommodated additional blood flow. Such defects may sometimes close spontaneously.

In small or moderate sized defects (0.5-1.0. cm. diameter) the symptoms are unusual in childhood and the murmur is heard at a routine examination after birth, since the right heart pressure in the first few days after birth is too high to allow the shunt to develop. The pulses are normal but the cardiac impulse shows evidence of left ventricular enlargement in moderate sized defects. The characteristic sign is a loud pansystolic murmur maximal in the fourth left intercostal space close to the sternum. It is often sufficiently loud to radiate somewhat to all other areas, including the right of the sternum and there is usually a palpable thrill. The loudness of the murmur is no real guide to the size of the defect. Any hole between about 2 mm. and 1 cm. in diameter will produce a loud murmur and a softer murmur may be either due to a very small defect or a very large one associated with pulmonary hypertension, in the later case there will also be signs of pulmonary hypertension. A better guide in the middle range defects is the presence of left ventricular enlargement or a diastolic flow murmur at the apex, both of which indicate that the defect is large enough to allow at least half the left ventricular outflow to be shunted through the defect.

When the defect is large (greater than 1.0 cm. diameter) symptoms occur in infancy. About the sixth week of life the infant fails to thrive becomes breathless and frequently is admitted to hospital in severe heart failure. The infant looks anxious and sweats freely probably due to a combination of catecholamine excess and the high metabolic rate resulting from increased cardiac and respiratory work coupled with a reduced systemic blood flow. There is lower costal and intercostal recession and an enlarged liver. The cardiac impulse is hyperdynamic. On auscultation there is usyally the characteristic loud pansystolic murmur but frequently, owing to associated pulmonary hypertension, the murmur is quiet and short and there is a loud second sound in the pulmonary area due to pulmonary hypertension. At the apex there is also a low-pitched mitral diastolic murmur due to the high flow from the lungs passing from left atrium to left ventricle.

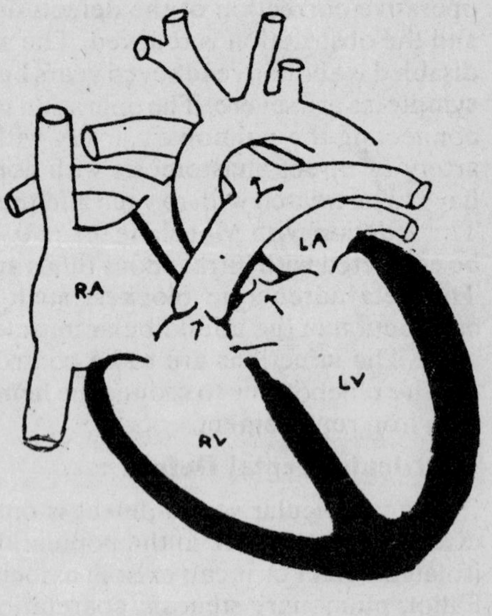

Fig.9.2 : Ventricular Septal Defect

Rarely a defect in higher portion of the ventricular septum may result in shunting of blood from left ventricle to right atrium. Many infants and children remain asymptomatic when the defect is isolated and small. Pansystolic murmur may be detected along the left sternal border during routine examination. The second sound is split. In half the number of infants the defect may close spontaneously during childhood. When the defect is small both the chest radiograph and ECG are normal. With moderate-sized defects the chest radiograph shows enlargement of the left ventricle and pulmonary plethora and the ECG shows an increase in voltage of the 'R' wave in leads V_5 and V_6 including left ventricular hypertrophy. In large defects with hyperdynamic pulmonary hypertension both ventricles are enlarged on the radiograph and the pulmonary vessels, particularly the central pulmonary arteries are large. The ECG shows hypertrophy of both ventricles demonstrated by tall 'R' waves in both right (V_1) and left (V_5 and V_6) ventricular leads. It should be noted that in all cases with a sizeable left-to-right shunt both ventricles have to pump the extra blood. When there is no pulmonary hypertension the extra load on the right ventricles is much less since the pressure is lower, where as in the presence of pulmonary hypertension the right ventricle has to contend with both a high pressure and a large volume.

The cardiac catheterisation reveals an increased oxygen saturation at the level of the right ventricle and it helps to differentiate ventricular septal defect from aortopulmonary windows, single ventricle, isolated large patent ducts arteriosus and truncus.

The condition may produce congestive heart failure and pulmonary vascular obliterative disease. The cardiac failure is treated medically. Antibiotic prophylaxis for infective endocarditis is necessary. The periodic examination of the children with VSD is necessary to note whether the defect has closed or diminished in size. The septal defect had to be closed during childhood and adolescence when the shunt is moderate to large left-to-right, under vision with cardiopulmonary bypass. Increased cardio-pulmonary vascular resistance contraindicates operative correction.

Patent Ductus Arteriousus :

The ductus arteriosus carries blood from the main pulmonary artery to the aorta in the foetal circulation bypassing the pulmonary circulation. The patent ductus arteriosus refers to persistence of a normal foetal vascular channel connecting the pulmonary artery to the aorta. The opening of the ductus on the pulmonary side is situated immediately to the left of bifurcation of the pulmonary artery and on the aortic side it is just distal to the origin of the left subclavian artery. The latter opening is larger than the former. This is a wide vessel and the main pulmonary artery, the ductus and the descending aorta appear as a continuous channel. When the lungs are expanded with air after birth the vascular resistance in the lungs falls sharply and the blood flow in the ductus is reversed. The flow of well oxygenated blood through the ductus stimulates it to constrict and normally the ductus is functionally closed within a few hours of birth. The duct can persist as a patent channel for some obscure reasons in pre-mature babies and it is a relatively common congenital anomaly and is frequent in females. There may be history of maternal rubella in the first trimester of pregnancy. The incidence is frequent in those born at high altitudes, premature babies, hypoxia due to respiratory problems or other cardiac abnormalities. In many cases, however, there is no obvious reason for the persistence of a patent ductus. The condition occurs frequently as an isolated anomaly, however, it can co-exist with other anomalies like coarctation of the aorta, VSD, pulmonary stenosis and aortic stenosis. In situations of pulmonary atresia or aortic arch anomalies the persistent ductus plays a vital role in the maintenance of pulmonary or systemic blood flow.

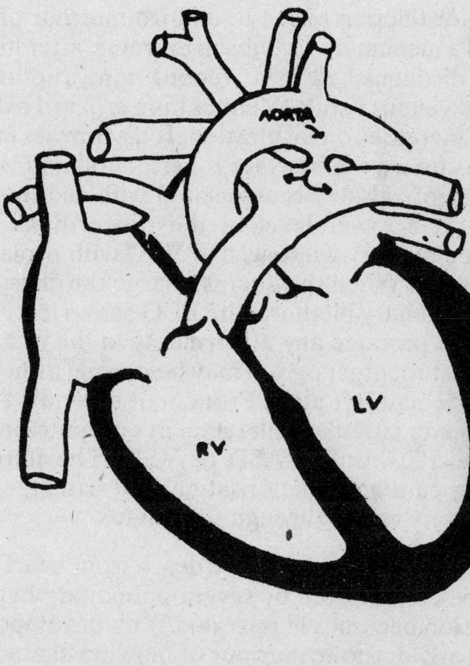

Fig.9.4 : Patent Ductus Arteriosus

The clinical picture depends on the size of the duct. When this is large symptoms occur in infacny, usually starting at two or three months of age. The infant fails to thrive and is noted to be breathless particularly on feeding. On examination there is tachypnoea, in drawing of chest walls due to the inspiratory effort required to ventilate the lungs which are abnormally stiff owing to the large volume of pulmonary blood. There is development of right heart failure. The pulses are collapsing due to the high systolic output from the left ventricle and the run-off into the pulmonary arteries which continues in diastole. The palpation reveals a hyperdynamic heart and auscultation a murmur, maximal in the pulmonary area which may be continuous or just systolic. The absence of the diastolic element is due to elevation of the pulmonary artery pressure so that the flow is mainly in systole.

Generally a small patent ductus exists without symptoms in infancy and childhood. It does not affect the growth and development. The existence of a small patent ductus in child may be recognised during routine examination by the presence of characteristic murmur. The characteristic continuous murmur is heard in the pulmonary area. The term 'continuous' implies that the murmur continues from systole into diastole in contradistinction to the to and fro murmur of aortic valve disease and is sometimes called a machinery or Gibson murmur, after its discoverer. A continuous murmur has to be distinguished from venous hum, rupture of sinus of valsalva and pulmonary arterio venous fistula. Venous hum is heard over the base of the neck on the right side and it increases on inspiration. It disappears in supine position. In pulmonary arterio venous fistula the murmur is peripheral and is associated with cyanosis. The rupture of sinus of valsalva is associated with sudden onset of continuous murmur and it is heard at a lower level of the precordium. PDA is difficult to distinguish from aortopulmonary window, and VSD with prolapse of aortic valve cusp into the septal deficiency. When the ductus is large the chest radiograph show cardiac enlargement and pulmonary plethora, the ECG shows left ventricular hypertrophy. A small ductus does not produce any abnormality in the radiograph or electrocardiogram. In some the chest roentgenogram may be normal or in large ductus there may be enlarged left ventricle and left atria. Prominent ascending aorta and pulmonary artery. There is pulmonary vascular enlargement and pulmonary plethora. Prominent aortic arch is seen in PDA unlike ASD or VSD. The fluroscopy reveals pulsating aortic knob. During cardiac catheterisation, the catheter will enter the descending aorta from pulmonary artery through the ductus.

A large ductus may cause death from heart failure in infancy and if left untreated, may be complicated by severe pulmonary hypertension so that cyanosis occurs and the lesion becomes in operable. With development of pulmonary hypertension, there is an early diastolic murmur of blowing character of pulmonary incompetence. With the reversal of shunt, the unsaturated blood from the pulmonary artery reaches the descending aorta and produces differential cyanosis. The toes exhibit cyanosis and clubbing and the fingers remain acyanotic. A small or moderate sized ductus may cause heart failure in adult life and may be subject to endocarditis or aneurysm formation. The operation is advised as soon as the diagnosis is established. The operation is performed through the left chest and the duct is either ligated or divided and sutured. After ligation of a fairly large ductus about 1 in 100 recanalises, but the alternative operation of division and suturing has a slightly higher risk. Following operation the cardiovascular signs return to normal within short time.

The Prostaglandins, the Potent Vasoactive substance is needed to maintain the patency of ductus in foetal life after birth oxygen triggers the closure of ductus. The functional closure in a term baby occurs within 24 hours while anatmical closure may take several weeks and completed by three months of age. The incidence is much higher among preterm infants with hyaline membrane disease. Over two-thirds of cases close spontaneously within 72 hours of treatment with diuretics especially those without hyaline membrane. If decongestive therapy fails then Indomethacin 0.2 mg. per kg. orally every 12 hourly to a total of 3 doses is most effective. But it is contra indicated in the presence of jaundice, bleeding and renal shut down conditions.

Coarctation of the aorta :

A condition in which the aorta is constricted just distal to the origin of the left subclavian artery, the site Corresponding to the insertion of ligamentum arteriosum (or ductus arteriosus). Occasionally the constriction may occur proximal to the origin of the left subclavian artery. The condition is due to a defect in the development of the media of the aorta. During intrauterine life very little blood flows in the portion beyond the subclavian artery since almost all the blood in the descending aorta comes from the pulmonary artery via the ductus arteriosus. There is thus little stimulus to grow in this area and this is probably one reason why coarctation occurs most commonly in this area. This is referred to as the preductile or infantile type. The other type is slightly lower, beyond the point where the ductus joins the aorta and is termed the post-ductal or adult type.

The coarctation of the aorta occur next in frequency to ventricular septal defect and PDA. There is a greater preponderance of its incidence in males. The condition is frequent in patients with Turner's syndrome. Almost half the infants born with coarctation of the aorta develop symptoms in infancy, beginning at one to four weeks of age. The site and extent of obstruction and coexistent cardiac anomalies determine the clinical manifestations. The common associated anomalies are hypoplasia of the junction of the aortic arch, bicuspid aortic value, PDA, VSD, ASD, aortic stenosis, mitral valvular disease, transposition of great arteries with VSD or Berry aneurysms of the circle of Willis. The obstruction to the flow in the aorta causes increased resistance to the left ventricular output. There is a gradual development of collateral circulation between the branches of proximal aorta and the branches of the distal aorta. In severe cases may present with cardiac failure during first 1-3 weeks of infancy. In many instances breathlessness on feeding is the usual symptom but in some babies present with 'failure to thrive'. Examination reveals rapid, laboured respirations and enlargement of the liver. The femoral pulses are absent or very weak and the brachial pulses bounding. Occasionally the left subclavian artery originates at or beyond the obstruction giving rise to an absent or diminished pulse in that arm. In infants there are no murmurs. Patients who remain well in infancy are usually picked up at routine examination. Coarctation is a condition which is still missed even into an

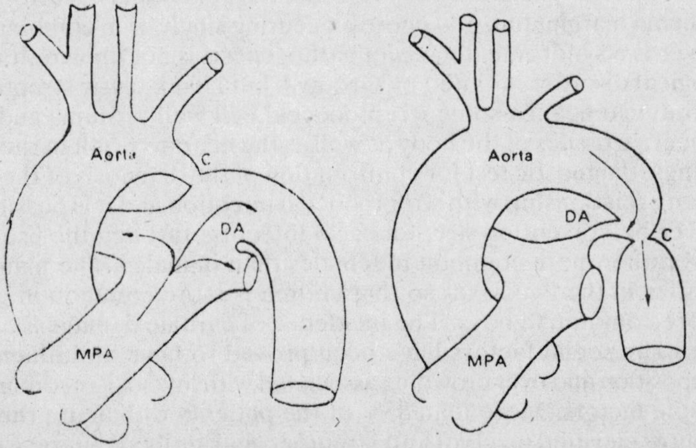

Fig.9.5 : Tye of coarctation — A : Infantile or preductal, B : Adult type, MPA = main pulmonary artery; DA = ductus arteriosus; C = Coarctation. (Courtesy of Macmillan Publishers)

adult life, those failing to make palpation of femoral pulses as a part of the routine examination of every child. The blood pressure in the upper limbs is increased, sometimes as high as 200/110 mm. Hg. but more typically 130/70 mm. Hg. to 160/90 mm. Hg. The ventricle is palpably enlarged and sometimes there is an apical systolic murmur due to functional mitral regurgitation; usually, however, there are no precordial murmurs, but a short systolic murmur over the back between the scapulae, due to the blood flowing through the constriction. Over the age of five to six years collateral vessels between the scapulae and the spine are felt pulsating or heard to give a soft continuous murmur. Coarctation of aorta is diagnosed on the basis of weak or absent femoral pulse, hypertension in the upper extremities and presence of collateral vessels. ECG may be normal or show evidence of left ventricular hypertrophy. X-ray of the chest shows prominent left ventricle. There can be central indentation along the margin of the aorta by coarctation with pre — and post-stenotic dilatation above and below it, giving a configuration of the letter '3'. There is notching of the ribs in their undersurface from erosion by the dilated internal mammary artery. But this is not a sign before 10 years of age. Cardiac catheterisation helps in determining the coexistent cardiac anomalies. The site and extent of coarctation is determined by aortography.

The preductal coarctation may be fatal during infancy from cardiac failure. The post ductal coarctation is a gradually progressive disease. The development of collateral vessels between the branches of subclavian artery, scapular artery, intercostal arteries and internal thoracic arteries with the distal vessels determines the speed of the progress of events. There is the likelihood of complications like congestive heart failure, aneurysmal dilatations of proximal aorta and of cerebral vessels, rupture of aorta or cerebral vessels and infective endocarditis or endoarteritis.

The children with coarctation have to be restricted from strenuous excercises. Antibiotic prophylaxis is needed when there is danger of infective endocarditis. The condition needs surgical correction. The coarctation is to be resected and end to and anastomosis is to be performed. A prosthetic tubular dacron graft may be necessary if the resected segment is long. During the post operative period, there can be sudden development of hypertension, abdominal distension and leucocytosis. The condition is associated with mesenteric arteritis. The blood pressure has to be promptly treated, otherwise there is danger of gangrene of the intestine.

Rheumatic Fever and Disorders of Rheumatic Valvular Diseases

It is a part of acute rheumatism, the others are rheumatic carditis, rheumatic nodules, erythema marginatum and chorea, occuring singly or in combination. Further rheumatic fever is a syndrome, the exact pathogenesis is not known. It appears to be an immunological disorder initiated by Group A beta haemolytic streptococcus. The antibodies produced against some streptococcal cell wall proteins and sugars react with the connective tissues of the body as well as the heart to result in rheumatic fever. There is no single diagnostic test for confirmation of the diagnosis of rheumatic fever. There is a strong relationship with streptococcal infection and it is possible to prevent rheumatic fever by preventing streptococcal infection through the use of penicillin. The disease is rather more common in females than in males. The manifestations of the disease differ in the two sexes so that chorea is more common in girls, whereas arthritis is more common in boys. The incidence of cardiac damage is about equal in the two sexes. The social factors have been proved to have an influence. Heredity genetic predisposition and over crowding associated with low socio-economic conditions are predisposing factors. More than 85% of the patients with acute rheumatic fever consistently show elevated levels of anti-streptococcal antibody titers. Although these features indicate the association of rheumatic fever with streptococcal infection.

Streptococci have nerve been isolated from rheumatic lesions in joints, heart or the blood stream. Considerable evidence now suggests that the rheumatic fever is an antigen-antibody reaction. Following streptococcal sore throat there is a latent period of 10 days to several weeks before the onset of rheumatic fever. This latent period is similar to the other antigen-antibody diseases like serum sickness.

The illness of rheumatic fever which may include arthritis, carditis, rheumatic nodes and erythema marginatum, is usually preceded by a throat infection but this may be so mild as to escape attention. Then after an interval of 10-21 days, rheumatic manifestations may develop. The main complaint is fever together with pain in the affected joints. The inflammation of the joints may cause no more than this, but in more severe cases there is tenderness, swelling, heat and perhaps synovial effusion. In some cases the fever settles in about a week but in others it lasts longer. There is tachycardia and the sedimentation rate is considerably raised and remains so as long as the disease is active. The circulating C-reactive protein can be demonstrated. More than 85% of the patients with acute rheumatic fever consistantly show elevated level of anti-streptococcal, antibody titres. The ASO titres above the value of 200 units/ml. is of diagnostic significance, though an increased ASO titre does not provide evidence of rheumatic fever but only of a recent streptococcal infection, yet a value below 50 units/ml. exclude rheumatic fever. The treatment with salicylates usually brings the temperature down and relieves the pain. Acute attack of rheumatic fever often leads to some degree of anaemia, so associated fever, joint pain and aching of bones, abdominal pain often misdiagnose as leukaemia, Rarely acute abdominal pain becomes difficult to differentiate from acute appendicitis in children.

The diagnosis of rheumatic fever is usually made with regard to the 'modified' Jones criteria'. These are the manifestations of rheumatic fever into major and minor groups. Two major or one major and two minor manifestations, together with evidence of recent streptococcal infection are required to diagnose acute rheumatic fever. Major criterias are carditis, polyarthritis, chorea, erythema marginatum, subcutaneous nodules and the minor criterias are fever, arthralgia, previous rheumatic fever, increased ESR or C-reactive protein, blood leucocytosis and prolonged P-R interval in electrocardiogram.

The significance of rheumatism depends upon the extent to which the heart is involved. The rheumatic carditis is a pancarditis involving the pericardium, myocardium and the endocardium. The carditis occurs in 50-60 percent of patients of acute rheumatic fever. It is an early manifestation of rheumatic fever so that by the time a patient seeks help he already has evidence of carditis. Almost 80% of those patients who develop carditis do so within the first two weeks of the onset of rheumatic fever. In pericarditis there is precordial pain which may be quite severe. On auscultation a friction rub is present. Clinical pericarditis is seen in 15% of those who have carditis. The ECG may show ST and T changes known as 'Pardae' wave. As a rule the rheumatic pericarditis is associated with small effusion and does not result either in tamponade or constrictive pericarditis. In myocarditis some degree of cardiac enlargement takes place and the maximum cardiac impulse becomes prominent and more diffuse than normal. With cardiac dilatation, the impulse is diffuse and feeble, as opposed to the thrustful apex beat of left ventricular hypertrophy or the slapping impulse of right ventricular hypertrophy, very rarely, congestive cardiac failure may occur. As the acute condition heals, the maximum cardiac impulse return to its normal position. The tachycardia is out of proportion to the rise of temperature but the finding of increase sleeping pulse rate as both diagnostic and prognostic importance in children. The disturbances of rhythm due to not only involvement of myocardium but also involvement of conducting tissue is present. Thus some degree of heart block may be present with increasing of P-R interval upto various grades of block and also Wenckebach phenomenon that is gradual increase of P-R interval and then subsequent drop beats occur. Also drop beat should be differentiated from multiple extra systole which may be present. So the diagnostic features of myocarditis are (i) cardiomegaly, (ii) soft 1st sound, (iii) protodiastolic gallop (S_3), (iv) CCF and (v) carey comb's murmur – delayed diastolic murmur heard with myocarditis in acute rheumatic fever. Most probably it is due to increased flow in diastole secondary to mitral regurgitation across inflamed rigid cusps.

The endocarditis is represented by a pansystolic murmur of mitral regurgitation murmur. Pathologically mitral valve is involved in 100 percent of cases of rheumatic fever who have carditis. Clinically, however, 5 to 8% patients may present as pure aortic regurgitation. Thus almost 95% patients will have mitral regurgitation murmur, a quarter of them also having an aortic regurgitation murmur, only 5% as pure aortic regurgitation. The tricuspid valvulitis resulting in tricuspid regurgitation occurs in 10 to 30 percent of cases. As isolated tricuspid valvulitis as a manifestation of acute rheumatic endocarditis does not occur. The clinical evidence of pulmonary valve involvement in acute rheumatic fever is never seen.

As mitral stenosis develops progressive enlargement of the left atrium occurs, followed later by hypertrophy of the right ventricle. The left atrial enlargement is demonstrated by barium swallow in right oblique anterior X-ray as backward identation in the course of esophagus. At least 2–5 years are necessary after an acute attack of endocarditis to reflect clinically the right ventricular hypertrophy, which is eventually revealed as left parasternal heave and the apex beat mainly due to pushed left ventricle becomes a slapping type but with no actual movement of the over lying ribs. On auscultation a localized diastolic murmur is heard at the apex with the patient lying on the left side or on exercise and better heard with a bell rather than the diaphragm of the stethoscope. This diastolic murmur is often presystolic but occasionally mid-diastolic with presystolic accentuation, ending with short, loud first sound. It may be associated with palpable diastolic thrill. The second sound is likely to be accentuated in the pulmonary area while the apex near the mitral area may have a 'opening snap'. The mitral regurgitation may frequently be evident before mitral stenosis has progressed to a perceptible degree. When there will be clinical evidence of left ventricular enlargement and a pansystolic murmur radiating towards axilla and in 10 percent of cases palpable systolic thrill on mitral area.

In aortic regurgitation there is left ventricular hypertrophy, the apex is forceful, down and outwardly displaced which usually moves the overlying ribs. There is progressive peripheral circulatory changes, evident in an increasing difference between the systolic and diastolic blood pressure (130/50 mm. of Hg.) and together with the pulse may take on a collapsing character, marked carotid pulsation and capillary pulsation is visible in the nail beds. A characteristic soft high pitched early diastolic murmur which may be best heard at the base, or in the new aortic areas on left 2nd and 3rd intercostal space near the sternum. The murmur is continuous with the second sound, with alteration of two-beat rhythm of heart sound, better heard by a diaphragm and patient holds its breath in full expiration. The murmur being of high frequency and the character has been likened to a whispered 'R'. The rheumatic stenosis rarely develops and rheumatic tricuspid lesions are not usually detectable in childhood years.

Treatment :

There is no specific treatment. The management is mostly symptomatic combined with suppressive therapy. Besides bed rest, regulated diet, the sheet anchor is introduction of penicillin after obtaining throat cultures, Initially the patient is given therapeutic doses of penicillin 4000,000 unit of procaine penicillin I.M. twice daily for 10 days. This is followed by prophylactic penicillin of long acting type 1.2 mega units every 3rd week. As suppressive therapy both aspirin or steroids are given. Since untreated rheumatic fever subsides in 12 weeks in 80% of the patients of either of the two agents is given for 12 weeks. The steroids are a more potent suppressive agent as compared to aspirin. However, there is no proof that the use of steroids results in less cardiac damages as compared to aspirin. The total duration of course for the suppressive agent, aspirin or steroids is 12 weeks. With aspirin the full doses in the order of 100 mg./kg. body weight are given for 10 weeks and a blood salicylate concentration is maintained in the range of 25-30 mg. per 100 ml. is appropriate. After 10 weeks of full doses of aspirin, it is tappered off in next two weeks. Full doses of steroids are given for three weeks and then tappered very gradually in the next nine weeks. The prednisolone is used commonly as 60 mg./day, for patients weighing more than 20 kg. and 40 mg./daily for patients weighing less than 20 kg. This is continued for 3 weeks and then reduced to 50 mg. daily for 1 week and then 40 mg. daily for another week. Following this the reduction in dose is by 5 mg. weekly till it is finished.

It is necessary to emphasize that there is no primary prevention of rheumatic fever. Secondary prevention consists in giving long acting penicillin. Ideally penicillin prophylaxis should be continued as life long procedure less than the ideal would be continue it till the age of 25 years. The least satisfactory approach is to give it for 5 years from the last attack of rheumatic fever.

References

1. Committee of the American Heart Association, Jones Criteria (revised) for guidance in the diagnosis of rheumatic fever. Circulation 32, 664, 1965.
2. Jordon, S.C. & Scott, O. (1974) : Heart Disease in Paediatrics; London, Butterworth.

Hypertension in childhood

As essential or idiopathic hypertension in childhood is extremely rare, a diligent search for a primary cause must be made. Elevation of systolic pressure, consistently over 130 mm. of Hg. and diastolic over 90 mm. of Hg. is said to be hypertension in childhood ages. The taking of the blood pressure is important, although often difficult in infants and children. It is important to use a cuff which cover two-third of the length of the upper arm and the auscultatory method is the best in all except very small infants when the 'flush' method is used; before inflating the cuff a crape bandage is wrapped firmly round the arm causing the skin to blanch. When the cuff is inflated and then gradually released a sudden flush indicates a value slightly less than the systolic pressure. The blood pressure varies with age.

Table 1.

Blood pre sure at various age group.

Age	Systolic mm of Hg.	Diastolic mm of Hg.
Birth	65—95	30—60
5 years	80—110	45—65
10 years	90—120	50—70

Rakesh Agarwal et al observed blood pressure pattern in school children of one thousand six hundred ninety two apparently healthy school children between 5 and 15 years. Blood pressure readings were taken to determine the mean BP subjects belonging to low, middle and high socio-economic group. Mean value with standard deviation were worked out in the respective age group. Factors such as sex and community did not make any significant difference. Values, however, showed a proportional increase with regard to body weight per cm. The measuring B.P. in children is known to give an early idea of detection of kidney diseases, for endocrinal an certain central nervous system pathology. The present study indicates that blood pı essure shows an upward trend with increase of age between 5 and 15 years being 96.5 ± 56 mm of Hg. at 5 years, 115.5 ± 45 at 15 years in males with an annual increment of approximately 1.5 mm. of Hg. The mean diastolic pressure in male children was 64.5 ± 7.5 mm. of Hg. at 5 years which may increase to 77.8 ± 5.2 mm. of Hg. at 15 years. The mean systolic and diastolic pressure in females was 97.8 ± 6.5 and 64.8 ± 6.8 respectively at 5 years which may increase to 115.9 ± 5.8 and 76.7 ±7.9 mm. of Hg. respectively at 15 years. Through the mean systolic and diastolic B.P. are higher by 1.5, 0.5 mm. of Hg. in female children respectively, the differences are statistically insignificant. Our observations suggest that annual increment is 1.4 mm to 2 mm. between 4 and 9 years, 9 and 12 years and 13 and 15 years respectively. The increase in annual increment at 13 years may be attributed to the growth spurt which occurs in three years.

Elevation of systolic pressure is found in arteriovenous shunt lesions, in thyrotoxicosis and hyperkinetic circulatory states. It is well tolerated and in most instances relatively easily treated. The diastolic hypertension on the other hand is less well tolerated and may be transient as in acute nephritis, more established as in chronic renal disease or periodic and later sustained as in phaeochromocytoma. The renal disease is the commonest cause of hypertension in childhood. Moreover, early urinary infections if not properly treated might one day present as a case of hypertension in later life. In new born examination, if there is any deformity of the ears and also presence of one umbilical artery instead of two in umbilical cord stump, one should examine a sample of urine to detect evidence of congenital anomalies related to kidney and excretory tracts and thereby precipitate infection and later on undetected renal hypertension.

Table 2.

Secondary causes of hypertension.

Cause	
Renal	Acute glomerulonephritis
	Chronic glomerulonephritis
	Chronic pyelonephritis
	Polycystic kidneys
	Renal tumours
Vascular	Coarctation of the aorta
	Reneal artery stenosis
Endocrine	Phaeochromocytoma
	Neuroblastoma
	Cushing's syndrome
Drugs	Cortisone
	Antidepressants

Hypertension may be associated with raised intracranial pressure from whatever cause, including encephalitis, and bulbar poliomyelitis. Other syndromes in which hypertension is a feature include familial dysautonomia in which postural hypotension, even causing syncope is fairly common. Hereditary acute porphyria may present with abdominal pain, paralysis and sensory and mental disturbances. Approximately half the patients have mild to severe hypertension in the acute phase. Hypertension is a features of pink disease (acrodynia) thought to be related to mercury ingestion. The renal damage from lead poisoning also causes hypertension. The mechanism of the production of hypertension in Turner's syndrome (gonadal agenesis) is uncertain although obviously the frequently associated coarctation of the aorta will play a part.

A raised blood pressure may be found on routine examination, or when symptoms of headache, vomiting or heart failure occur.

Failure to find a remediable cause means rapid deterioration or, at least a life time of taking hypotensive drugs. Investigations should include urine microscopy for white cells or organisms (infection) or casts, renal cells and protein (glomerulonephritis) urinary catechlomine (phaeochromocytoma), Regitin Text (phaeochromocytoma) intravenous pyelogram to find out structural defects (hydronephrosis), renal size, differential excretion rates, angiography (renal artery stenosis). Phaeochromocytoma, neuroblastoma, Renography (by Retrograde pyelography and micturating cysto-urethrogram to detect bladder neck obstruction and ureteric reflex from bladder to ureters.

Hypertension alone is expected in about half those presenting with acute glomerulonephritis, but in many children this may be transient or of moderate degree which does not require treatment with hypotensive drugs. Severe or rapidly progressive hypertension should be controlled with phenobarbitone (5-10 mg./kg.) and reserpine (0.1 mg./kg./every six hours, orally. In addition pentolinium tartarate (0.1 mg./kg./day) may be given intramuscularly. The convulsion of hypertensive encephalopathy may be controlled with diazipam (0.25 mg./kg. intravenously) or paraldehyde (0.2 ml./kg. intramuscularly).

References

James, J.A., Lieberman, E., and Fine, R.N. (1976) : Renal Disease in Childhood, 3rd ed., ed., St. Louis, Mosby.

Agarwal et al : Blood Pressure in School Children, Indian Paediatrics, Vol. 19, July, 1982.

CHAPTER – TEN

DISEASES OF KIDNEY

The kidneys cannot be heard; they do not murmur or wheeze. After the first few days of life they cannot be felt very well. Until recently they were rarely seen until too late; but now, through biopsy followed by light or electron microscopy and also by various radiological investigations including renal scan they are beginning to be seen during life and we are learning much more about how they function. In clinical practice their performance is judged mainly by their two important functions, excretion and homeostasis.

Infection of the Urinary Tract :

Infection of the urinary tract is common in childhood, and it is important to be sure what is meant when it is diagnosed. The presence of pus cells in uncontaminated specimens of urine does indicate an inflammatory process but does not necessarily mean bacterial infection in the urine. By a urinary tract infection is meant a condition in which actively multiplying bacteria persist in urine within the renal tract. This is diagnosed by the demonstration of pus cells, and a significant bacteriuria, a variable amount of protein may also be detected together with some red cells. The two most important among the list mentioned above are significant pyuria — more than 6 cells per high power field and on cultures of two consecutive clean specimens and ideal mid stream specimen, a pure growth of 100,000 organisms/ml. or more is obtained.

They are present more commonly in females than males in the ratio of about 6 : 1 with the exception of the neonatal period when the sexes are equally affected. The inflammatory changes are rarely limited to one part of the renal tract. The only known aetiological factors are those that impair or obstruct the flow of urine, for example, urethral valves. The organisms, most frequently responsible for urinary infections, are those of the E. Coli group, and less frequently those of the proteus, pseudomonas and klebsiella groups, strepto faecalis and other Gram positive organisms may also be found. Infections are seldom localized to a particular part of the urinary tract so that the terms cystitis and pyelonephritis are rarely applicable. Moreover, screening studies have shown that 1-2% of girls of school age may have a significant but asymptomatic bacteriuria. Acute pyelonephritis is the term used to describe bouts of infection involving renal tissue. It may be suggested by colic pain, fever and frequency of micturiction; and is occasionally with very high temperature associated with irritability, anorexia, meningism and even febrile convulsion. The gastrointestinal disturbances may dominate the clinical picture in the infant, vomiting may be severe and mimic the projectile vomiting of pyloric stenosis and occasionally this may be accompanied by diarrhoea suggesting gastro-enteritis. The older children are more likely to have frequency and urgency of micturition together with dysuria but there is usually less constitutional disturbances than in the infant. The lumbar pain and tenderness over the renal angle may be present. Without the treatment and providing that abscess formation in kidney, parenchyma does not take place and generalised septicaemia do not occur, the clinical course is relatively short. The symptoms may subside after about one week but the urinary changes may be detected for about three weeks. In chronic pyelonephritis, the infection may persist for months or years and is not associated with such onset of clinical symptoms like an acute type. It may be detected by routine discovery of proteinuria but sometimes may also present with failure to thrive or unexplained pallor and anaemia. Irregular fever accompanied by detection of pus cells in the urine may occur at intervals. Ultimately chronic pyelonephritis will result in renal failure and hypertension. The diagnosis depends on the combination of significant numbers of white cells with bacteria. In normal urine a few white cells may be found and a small number of bacteria may be grown. The numbers accepted as significant, vary according to the patient's sex, the method of collection and the pathological examination too, a number of bacteria exceeding 10,000/ml. of urine is suspected and more than 100000/ml. usually evidence of infection. Now in every child bacteriologically proved infection, should be further investigated by X-ray methods, even one attack in a male child and more than 2-3 attacks in a female child within a very short time. An intravenous pyelogram indicates the degree of kidney damage and the presence of malformations or obstructions. A micturating cysto urethrogram outlines the lower urinary tract as well as the upper, and demonstrates reflux from bladder to ureter.

The main principles of treatment are the eradication of the infection and prevention of recurrences. The plan of treatment depends on the age of the child, clinical condition, presence of complication, structural abnormalities and the type of organisms. Pending information concerning the sensitivity of the infecting organisms to antibacterial agents, treatment should be given with ampicillin (50 mg./kg./day) or co-trimoxazole (sulpha methoxazole 20 mg./kg./day plus trimethoprim 4 mg./kg./day). The sulphonamides (100 mg./kg./day) are effective agents for the treatment of many urinary tract infections and sulphadimidine and sulphadiazine are used for this purpose in view of their high solubility and less crystalluria. Nitro-furantoin (5 mg./kg./day) and nalidixic acid (50 mg./kg./day) are effective agents that may have a place in treatment depending on the sensitivity of the infecting organisms. The other drugs available include cephaloridine, colistin, gentamicin and kanamycin but these have the disadvantages of relatively high cost and the need for parenteral administration. The length of treatment has been much discussed and has tended to become progressively longer, for the first infection upto 2 weeks and for repeated infections, repeated cultures are necessary to monitor the progress of the treatment and the sensitivity of the respective organism and some times the treatment continued even more than 3 to 6 months period. Where a congenital malformation of the urinary tract is present or ureteric reflux has been demonstrated, treatment extending over several years may be necessary. The obstruction must be corrected. The associated surgical correction is required for stones, bladder diverticula etc. Children with ureteric reflux needs special consideration. In chronic or recurrent urinary tract infections, cyclic therapy with a series of drugs may have to be employed in order to prevent the emergence of resistant strains. Care should be taken with potentially toxic drugs in that the impaired renal function that results from pyelonephritis may allow dangerous retentions of the drugs with normally safe dosage.

Nephritis :

It is a generic term to include several diseases of different aetiology and course, but all with the potential to develop chronic stages and subsequently to renal failure.

Acute glomerulonephritis is an acute inflammatory disease of the kidney a sequel of streptococcal throat or skin infection probably due to hypersensitivity to extra renal infection and is characterised by haematuria, edema and mild hypertension.

The children of both sexes are affected, with a slight preponderance of males. It is rare in young children but no age is exempted but it occurs mostly in between 3-10 years of age. The responsible organisms are one of the nephritogenic strains of Lancefield Group A — haemolytic streptococci which belong to Griffith phage type 12 and to lesser extent to types 4 and 49. Acute nephritis usually follows 7 to 15 days after an episode of sore throat or impetigo due to streptococci. The antigens in the cell walls of these nephritogenic strains are chemically and immunologically similar to the antigens in the basement membrane of the glomerular capillaries. It is accompanied by a rise in the anti streptolysin-O (ASO) titre and a fall in the serumcomplement. The kidneys are slightly enlarged and pale and may have scattered punctate haemorrhagic lesions. On microscopy the glomeruli are seen to be especially involved with proliferation of the endothelial and mesangial cells of the glomerular tuft and polymorphonuclear infiltration. There is epithelial crescent formation and adhesion of inner cell walls with capsular walls take place and obliteration of glomeruli capsule might result. The renal tubular changes are minimal and non-specific. The glomerular filtration rate is diminished and the total body water as well as plasma volume and interstitial fluid are increased paripassu with the absorption of sodium. Water is absorbed passively resulting in circulatory overload, congestion and edema. There is anaemia due to haemodilution, ineffective erythropoietin and also due to lowered life span of erythrocytes.

The onset of acute glomerulonephritis is sudden, usually with fever, puffiness of the periorbital region and edema of the dependent parts. The urine is smoky brown due to haematuria and due to presence of haematin. Urinary output is reduced. Non-specific signs include loss of appetite, headache, vomiting, fatigue and irritability. Blood pressure is elevated and may even cause hypertensive encephalopathy. There might be left ventricular strain and pulmonary congestion leading on in some cases heart failure, more so due to salt and water retention. Papilledema is present occasionally. In a very few patients may develop acute renal insufficiency and may die of uraemia.

The urine examination reveals haematuria with both red cell casts and hyaline and epithelial casts, moderate amount of proteinuria and raised specific gravity.

The blood shows anaemia, blood urea nitrogen and creatinine are elevated serum albumin is slightly reduced. B_1C globulin is low and ESR is high. The evidence of streptococcal infection is detected by culture of throat swab and high ASO titre in blood.

This type of acute nephritic syndrome might occur in other condition which should be differentiated such as Henoch Schonlein purpura with acute nephritis, thrombocytopenia, haemolytic uraemic syndrome and hereditary nephropathies.

The course of this illness where recovery is usual in children, more than 90 percent of cases. The gross haematuria diminished in 2 to 3 weeks but blood and RBC persist in urine for 8 to 12 weeks and very rarely 6 to 12 months, which can be detectd microscopically. The oedema and raised blood pressure persist for 3 to 4 weeks. The patients with persistent haematuria of over 6 months duration are likely to develop chronic glomerulonephritis. More than 5% die in acute stage with complications of uraemia, heart failure and hypertensive encephalopathy.

There is no such specific therapy for the disease process as such. Penicillin should be given to eradicate any persistent streptococcal infection and should be continued till proteinuria disappears. The bed rest promotes early recovery and diminishes the risk of pulmonary oedema and hypertensive crisis. A strict daily record of the child's intake and output of fluid together with the weight and blood pressure, should be kept. The fluid intake should be restricted during the oliguric phase to a volume to the sum of the urine output and the insensible loss during the preceding 24 hours, as 300 ml/M^2 of the body surface plus the amount equivalent to the urine passed. Intake of salt and protein is also restricted. If diuresis is adequate, gradually normal diet and water are allowed. Fruit juices and other foods with a high potassium content should be avoided. After diuresis the fluid intake may be increased but protein should not be reintroduced into diet until the blood urea begins to fall. The children who are vomiting during the oliguric phase needs I.V. fluid and 20% dextrose or fructose may be used. The hypertension is treated with reserpine (0.04 to 08 mg./kg. I.M. once or twice daily) hydralazine (0.2 to 0.6 mg./kg. I.M. or by mouth 4 hourly) or methyldopa (15-60 mg./kg./day). The convulsions of hypertensive encephalopathy may be controlled with diazepam (0.25 mg./kg. I.V.) or paraldehyde (0.2 ml./kg. I.M.). The hyperkalaemia of more than 7 meq./litre should be treated by the use of an ion-exchange resin such as Resonium — A, rectally or by mouth, but peritoneal dialysis may be needed if this is not tolerated. The cardiac failure may be treated with digitalis and furosemide.

Nephrotic Syndrome :

The nephrotic syndrome is defined with the characteristic features of massive proteinuria (5 gm. in 24 hours) hypoalbuminaemia (2 gm. in 100 ml.), generalised oedema and hypercholesterolemia >300 mg. in 100 ml.). There are several distinct clinical types of nephrosis such as primary, secondary and congenital nephrosis. Primary type is further subdivided on the basis of histological findings into those with (a) minimal lession (74 percent) and (b) significant lesion (26 percent) on light microscopy. The histological changes in the later may be proliferative or membranous type. The membranous type is extremely uncommon (1.5%).. The secondary nephrosis may be secondary to other systemic disorders such as amyloidosis, systemic lupus erythromatosus, Henoch Schonlein vasculitis, post streptococcal glomerulonephritis (complement levels are low) and hypocomplementaemic persistent nephritis, hereditary nephropathies, metabolic disorders like cystinosis, toxic reactions due to drugs, e.g., mercury and tridione and quartan malaria due to plasmodium malaria, diabetes which is rare in children (nephropathy in diabetes take several years to develop). Secondary nephrosis collectively account 3.5 percent. In infantile microcystic disease or congenital nephrosis very rare in children. Onset is below one year of age and proximal tubules shows cystic dilatation. Response to treatment is poor.

The minimal lesions of the primary type occurs in children aged one to seven years, more in male child. Onset may be preceded by a viral upper respiratory infection or after an attack of diarrhoea and is frequently insiduous but can be abrupt and is characterised by oedema which increases in extent and degree until it is generalised and gross. The oedema firstly appear on face, the eyes appear puffy and periorbital oedema, later the oedema starts appearing on the dependent parts. The oedema pits on pressure. Ascitis, hydrothorax and hydroceles may develop. Intestinal oedema causes anorexia and malabsorptive diarrhoea. Blood pressure is usually normal. A considerable weight gain is associated with oedema. The urinary output is diminished. The urine contains a large amount of protein upto 10 G./day and has a high specific gravity. The proteinuria is selective in that it comprises plasma proteins of low molecular weight. Sometimes red cells and casts as granular, hyaline and fatty may be seen on microscopy. The blood cholesterol is raised, values of 350-1000 mg./100 ml. may occur. The plasma albumin is grossly reduced, often to 1-2 G/100 ml. and there is an associated fall in protein-bound fraction of the serum calcium. Electrophoresis of the plasma protein and gammaglobulin shows in addition to the decreased albumin increased α_2 and β lipoproteins, greatly increased and fibrinogen present in large amounts as also to the elevation of beta/alpha lipoproteins ratios but the serum complement is normal. The blood urea is not usually raised but ESR is very high. The child is more prone to infections and peritonitis is a usual complication. It should be suspected if there is abdominal pain, tenderness and abdominal wall oedema. Rigidity may not be present.

The nephrotic syndrome should be differentiated from kwashiorkor, cardiac failure, cirrhosis of liver and hypothyroidism from their clinical features and relevant investigations.

The course of the disease may be prolonged and there might be intermittent remission. Permanent remission reported after an attack of measles. About 70% of affected children will achieve a lasting remission but about 20% have a longer course extending over 10-20 years in which persistent proteinuria, episodes of oedema as an inconstant feature. A small group of children may run a rapidly progressive and fatal course of 1-5 years duration with presistant oedema, increasing hypertension and impaired renal function.

The symptomatic and supportive therapy includes bed rest when there is generalised oedema. The diet should be rich in protein. Salt and other sodium compound should be restricted. The infection should be kept under surveillance and preventive treatment should be started promptly. Initially for 1-2 weeks before corticosteroids, general diuretics like Furosemide and Spiranolactone should be tried. The check X-ray of the chest should be done to exclude associated tuberculosis. Urinary infection, if there is any, should be properly treated. The renal impairment should be investigated by blood urea and creatinine level estimations. Low salt albumin or dextran infusion may be given to expand blood volume.

The corticosteroids are the main sheet anchor of treatment. It is thought to be justifiable to treat all children with an initial course of prednisolone in high dose (50 mg./day) for a period of 10 days and subsequently tapered off during the next four weeks. Of the initial group 30-40% will have a permanent remission; about half will respond initially but will subsequently relapse, while the remainder will be resistant to treatment with steroids.

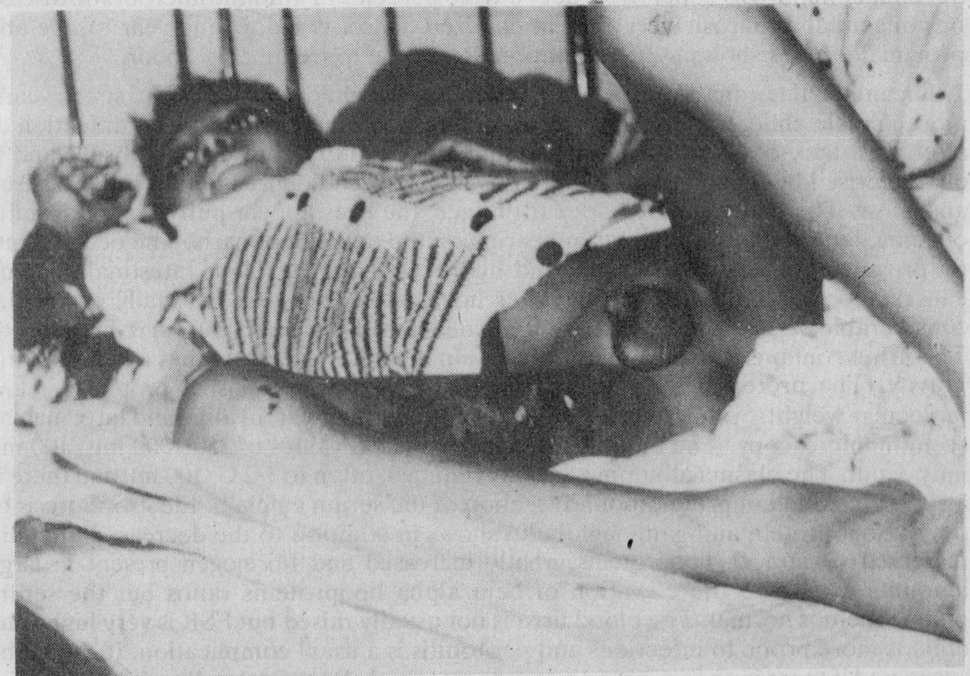

Fig.10.1 : Nephrotic Syndrome, frequent relapses of chronic nephritis and renal failure.

The children who relapses after an intial response to steroid therapy and the third relapse within 12 months should be treated with cyclophosphamide (2.5 mg./kg./day) given in conjunction with steroids for two months after which the steroid dosage is tappered off. The children on prolonged steroid therapy may develop hypertension, peptic ulcer and overt infections. The usual side effects of cyclophosphamide therapy are alopecia, bone marrow depression and haemorrhagic cystitis and gonadal deficiency.

Renal Failure :

The kidneys in renal failure cannot perform their normal function of excretion of metabolic end products and control of the concentration of the body fluids. In acute renal failure the onset is sudden and the renal functions recover spontaneously with or without treatment. Chronic renal failure develops over a long period, the number of functioning nephrons is reduced and complete recovery of the renal function does not occur.

Acute renal Failure :

Acute renal failure is said to occur when the kidneys become unable to excrete nitrogenous and other waste products or to maintain water and electrolyte homeostasis over a short period of time — usually hours or days. It usually follows a stereo typed pattern but in a few cases the onset may be over a period of weeks and some of the features of chronic renal failure may be seen. Acute renal failure is by its nature decompensated in that a steady state is not reached and there is a progressive accumulation of metabolic waste materials until recovery occurs or extra renal means are used, for their removal. The urine volumes listed below are often described by special terms.

Volume/24 hours :	O-Absolute Anuria
	<200 ml. Anuria
	200-800 ml. Oliguria.

These figures are relative and only apply to normal sized adults. In children the urine output to less than 10 ml./kg. of body weight or 400 ml./M^2 of body surface per day.

The etiological factors of acute renal failure may be classified as :

Pre-renal causes :

Severe hypovolemia due to diarrhoea, vomiting, burns, haemorrhage, shock due to septicaemia and congestive cardiac failure.

Renal causes :

(i) Acute glomerulo nephritis.

(ii) Acute tubular necrosis —

This may be either to severe ischaemia from hypovolumic injury to renal vessels, spasm of vessels and circulatory insufficiency or secondary to toxic damage to tubules from poisoning with mercury, arsenic, lead, sulphonamides, potassium chlorate and diethyleneglycol etc. Even in toxic damage, the ischaemia supervenes.

(iii) Haemolytic uremic syndrome.

(iv) Bilateral renal vein thrombosis.

Post-renal causes :

Obstruction to the outflow by clots of pus, blood, crystalluria, haemoglobinuria and formation of hematin casts in the collecting tubules (due to drug induced anaemia G6PD deficiency, mismatched transfusion and black water fever) and retroperitoneal fibrosis.

Normally the renal blood flow is approximately 500 ml./minute. This is in excess of metabolic requirements, as evidenced by the low arteriovenous oxygen difference. In periods of stress where a greater proportion of the cardiac output is required elsewhere (as in fright and heavy exercise) or when total cardiac output is reduced (shock, hypotension and cardiac failure) renal blood flow is severely reduced. As well as the total being reduced a redistribution occurs with a larger proportion perfusing the inner or juxta medullary part of the cortex. This is a 'normal' reflex in response to abnormal conditions and although it causes an immediate fall in GFR, renal function and urine output; it is not harmful unless very severe and prolonged.

In the initial phases there is a very marked oliguria or even complete suppression of urine. The phase lasts for a few days (about 3-7 days). The renal blood flow is reduced to about 2/3 of the normal but the glomerular filtration rate falls to less than 1 percent.

Clinically the child looks pale because of anaemia and hemodilution. Anaemia results from bone marrow depression and hemolysis. Overhydration manifest with oedema, raised JVP, tachypnoea and rales over the lung bases. They also have headache, nausea, vomiting and mental dullness. Breathing is often deep and sighing due to associated acidosis. Hiccup, vomiting, diarrhoea, clouding of consciousness and coma point out to elevation of blood urea levels. Potassium and phosphates due to the breakdown of the muscle proteins, catabolised for the energy needs. Bicarbonate level falls and the pH of the blood is reduced. There is fall of serum sodium and chlor ide due to increase extracellular water. ECG shows tenting of T waves, flattened P and depressed ST segment. After a few days the diuretic phase starts and the volume of urine may exceed 50 ml/M^2 of the surface area per day. Initially the urine is a pure ultrafiltrate of plasma but a few days later the kidneys regain the capacity to reabsorb salt and concentrate urea. The general condition of the child improves, urine flow increases. Unless a close watch is kept on the electrolyte disturbances in diuretic phase, usually lasting for a week, during which large amounts of water and electrolytes, particularly potassium may be lost. The patient may get dehydrated of these lesions are not adequately replaced.

The first line of treatment should be that of the cause — volume replacement for hypovolumic shock, appropriate antibiotics for sepsis and other supporttive measures. If after investigations are completed, it is concluded that the patient is in acute renal failure and that pre-renal elements and obstruction have been excluded or corrected therapeutic endeavour should be directed towards keeping the patient alive and well until renal function returns.

The following are some of the important aspects of patient management : In acute renal failure due to pre-renal causes, circulating blood volume is restored by I.V. infusion of Ringer lactate solution or isotonic saline 20-30 ml./kg. of body weight are given in one hour keeping a close watch on JVP so that central venous pressure should at no time exceed 5 cm. of H_2O. In shock due to haemorrhage or in burn 10-20 ml./kg. of body weight of blood is administered. If oliguria persists 0.5 gm. of manitol per kg. of body weight in a 20% solution is administered over the next 20 minutes. If the renal failure is reversible, the urine excretion increases by 6-10 ml./kg. in the next 1 to 3 hours. If there is no increase in urine flow, further administration of mannitol is withheld. If no effect, the diuretic furosemide may be administered in a dose of 1 mg./kg. I.V.

If the anuria persists or if the cause of renal failure is renal in origin due to parenchymal involvement, management will follow in this schedule. The child is weighed daily and intake output chart is maintained. The daily weight should be maintained, preferably the child will loss weight of 1 to 2 percent every day. The fluid intake both oral and intravenous should not exceed 300 to 500/M^2 of surface area per day plus the amount lost in urine, stools or vomitus, with initial oedema only insensible losses of water is allowed, no extra amount for urinary loss. I.V. fluid will be 25% dextrose without sodium or potassium. Extra calories should be provided from CHO source so that the body protein are not catabolised for the energy needs.

Excessive Na salts are withheld even when serum sodium level is low. 1-2 m mol./kg./day can be given. The acidosis is treated by adequate calories. Sodium bicarbonate or lactate should be used, so that there is no excess sodium. If necessary severe acidosis is treated by ion exchange resin in a dose 1 gm./kg. orally or per rectum. Calcium gluconate 10% solution 0.5 mL/kg. is used to counteract the effect of hyperkalaemia. Hepatic glycogen is restored by using 25% glucose solution I.V. followed with 0.5 units of insulin for every gm. of glucose administered. Dialysis is necessary in severe hyperkalaemia. CCF is prevented by regulation of water intake. Digitalis and diuretics should be used judiciously when needed. Hypertension is treated with bethamidine (0.2 mg./kg./day) or methyldopa (10 mg./kg./day) together with appropriate diuretics, given I.V. over 5 to 10 minutes. Peritoneal dialysis is used commonly because it is easier and convenient. Indications of dialysis include blood urea level 300 mg./dl., potassium 7 mg./dl., increasing acidosis, CCF and clinical deterioration.

Initially each cycle of the exchange of dialysate is 20 ml./kg. increased later to 40 to 50 ml./kg. per exchange cycle. Initial loading fluid is not removed. The fluid is allowed to run fast, equilibrated for 20 minutes and then drained for 15-20 minutes.

At every fifth cycle, the abdomen is allowed to drain dry. The dialysis is carried on for 36-72 hours. The composition of the standard dialysing solution is Na 140 mEq./L., Chloride 101 mEq./L., Cal. 4 mEq./L., Mag. 1.5 mEq./L., and acetate 45 mEq./L.

Reference

Reference

The Mechanism and Management of the Renal Failure : Education Service : Hoechst in Lancet 11, 7767, 8th July, 1972.

James, J.A. Liebuman, F., R.N. (1976) : Renal disease in childhood, 3rd ed., St. Louis, Mosby.

CHAPTER — ELEVEN

CENTRAL NERVOUS SYSTEM.

Meningitis :

The term itself is an inflammation of membranes covering the brain and spinal cord due to various infective agents. Although it is customary to speak of meningitis, no central nervous system infection is completely tissue-specific thus, meningitis may more properly be termed meningo-encephalitis and in the encephalitis there is some meningeal involvement. The early diagnosis and prompt management are of paramount importance not only to prevent mortality in children but also to prevent permanent morbidity with various neurological sequelae and mental retardation.

The common types of meningitis may result due to acute bacterial infection as Meningococcus, Pneumococcus, H. Influenzae, Streptococcus, Staphylococcus, E. Coli., Proteus, Pseudomonas — Aerogenus, Klebsiella, etc. The various virus also lead to aseptic meningitis such as poliovirus, coxsackie, ECHO, adenovirus, mumps virus, varicella, lymphocytic choriomeningitis. There are also tuberculous meningitis which is very common under 5 years of age with primary complex in the lungs. The rare forms are due to mycotic organisms such as histoplasmosis, torulosis, and other fungi, and protozoal-toxoplasmosis, amoebiasis. The syphilitic meningitis which is of granulomatous type may occur in children as a late manifestation of congenital syphilis.

Acute pyogenic meningitis :

Acute bacterial meningitis may result from bacteraemia or septicaemia where the pyogenic bacteria have gained entrance to the meninges via the general blood stream or from secondary to localized in or near the meninges as for example, cerebral abscess, ear or sinus infection or osteomyelitis of the skull or spine. The entry may also result from congenital defects such as meningocele or dermal sinuses and these should be carefully searched in the neonatal meningitis. The children and specially the infants in the first year of life, are particularly susceptible because of the relatively high vascularity of their brain and the low levels of immunity to some organisms especially H. Influenzae. The commonest bacteria found to be responsible for acute pyogenic meningitis are haemophilus influenzae, Neisseria meningitidis and diplococcus pneumonia. Less common agents include streptococci, staphylococci, escherichia coli, pseudomonas pyocyanea, salmonella and listeria monocytogenes. In the neonatal period and early infancy, escherichia coli, monocytogenes, streptococci and staphylococci are the usual organisms.

In the following section, features common to all types of purulent meningitis are outlined :

The subarachnoid space is filled with creamy pus. The lepto meninges are infiltrated with inflammatory cells.

Initially the ependymal surface appears normal but later the cortex of the brain shows proliferation of the microglia.

The ependymal are destroyed and purulent exudate collects at the base of the brain. This may block the foramina of Luschka and Magendi and result in internal hydrocephalus. The thrombophlebitis of the cerebral vessels may occur leading to infarction and neurological damage. If the patient survives, the purulent exudate organises resulting in fibrosis. The permanent neurological sequelae result from infection, necrosis and hydrocephalus. The onset is usually sudden, with vomiting, headache, high fever, photophobia and neck rigidity and kernig sign positive. A frank convulsion may occur early or late in the disease.

They appear to be a bad prognostic sign. On examination, the child is drowsy but presents disturbances and is often irritable and with a high pitched cry. The meningeal irritation is shown by presence of neck rigidity, Kernig's sign positive, that is straight leg raising is limited. The tripod sign and inability to kiss the knees are present. The pupils may be small or unequal and cranial nerve palsies especially the sixth nerve, with internal squint on one or both sides occur occasionally. When the anterior fontanelle is open it may bulge indicating raised intracranial pressure. In meningococcal meningitis; the features of toxaemia, shock, purpuric rashes overshadowed the picture of those of meningitis. This may further associated with sign of acute peripheral circulatory failure with restlessness going on to coma.

The classical picture of meningitis may not be there due to previous administration of antibiotics due to primary respiratory or other pyrexial illness which may precede it. In such cases not only the clinical but also the bacteriological diagnosis may be obscured but only clinical suspicion of meningitis in a sick child may help in establishing the diagnosis. The meningitis in the first month of life is not uncommon and is present in a quarter of the cases of septicaemia. Premature infants are especially liable, probably because of their susceptibility to infections and increased permeability of their blood-brain barrier. The infections of the maternal genital tract, birth trauma and prolonged labour after premature rupture of membranes may all be predisposing factors. The disease may be insidious in its onset and non-specific in its features such as meagre symptoms as fever, poor activity, feeding difficulties, grey appearance, cyanosis or dyspnoea, jaundice, vomiting and convulsions are common presenting symptoms or even simply failure to thrive. High fever and signs of meningeal irritation are often absent. A tense fontanelle may or may not be present. If the diagnosis is delayed, enlargement and retraction of the head may follow.

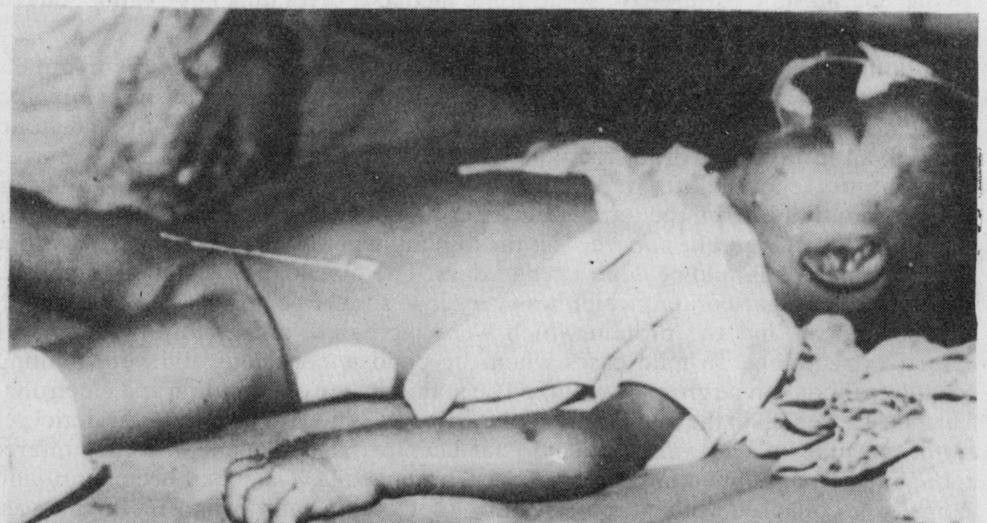

Fig.11.1 : Meningococcal Meningitis

The lumbar puncture is indicated whenever the suspicion of meningitis in a child is made and in fact the diagnosis of meningitis should constantly be borne in mind by every paediatrician especially in children who are acutely ill. The CSF in pyogenic meningitis is under raised pressure and cloudy with increase white cells which are mainly polymorphonuclear. The organisms are often seen on gram-stained smears, and grown on suitable culture media. The protein content is often raised and the sugar greatly reduced or absent. The blood culture is also helpful whenever possible before treatment is started since they may yield bacteria when the CSF is sterile.

The children with fever and signs of meningeal irritation may be suffering from (i) Pyogenic meningitis, (ii) Tuberculous meningitis, (iii) Viral or aseptic meningitis or from rare organisms, (iv) Meningism or meningeal irritation secondary to an infection elsewhere, such as ascariasis pneumonia, tonsillitis, otitis media or acute pyelitis. In this, the CSF is normal only the pressure might be increased. The neck rigidity might be associated with posterior fossa or cervical cord tumour or abscess but here the head stiffness is persistent besides other neurological features. The various forms of meningitis should be diagnosed by CSF findings but the type sometimes can be suspected from the clinical picture. For example, drowsiness is common in bacterial than in aseptic meningitis or meningism and the onset of tuberculous meningitis is usually more insiduous than in pyogenic forms.

The treatment of pyogenic meningitis should be prompt, thorough and is possible with specific and adequate antibiotics and chemotherapeutic drugs. The treatment also includes of associated circulatory failure and symptomatic measures, such as sedatives for convulsions and maintenance of electrolytes specially potassium and fluids, etc.

The choice of drug depends on the bacteriological diagnosis based on the CSF examination. Whenever clinical diagnosis is made, lumbar puncture is done preceding treatment; a cell count and a gram stain should be prepared from the centrifuged sediment of CSF smear. The organisms may be identified from the direct smear but in some cases either no bacteria is seen or their morphological character is misleading, so the CSF must be cultured on appropriate media. It takes time but treatment never awaits these results. A blood culture also be asked for.

In doubtful cases or before the specific culture report is available, the treatment must be started at once with triple therapy, a combination of sulphadiazine, ampicillin and chloramphenicol. The drugs must be given intravenously for first 48 hours through an intravenous drip. The chloramphenicol and sulpha are better absorbed through intravenous route. In all cases of pyogenic bacterial meningitis, the drugs must be continued until the temperature has been normal and the CSF sterile for at least four days. Generally two weeks is the minimum period of treatment. The second lumbar puncture should be done after 14 days. The biochemical criteria of improvements are the sugar content which was very low, should be normal and cells mainly the polymorph and the protein which were increased, are greatly reduced with effective treatment. In mild cases when the child is conscious and not vomiting, adequate fluids can be given by mouth. The maintenance of hydration and electrolyte balance is essential in the management of meningitis. The Waterhouse — Friderichsen syndrome due to acute bilateral adrenal haemorrhage is a picture encountered though rarely, in fulminating meningococcal septicaemia. The infant becomes rapidly comatose, collapsed with purple mottling of the skin, and cyanosis. In this case hydrocortisone and plasma are required to pull up the patient from extreme degree of shock.

The adrenergic agents such as noradrenaline, may be needed to combat hypotension and severe shock, the rate of infusion being carefully adjusted to maintain a normal blood pressure. To combat both restlessness and frank convulsions, the following anticonvulsive drugs are used such as paraldehyde which is safe and effective (0.2 ml./kg. intramuscularly), phenobarbitone (5 mg./kg. I.M.), or diazepam (0.25 mg./kg. I.V. or I.M.), phenytoin 3 mg./kg. I.M. or I.V. may be given to build up rapidly adequate blood levels. The care of the unconscious or semiconscious child with meningitis must include the avoidance of aspiration by proper nursing on his side and frequent suction, the maintenance of nutrition and detection of urinary retention. The surgical treatment may be indicated for primary conditions such as associated mastoiditis, empyema and osteomyelitis etc. The subdural effusion, which is commonest with H. influenzae meningitis, should be suspected when vomiting or pyrexia persists after adequate antibiotic therapy and persistence of bulged anterior fontanelle with increase of head size. The maximum occipitofrontal circumference of the skull should be recorded daily and also when doubt arises skull X-ray may suggest the presence of 'sterile pus' as effusion in the subdural space, which again is confirmed by subdural taps. The EMI scan, if available, will also help and demonstrate the presence of fluid.

Apart from neonatal meningitis where the outlook is grave, the prognosis in meningitis has vastly improved in the last two decades with modern specific antibiotic therapy aided by supportive therapy as outlined above. The significant reduction in mortality rates from pyogenic meningitis has unfortunately been followed by an impressive increase in the morbidity and serious neurological handicap among the survivors. The important among the complications are subdural effusions, hydrocephalous, recurrent convulsions, and other neurological sequelae ranging from minimal brain dysfunction syndrome to gross mental retardation, deafness and hemiplegia.

Encephalitis :

Encephalitis means inflammation of the brain and could result from infection with viruses, bacteria, rickettsia and many other agents. The bacteria causes localising lesion of the brain but viruses usually cause diffuse disease often accompanied by lymphocytic meningitis and myelitis. This may be viral in origin or follow viral exanthema or vaccination. These two different types of response of the nervous system to systemic virus infections are used to classify encephalitis into acute viral and post infectious. In the first type, an inflammatory reaction to the virus is greatest soon after it enters the brain whereas in the second, post-infectious type, virus particles have disappeared following a cellular response with perivascular destruction of myelin. The post-infectious encephalitis represents an allergic reaction to the virus, which is usually not isolated in fatal cases. Although there may be some overlap in individual cases, this division into two types is a useful one.

The encephalitis primary or post-infectious may be associated with convulsions and disturbances of consciousness deepening into coma. The cerebral form of malaria, as well as other protozoal infections such as trypanosomiasis and toxoplasmosis, may present in the same way.

It is preferably not to include bacterial infections in the term encephalitis, reserving this for cases of proved or presumed viral etiology, regardless of whether CSF shows an increase in cell count (simple CSF changes are not constant). The word encephalopathy is sometimes loosely used as a synonym for encephalitis, but it should be reserved for cases not of infective origin.

The acute viral encephalitis due to arbor viruses include St. Louis, Japanese-B, Murray Valley and eastern and western equine encephalitis transmitted by an insect vector.

The encephalitis due to arbor viruses has long been recognised in Japan outbreak occured as early as 1871. But the viruses of JE was isolated only as far back in 1936. The virus is transmitted to man by the mosquito culex tritaeniorhynohus and it breeds in rice fields. Several epidemics of this disease have been known to occur in India from time to time. Recently JE Encephalitis occurred in India followed the localities nearer the river belts such as in Andhra Pradesh and Karnataka, the Krishna and Godavari river belts, then also at Jamshedpur, Patna in Bihar along Ganges and Subarna Rekha, then at Bankura in West Bengal. From all the places, the cases those who had chance of admission in hospital, some of them are followed up in Pune Virus Research Laboratory where the JE virus could be isolated. In Bangalore, Neurological Research Institute some of the cases, the post-mortem study of brain tissue demonstrated the typical brain changes due to arbor virus infection. In Patna outbreak which were clinically diagnosed as encephalitis and admitted in medical college as JE encephalitis type, followed up and investigated. The virus was not isolated. 17 cases died out of 50 (34% mortality) and 33 left with residual mental changes. The epidemiological study of this recent cases showed that the virus disseminated-pig-mosquito-pig cycle. The pigs infestation are now known to be good indications of the prevalence of the virus in any given locality. The clinical presentations of these cases should be differentiated from meningitis specially tuberculosis, cerebral malaria and Reye's Syndrome (encephalopathy and fatty degeneration of liver).

The neurological complications and sequelae were mainly of various central nervous system involvement, leading to the most crippling conditions including various degrees of mental derangements. This epidemic in India presented a great public health problem and not only from increasing mortality but also the morbidity from the dreadful diseases. However, research is going on to find out successful vaccine which will be able to prevent the attack of JE and moreover preventive measures should be sought to destroy the insect vector culex and also irradication of the JE infection of the intermediate host-pig.

Acute Anterior Poliomyelitis :

Acute anterior poliomyelitis is a viral illness of paralytic nature which may destroy the anterior horn cells of the spinal cord and cause paralysis of limbs, trunk, respiration and swallowing. Some patients remain permanently paralysed after the acute disease. The estimated number of children with untreated severe residual paralysis reach several millions and 90% of all acute cases still occur in those under 5 years.

Usually infection with the virus causes only a mild febrile illness, but in severe cases damage to anterior horn cells results in flaccid paralysis of varying severity and distribution.

Infection with each of the three strains of poliovirus is thought to confer a lasting immunity. Specific for that type, but ineffective for others, so that the rare second attacks of the paralytic disease are probably due to infection with another type.

There are three enteroviruses besides polio, the other two are ECHO and coxsackie. The man is the only known reservior of the poliovirus which can be recovered from the stools of patients and symptomless carriers as well as from sewage during epidemics, and sometimes also from flies, water, milk and food. The faeco-oral transmission is the main source of spread and greatest in conditions of poor hygiene. The epidemics of paralytic poliomyelitis are commonest in summer and autumn, but may occur throughout the year. The geographical variation occurs. It is known as a civilised disease. The paralytic cases are greatly outnumbered by ill, non-paralytic cases and the symptomless carrier state even is more commoner. The paralysis occurs more in elderly children and countries with poor hygiene,the young groups are more affected with non-paralytic disease and in an occasional case of infantile paralysis but a lasting immunity in the general population.

These stages occur in the classical course of poliomyelitis, one or more of which may be present. The initial illness develops after an incubation period of between 7 and 21 days during which virus is present in stools and throat. Then there is sudden high rise of temperature with viraemia with general symptoms simulating an infectious disease. These symptoms last from a few hours to a few days and that might and with paralysis or aborted as like any other infectious disease like typhoid or influenza in tropical countries. Sometimes meningitic illness follows the initial symptoms giving the disease a bi-phasic character. To be differentiated by other meningitic illnesses or simple meningism associated with various illnesses in children. There may be severe muscle pains and tenderness. The transient retention of urine may occur and constipation simulating typhoid. The history of febrile convulsion is rare instead the patient is aleart, reliance becomes a mood point of differential nature with other meningitic and encephalitic conditions.

At this stage the neck rigidity or stiffness without such signs of meningeal irritations are diagnostic points. The CSF changes occur but not invariably present. The cell count is increased upto several hundreds with a variable proportion of polymorphonuclear cells. The protein level is slightly raised. The cell count returns to normal in the course of a week or two, the polymorphonuclears decreasing before the lymphocytes. The protein level gradually rises but the sugar is normal and culture for bacteria negative, returns to normal in four to ten weeks. The meningitic illness may last between three and ten days, and may be followed by complete recovery, in which case it is described as non-paralytic or followed by paralysis, when it is referred to as the preparalytic type of poliomyelitis. The paralytic illness usually begins between the second and fourth day of the meningitic illness, when the fever of this phase may have begun to fall. The temperature rises again shortly before the onset of paralysis. In most cases paralysis is complete within 24 to 48 hours of its onset, but may continue to increase when the fever persists. Since it is due to damage to anterior horn cells, part of the lower motor neuron system, paralysis is of the flaccid type associated with loss or diminution of tendonreflexes and eventually with muscle wasting and often trophic changes in the affected limb. There is no sensory loss. The brunt of the paralysis may fall on muscles supplied by neurones in the spinal cord, brain stem or both and the clinical picture varies according to the emphasis of the paralysis. Thus there are three main clinical types :

1. **The spinal form :**

The groups of muscles are affected in a typically asymmetrical distribution. The paralysis tend to affect the legs more often and more severely than the arms and the arms than the trunk. The degree of respiratory muscles involvement will determine the immediate outcome. The muscle power begins to recover when the fever has fallen and most of the recovery which can occur has probably done so within three to six months. The severity of paralysis vary from monoplegia to quadruplegia with varying recovery of complete paralysis to a total and permanent residual paralysis of four limbs and trunk.

2. **The bulbar or brain stem form :**

In this form the motor cranial nerve nuclei in the medulla including the centres for respiration and circulation are affected most, so that the illness is severe and the mortality very high.

The paralysis of the palate, pharynx and larynx impairs the swallowing and coughing mechanisms with risk of suffocation from inhaling food or secretions. The palatal weakness may be first detected by the nasal speech. The facial palsy and squints may occur. The involvement of the respiratory centre causes shallow, irregular breathing and sudden respiratory failure may follow. The peripheral circulatory failure and hyperpyrexia are other serious complications.

3. **The bulbo-spinal form :**

The bulbar poliomyelitis often occurs in combination with the spinal form and the association of swallowing and coughing difficulties with respiratory insufficiency due to intercostal and diaphragmatic paralysis and involvement of the respiratory centre produces a dangerous situation with a severe prognosis.

A rare cerebral or encephalitic form of poliomyelitis is also recognised with irritability, drowsiness, delirium and stupor. This must be distinguished from the mental changes resulting from hypoxia and hypercapnia with respiratory insufficiency in paralytic cases of the disease.

The initial illness cannot usually be distinguished from ordinary influenza or other mild fevers, although its occurrence during an epidemic may suggest that it is due to poliovirus.

The meningitic illness may be differentiated from other types of aseptic meningitis by the muscle tenderness that is often present. The lack of drowsiness and the CSF change with normal sugar and failure to detect bacteria help to distinguish the meningitic illness of poliomyelitis from bacterial meningitis. The paralytic type must be distinguished from other cases of flaccid paralysis. Acute infective polyneuritis (the Gullian-Barre Syndrome) is the common condition most liable to be confused. In polyneuritis, paralysis is more often symmetrical and distal than polio. There may be sensory symptoms and CSF changes showing a high protein with a normal cell count albuminocytological dissociation. The ECHO and coxsackie virus may sometimes produce a clinical and pathological picture indistinguishable, except virus study from non paralytic poliomyelitis. The pseudoparalysis in young children due to inflammatory and other diseases of bones or joints may be confusing, acute rheumatic fever, scurvy and osteomyelitis may have to be differentiated from acute poliomyelitis. Bone injuries may at times mimic paralysis of a limb as in some cases of fractured clavicle or epiphyseal injury.

The diagnosis is mostly clinical and in some cases of doubt then isolation of virus by tissue culture from stools and nasal washing and the detection of a rising titre of antibodies in the serum during convalescence will often allow a definite aetiological diagnosis to be made.

The mortality rate is highest in bulbar and bulbo-spinal types. In this group the prognosis depends upon the availability of modern scientific methods of assisting respiration and good nursing in an well equipped hospital.

The cranial nerve paralysis usually recover completely in the survivors. The patients with limb weakness about half recover completely and half have some permanent deficit. A little recovery can be expected in muscles without movement after 4-6 weeks time.

The treatment is largely symptomatic and anticipatory, since no drugs are effective against poliovirus. The wide-spread use of polio vaccines has resulted in the virtual disappearance of the disease in countries with effective immunization programme. It is now recommended that three doses of oral poliovirus vaccine (OPV) a mixture of attenuated strains of all three be given in the first year of life, starting at four to six months of age, three doses with intervals of six to eight weeks between doses and with further booster doses at 2-2½ years and next at five years or school entry, and the three early doses of OPV are conveniently given at the same time as tripple (DPT) vaccination.

The meningitic and paralytic cases should be admitted to a hospital with facilities for dealing with possible acute emergencies. Best will be in an isolation hospital until three weeks after subsidence of fever and the excreta should be disposed of antiseptically. The complete bed rest and minimal disturbances are needed in the early stages. The analgesics may be needed for muscle pains. The paralysed muscles must be positioned to relax and this type of management should be better conducted under the supervision of a physiotherapist. A careful watch must be kept on respiratory involvement. As paralysis of intercostal muscles and diaphragm can occur rapidly, so a machanical respiratory and staff experienced in managing this emergency should be ready at hand. In bulbar cases the most immediate damage is suffocation by aspiration of pharyngeal secretions, a clear airway must be maintained. Here also staff who can deal with respiratory emergencies should be incharge, best is an intensive care unit with the help of an anaesthetist who is competent enough to do intubation when necessary.

During recovery the patient must be weaned slowly from his dependence on the artificial respirator and repeatedly assured. Some patients will continue to need periodic or partial assistance with respiration for short or long periods.

The management as a whole is of a team approach for acute poliomyelitis cases. This spirit is also needed during rehabilitation which may continue for years together. The paediatrician is a collaborator between the orthopaedic surgeon, physiotherapist, neurologist and not the least the social worker cum psychiatrist. The child's residual disability may proven attendance at an ordinary school and careful thought must be given to the most suitable educational placement.

Reference

Till, K. (1975) — Paediatric Neuro Surgery for Paediatrician and Neuro-Surgeons, Oxford, Blackwell.

CHAPTER – TWELVE

PAEDIATRIC EMERGENCIES

The child patient is a problem to all practitioners because without any co-operative history from the patient, only from the clinical symptoms and signs, one should have to manage. Moreover, if it is a medical emergency in a child then one confronts with double or tripple handicaps because, the patient is a child, least co-operation and thirdly the parental anxiety sometimes makes the attendant physician more perplexed to come to diagnosis and further more the total management of the case.

With this background, let us recapitulate the important and common childhood emergencies which a physician should handle, may be on the spot management or referral to a specialist for further diagnosis and management.

The following conditions one should enumerate as commoner medical emergencies in childhood period :-

(i) Convulsive disorders in childhood.
(ii) Fluid and electrolyte dehydration after gastro-enteritis.
(iii) Accidental poisoning in childhood.
(iv) Respiratory distress may be stridor and/or dyspnoea.
(v) Hyperpyrexia in childhood.
(vi) Abdominal pain both medical and surgical causes, including abdominal distension.
(vii) Excessive crying specially in early infancy.
(viii) Retention of urine and stool.

Convulsive disorders in childhood :

The epilepsy and convulsion should, like fever be regarded as symptom than diagnostic entities, with a wide range to underlying aetiological factors. The word 'epilepsy' implies to a condition in which there is a tendency to recurrent attacks usually involving alternation in consciousness, together with a variety of other phenomena, motor, sensory and psychic. It is often demonstrated by organic brain disease, shown by electroencephalogram (EEG). This definition excludes patients who have one or two attacks transient in nature with biochemical abnormalities in new born period and with high temperature termed as 'febrile convulsion' in between 6 months and three years. These, sometimes, are best referred as convulsion. It is often necessary in a child to reserve judgement when there have been one or two convulsions since it is difficult to know whether this convulsion will recur or not.

The convulsions in the newborn period are common. It is associated with prolonged, traumatic and difficult delivery, neonatal asphyxia and hyperbilirubinaemia leading to kernicterus. In such cases the long term prognosis is poor, not only its repetitive nature but also for mental and motor development. The convulsion or fit may be feature of neonatal infection, leading to septicaemia and meningitis. Any doubt, lumbar puncture should help to establish the diagnosis. Already pointed out earlier a small but often remediable group of convulsion results due to biochemical abnormalities such as Tetany, due to low ionic calcium, hypoglycaemia due to low sugar and hypomagnesaemia. This is not too infrequently noted that pyridoxine dependency or deficiency associated with some inborn error of metabolism may present as neonatal convulsion. The neonatal convulsion usually in the nature of twitching, which is focal but sometimes tonic contraction might be seen, specially in neonatal 'tetanus' which is fatal in more than 90% of cases. Easily preventable by proper immunisation of the mother in the antenatal period by 'Tetvac' injections in 28, 32 and 36 weeks of pregnancy.

The febrile convulsions remain one of the commonest and least understood disorders of childhood. In certain families there is a genetic predisposition for the children between six months to 3 years, may extent upto 6 years in some percentage of cases, to react to common febrile illnesses with convulsion. Sometimes history of such attack was also presented in one of the parent or in siblings.

This tendency ceases after 6 years but in some (5 to 10%) it continues, so that later on it is diagnosed as epilepsy. Although, there is at least 5% mortality below 3 years of age and sometimes 10 to 15% of morbidity occurs in the group of 3 to 6 years. Analysing a few series of cases, it was noted that some cases turn to temporal lobe epilepsy in the later ages of childhood. This group is often benefitted by surgery than continuation with anticonvulsive drugs.

There might be associated extra cranial conditions such as Tonsillitis, Otitis media, Pyelitis to explain high rise of temperature but one should try to prevent the attack by early administration of anti-convulsive drugs like Diazepam, Phenobarbitone, Paraldehyde and Phenothiazone derivative to bring down the temperature quickly with other antipyretic drugs such as aspirin. Also teaching parents how to bring down the temperature with tepid sponging and to avoid injuring the child of his own tongue by putting a wrapped tongue spatula between the teeth and tongue clear the air ways, putting the child on a firm flat surface. These are preliminaries, the parent should take precautions before the physician attends the sick child. There is still controversy, whether all children who have one or two febrile convulsion should receive regular anti-convulsive drugs. In them more than 50% has no recurrence of fits. So it seems advisable to categories who should have 'risk' of developing recurrent fits or continuation of fits, after one or two attacks of febrile convulsion. The criterias again were observed in various series all over India, enumerated in this way. If the febrile convulsion occurs below 12 months of age, mostly in male child, prolong fit over 15 to 30 minutes, recurrence of fits within 8 weeks time, neurological deficits persisting after an initial attack, repeated attacks after phenobarbitone prophylactic use. The situation is not yet clear whether prophylactic phenobarbitone, will prevent further attacks. Each case should be judged by its own merit, so long more informations are available regarding the mechanism and aetiopathogenesis of so-called 'benign' nature of febrile convulsion.

Infantile Spasm :

It is also known as lightening attacks or salam attacks or major fit in the minor age group. They usually begin between the ages of five months and eighteen months with a peak at 7 months. A typical attack involves sudden flexion of the neck and trunk, with adduction of arms and lower limbs, often associated with a high pitched cry. If the body is in sitting posture over the mother's lap sudden forward bending results like the attitude of 'Salam'. Occasionally, there is extension rather than flexion, of the limbs and trunk. Typically, the attacks once established, occur in series of from 5 to 80 or more separated by a few seconds interval. Many such seizures occur each day. Gradually with the onset of spasm the child shows signs of growth failure and also failure of adaptive behaviours, loosing social awareness and the skills which he has acquired. This clinical picture is generally associated with typical EEG changes as hypsarrhythmia. It is like other forms of epilepsy associated with varied aetiology such as precipitated in those associated with perinatal injuries, those with inborn error of metabolism as phenylketonuria, neuro-cutaneous hereditary disorder as Tuberose Sclerosis and a few children develop infantile spasm after receiving diphtheria-tetanus-pertussis immunisation injection and it is thought to be the reaction of pertussis element in DPT immunisation.

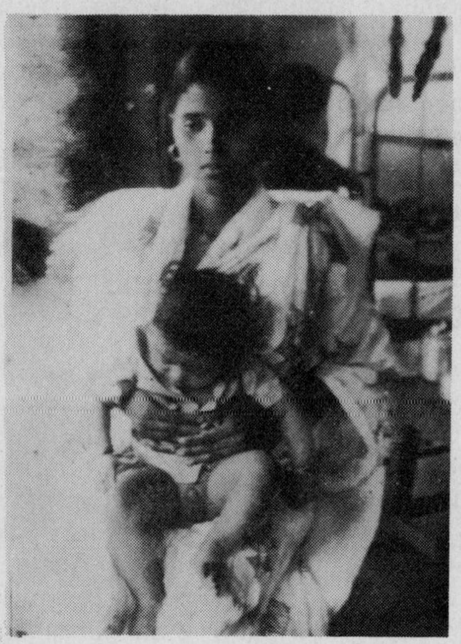

Fig.12.1(a) : Infantile Spasm on Mothers' lap

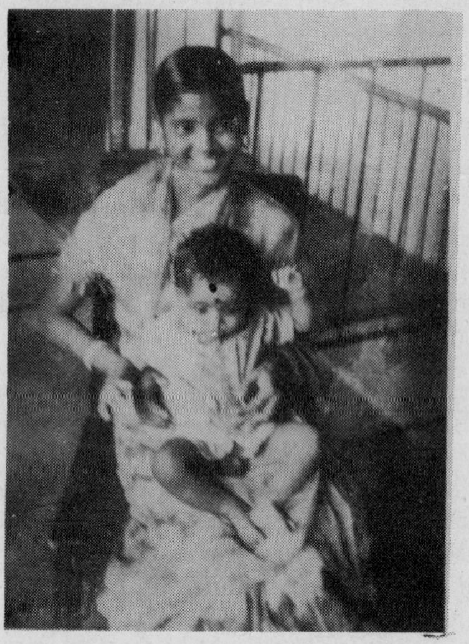

Fig.12.1(b) : Controlled with ACTH & Pyridoxine therapy.

The prognosis is bad, resulting mental retardation. It is said that anticonvulsive as Diazepam and use of AÇTH or cortisone in some cases, can prevent the series of spasm and thereby blocks the recurrent on-slaught of the brain. The prognosis depends, among other factors, on the aetiology, being best in the idiopathic group and worst in those grossly abnormal children in whom the spasms are only one problem among many.

Some patients only have convulsion which faced with rhythmically flashing lights and in others these are one among several provoking factors such as 'Television fits'. Also fits associated with worms infestation specially 'Ascariasis'.

The true fit to be differentiated with 'Breath Holding attack' or cry convulsion. The children are liable to hold their breath and becomes blue. This is common in between 9 months and 18 months and mostly prevalent in 'spoilt' child, who are more easily frustrated. Though alarming and often repeated, the prognosis is good. The EEG is normal.

The syncopal attacks in elderly children should be differentiated from fits. It is common in girls and they often occur while standing at school and in crowded surroundings.

The varieties of epilepsy, which are again classified as grand mal, petit mal, psychomotor or temporal lobe and Jacksonian or Focal epilepsy, could be well differentiated by EEG pattern. Sometimes the interpretation of the EEG in children is often difficult and it must always be considered in the context of the total clinical problem, rather than regarded as a diagnostic or prognostic test in its own right.

The typical epileptic fit of recurrent type, mentioned above, is generally not seen below three years of age. Moreover, an attack of epilepsy in the elderly children might be the first onset of idiopathic epilepsy but one should also exclude the possibility of space occupying lesion such as intracranial tumour, might present for the first time as epileptic fit or obscured head injury, subdural haematoma as birth injury might be a trivial one, which ignored by the playful child or generally ignored by the parents as well.

The investigations in a case of epilepsy or convulsion in a child should be guided by preceding clinical history which will include presence of family history of epilepsy, a grossly abnormal birth history or association with cerebral palsy or mental retardation. The skull X-ray and EEG are required in recurrent fits. The biochemical such as hypoglycaemia, hypocalcaemia, hypomagnesaemia and pyridoxine deficiency should be excluded by estimation from blood. In neonatal convulsion a therapeutic test with an injection of pyridoxine is advisable when fits are associated with mental retardation especially with a family history of previous presence of inborn errors of metabolism and should be excluded by aminoacid chromatography of blood and urine. The causes of focal epilepsy can be demonstrated by EEG or brain scan to help detection of intracranial tumour.

The anti-convulsive drugs are used in epilepsy, only a very few are available in India. The anti-convulsants can be divided into those effective in grand mal and those effective in petit mal. The former includes phenobarbitone, phenytoin and primidone. The latter includes ethosuximide and troxidone. The temporal lobe attacks often respond to phenobarbitone, phenytoin or primidone, alone or in combination. Valproic acid may become the drug of choice for treatment of grand mal and petitmal epilepsy.

The status epilepticus should always be regarded as an emergency. The drugs to be used are Paraldehyde, Diazepam and Barbiturates. In this case hospital admission is preferable and it is dangerous to defer treatment until this can be arranged as valuable time is lost. Sometimes intravenous alimentation needed to maintain the drug level of anti convulsion and simultaneously to maintain the nutrition of the child. The use of Diazepam (0.2 mg./kg. body weight) is often effective in the control of status epilepticus when given I.V. instead of intramuscular injection. In status epilepticus, it is a team approach consisting of an anaesthetist, biochemist, and not the least the paediatrician, needing active and expert management.

The second *common paediatric emergency,* i,e., the fluid and electrolyte dehydration after gastroenteritis has been dealt with in the previous chapter under gastroenteritis in infant and children.

Accidental poisoning in children.

The accidental poisoning in children is prevalent all over the world. The change of social culture and environmental changes has brought about a noticeable alteration in the pattern of poisoning seen now-a-days. In India, still now, more than 15 to 20% die of infectious diseases in hospital statistics besides malnutrition directly or indirectly are responsible in the rampant death with infectious diseases outside the hospitals. It has been stated that poisoning causes 0.03% deaths in children below 1 year of age, 0.16% in 1-4 year age group and 0.37% in 5-14 year age group according to the official report submitted to the Government of India. The hospital statistics observed periodically from different parts of the country indicate an incidence varying from 0.33% to 7.64% of total admissions. The poisoning is much more commoner in pre-school children. Among the group in between 2 to 3 years age, more than 50% has been reported and 80 to 90% are under 5 years of age. The pattern of poisoning varies according to the growth and development of the child. As the infant starts crawling at 10 months and walking around one to one and half of year of age, his activity and explorable curiosity increase and lead him to put everything into his mouth, later by 3½-4 years of age, the child's adaptive behaviour pursuadè him access to any unlocked drawer or cupboard within easy reach at home despite too many hurdles to reach the objects. By the age above 4 years, again the incidence of poisoning drops because due to more maturity of motor and scholastic development, the child is in a position to select things that taste good for purposes of ingestion. A preventive programme must be oriented with this background of child's motor and mental developmental achievements known to the observers. A 3 year old child can be made to understand and taught basic safety rules and prevented from sampling any odd objects he may come across. After the age of 4 years, education or guidance is the main factor in preventing programme.

The male children predominate over the females as they display a greater degree of activity, the incidence also tends to be hightened in socio-economic groups and in large families where the mother usually illiterate, is overburdened by duties and is more likely to be careless in storing potentially the poisonous substances or cup board of medicines out of the reach of her children.

In order of frequency, the commonest poisonous substances identified are (a) household (45-70%), (b) drugs (15-30%) and seeds (8-20%). The kerosene oil poisoning is most frequently incriminated since it is commonly used for lighting and cooking.

The incidence of kerosene poisoning ranges from 9% to as high as 60% of all cases in some series. The other household products include DDT, Flit-which contains pyretham, Tik 20 (Penitrothion), Varnish oil, Rodenticides (containing phosphorus), Caustic soda, various pesticides and, insecticides, phenol, acetic acids, the ointments for external use, the incidence of organophosphorus poisoning is increasing due to its use in pesticides for agricultural use.

Among the drugs, the opium poisoning is commoner due to its widespread use as an antidiarrhoeal and also a tranquiliser by parents and local quacks. The other drugs which are also tested, among them lomotil, phenothazine, barbiturates, iodine, dettol, aspirin, Iron, INH-in excess doses, prescribed by physicians or accidentally swallowed by the children and the overdosage or idiosyncrasy to the particular drugs have been reported as 20%. The seed poisoning is mostly seen above the age of 3-4 years and mostly in urban and rural areas. The common seeds are dhatura, castor oil seeds, etc. The principles of management of poisoning include removal of unabsorbed poison, hastening the elimination of absorbed poison and treatment of acute circulatory and respiratory failures. If available, a specific antidote should be administered and with impending renal failure, a dialysis may be indicated. Inspite of these early procedures, many children still die due to accidental poisoning. The deaths could largely be prevented by correct counselling to the parents and health education to our illiterate mothers regarding keeping the medicines out of reach of the children, always the households detergents and pesticides should be locked and moreover to be vigilant regarding the activities of 1-4 years group, because this is the vulnerable age group with their normal growth pattern and explorative inquisitiveness become the prey of accidental poisoning.

Respiratory distress may be as 'Stridor'and/or dyspnoea :

Under this heading, the three important respiratory conditions should be considered — (i) Bronchiolitis, (ii) Acute laryngo-tracheobronchitis and (iii) Bronchial asthma with status asthmaticus. No. (i) and (iii) have been discussed in their relative chapters. Here only the conditions associated with 'Stridor' should be discussed.

The term Stridor or croup is commonly present in six different conditions :-

(i) After foreign body inhalation and obstruction in the laryngo-tracheal tree.
(ii) Laryngeal diphtheria.
(iii) Acute laryngo tracheobronchitis.
(iv) Simple laryngitis : Spasmodic croup (Laryngitis Stridulosa).
(v) Laryngismus stridulus.
(vi) Acute epiglottitis.

It is necessary to differentiate between laryngeal diphtheria, laryngismus stridulus (a symptom of tetany), acute epiglottitis, acute laryngotracheo-bronchitis and obstruction by a foreign body. In laryngeal diphtheria, the constitutional upset is severe and there is presence of central cyanosis. An examination of the throat shows as a rule, accompanying pharyngeal diphtheria or nasal diphtheria. In laryngitis stridulus there is no evidence of accompanying infection. The associated signs of latent or overt tetany are found usually is association with signs of rickets and hypocalcaemia. In acute laryngotracheo-bronchitis there is a rapidly progressive condition. The bronchial or laryngeal obstruction from viscid secretion may cause an asphyxial death, unless a prompt tracheostomy or intubation is carried out. There may be both inspiratory and expiratory difficulty. In acute epiglottitis, there is commonly a preceding respiratory infection. The stridor is progressive, but in the early stage is indistinguishable from spasmodic croup. Laryngoscopy will reveal the obstruction of the airway by oedematous epiglottitis.

The spasmodic croup is caused by the same types of infection as other upper respiratory infections, but there is extension of the infection. There is congestion and swelling of the vocal cords. The spasm of the laryngeal muscles may occur as part of the attack. This type of croup most commonly occurs between six months and three years.

A foreign body in the larynx may be unsuspected by the parents but must be excluded by direct laryngoscopy in case of persistent stridor. Sometimes it may go down and causes blocking of the bigger bronchus commonly in the right middle lobe or lingula of left lung. There may be direct evidence of foreign body by laryngoscopy but indirectly one should suspect by visualising obstructive emphysema in checking radiological investigations.

The laryngitis specially of infective origin should be taken very seriously from management point of view. The children tend to tire suddenly and heart failure can occur. The provision of a high humidity is the most important aspect of treatment of all forms of infective laryngitis besides specific antibiotics. It is of bacterial origin which is very rare and proper timely management of diphtheria with anti-diphtheretic serum and penicillin injections. Those which are of viral aetiology which is commonly the source of infection, only symptomatic treatment is needed. Either a steam tent is made or the child is placed in an oxygen tent, with a humidifire attachment. A sedative such as phenobarbitone or chloral hydras should be given. The intubation is indicated in patients who continue to show acute spasm for more than a few hours and in whom cyanosis and increasing difficulty in inspiration develops.

Hyperpyrexia in childhood :

Hyperpyrexia, inspite of high environmental temperature and humidity occurs relatively infrequently in childhood years even in the newborn period. The hyperpyrexia of 41°C. (105.8 F.) or above may occur for a variety of reasons in the newborn, infancy and later childhood years. The over heating in an incubator is an important and obviously preventable cause. In very hot climates, dehydration may contribute to the syndrome of heat exhaustion unless steps are taken to control the environmental temperature and to provide the infant with an adequate fluid intake. In severe brain damage or severe cerebral malformations such as hydrocephalus, hyperpyrexia may develop as a result of dysfunction of the temperature regulating centre. Hyperpyrexia may occur in severe neonatal infection and in association with convulsions is a grave prognostic sign. Hyperpyrexia is also common in acute attack of malaria, though the diagnosis of malaria is best with difficulties. There are no specific signs, though the combination of a stringing fever, palpable spleen, mild jaundice and mild anaemia may suggest malaria. The malarial parasitaemia is so common in endemic areas that its presence may mask the primary cause of acute symptoms, in particular meningitis, acute urinary tract infection, infective hepatitis or amoebic hepatitis amongst many others. A mild attack of malaria may precipitate severe relapse of an underlying disease such as crisis in thalassaemia or miliary tuberculosis.

The hyperpyrexia which accompanies many infections should excite concern only if the child has a previous history of convulsion is showing 'preconvulsive' sign of disorientation, jerkiness or twitching, or is uncomfortable because of his fever. In these circumstances, it may be wise to use phenobarbitone or possibly diazepam as a prophylactic measure against convulsions, and to try tepid sponging, sponging with alcohol, fanning, or wrapping in a wet sheet, all of which will lower the temperature by evaporation and surface cooling.

The indiscriminate prescribing of aspirin as an antipyretic is not without its dangers. If, as is likely, the urinary output is low, the kidneys may not excrete salicylate adequately and the blood level will be correspondingly raised. The stomach shares in the general hyperaemia and the risk of gastric erosion and blocking is increased. And, finally, the spurious effect on the temperature chart when aspirin is given sporadically can obscure the true cause of the illness. If aspirin is used as an adjunct to temperature control it is most sensible to give soluble aspirin, to accompany it with plentiful oral fluids, and not to prescribe more than three doses at 4 hourly intervals without reasoning the whole clinical picture. The 'febrile convulsions' represent a smaller proportion of convulsions in tropical paediatrics than they do in temperate climate, and the warning never to make this diagnosis without first proving CSF normal by lumbar puncture, is particularly important.

Hyperpyrexia often accompanies other manifestations of malarial infection such as convulsions or collapse. The febrile child becomes drowsy and lapses into coma with or without convulsions in 'cerebral malaria' associated with plasmodium falciparum parasitic infection. There is usually no meningisms and the cerebrospinal fluid may contain a few lymphocytes and slightly raised protein level, but may be perfectly normal. The blood film usually shows a heavy infection of P. falciparum unless prior chloroquine treatment is already well underway. Immediate and effective therapy may save the child, who slowly recovers consciousness over a period of a week but may be left partly brain damaged. At the terminal phase of a severe P. falciparum infection, there is a short period of hyperpyrexia, diarrhoea or vomiting followed by the clinical picture of collapse, hypovolumia, cold extremities and signs of shock.

In case of acute neurological syndrome parenteral antimalarial therapy is started immediately I.V. or I.M. or both. The convulsions must be controlled by I.V. diazepam 0.5 mg./kg. or I.M. injection of paraldehyde 0.1 mg./kg. Intramuscular phenobarbitone (5 mg./kg. upto 60 mg.) can be given at the same time as paraldehyde to maintain control. The hydration and nutrition must be maintained either by nasogastric tube or if vomiting is severe, by intravenous infusion. Care must be taken not to over transfuse or overload with sodium. It is important, if possible, to monitor the plasma electrolyte disturbances, hypoglycaemia and metabolic acidosis. The hyperpyrexia itself may also be a compound problem and the rectal temperature must be measured at intervals. If the child remains in coma over 24 hours despite clearing of P. Falciparum parasites, reduction of cerebral oedema by intravenous manitol infusion may be tried (20 ml. of 20% solution/kg. given rapidly). Intramuscular dexamethasone 10 mg. daily for three to four days and anticoagulant and fibrinolytic drugs such as streptokinase have no proven value; there is a definite risk of haemorrhage with heparin. Recovery, if occurs, is often slow and may be incomplete. A fever rising rapidly above 39°C. (102°C) or a single reading above 39.5°C ((103°F) measured rectally is an indication for tepid sponging. Covering the patient with a damp sheet next to a fan can replace sponging. Chlorpromazine (1-2 mg./kg. upto 20 mg.) or soluble aspirin (60 mg./year of age upto 300 mg.) dissolved in milk or glucose water is also helpful. The care must be taken not to let the temperature fall below normal, especially in infants. Once the antimalarial therapy has began to reduce the parasitaemia the swinging temperature will begin to subside.

ABDOMINAL EMERGENCIES

An acute abdominal pain is an emergency in newborn and childhood periods. There are various causes. It is not always to be sure that the infant has a pain because he cannot tell you exactly where he feels it. The mother can recognise crying which is due to pain rather than to her baby's anger or desire for company. The infant with pain in the abdomen cries, draws up his legs and clenches his feet, if pain is due to anal fissure he cries when passing stool and becomes constipated. The other child with pain tends to lie still and may go pale. The important causes of acute abdominal pain are enteritis, intussuception, appendicitis, mesenteric adenitis and strangulated inguinal hernia. Pyelitis may also cause pain, which in children can be diffused or rather

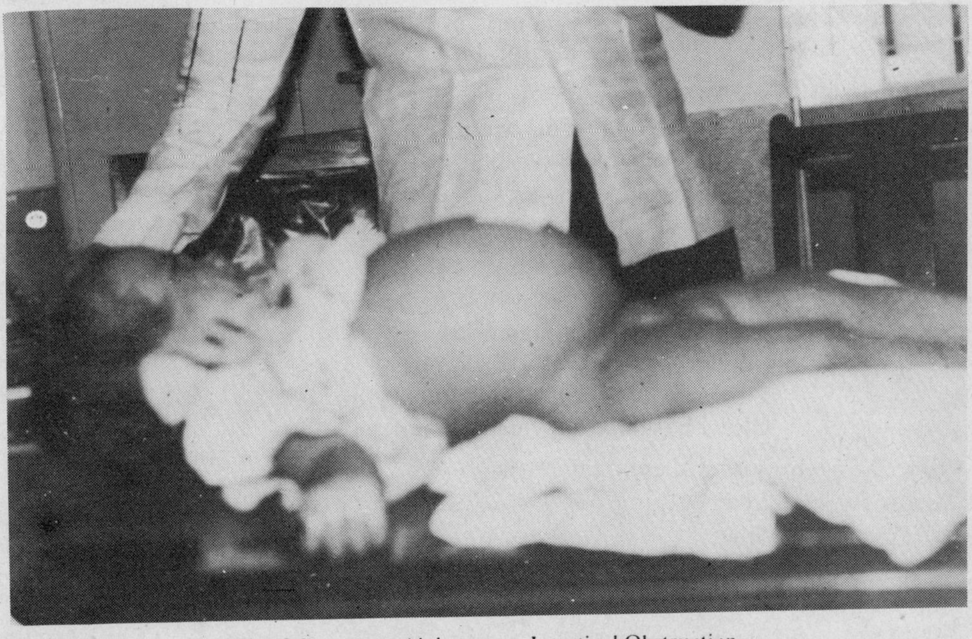

Fig.12.2 : Acute Abdomen — Intestinal Obstruction.

localised than in the loin. Diabetes with ketoacidosis for the first time might present as acute abdominal pain, pneumonia and anaphylactoid purpura may present with abdominal pain and are diagnosed from the general examination in all children with abdominal pain. Observation must be continued until a definite diagnosis is made or the pain subsides.

The aerophagia leading on to wind and colic is very common in between 2-3 months of age in most of the artificially fed babies. The babies may swallow large quantities of air for various reasons, they suck too hard, too fast or too long at breast or bottle. The child improves with proper technique of bottle feeding and burp up the swallowed air by patting on the back in up right position.

Sometimes with pylorospasm, it improves with an anti-cholinergic drug. The recurrent common abdominal pains of childhood are mostly due to emotional disturbances and are not due to organic disease. What is more, the list of organic causes does not include recurrent appendicitis but in our country it is very common with worms such as ascariasis. All the same, there is nothing to stop a child with emotional disturbances from getting infested with ascariasis and acute appendicitis, just like any other child. If this happens one should be alert to diagnose by finding out the differences in the pattern of the attack. By and large, recurrent abdominal pain follows a typical pattern. With an attack of acute appendicitis, the pattern is different, so as with ascariasis, often history of passing worms in the past. The diagnosis of various organic causes should be assessed during an attack, on the spot.

The abdominal distension in the younger infants and children sometimes possess a great threat to the clinicians as an acute emergency. The important causes are enumerated below :-

1. Acute or Subacute :

   (a) Intestinal obstruction

   (b) Peritonitis

   (c) Ascitis : The commonest causes are malnutrition, nephrosis, tuberculosis, peritonitis and cirrhosis.

2. Recurrent :

   (a) Air swallowing : This occurs in infants with crying or violent sucking. It occurs also in older children with crying or emotional disturbances.

   (b) Constipation : If severe, acquired or congenital megacolon (Hirschsprung disease).

3. Subacute or Chronic :

   (a) Malabsorption.
   Malnutrition with diarrhoea.
   Coeliac disease.
   Fibrocystic disease of pancreas.
   Disaccharidase enzyme deficiency.

   (b) Visceral enlargement :
   Liver
   Spleen
   Kidney
   Bladder — distended.

   (c) Tumour or cyst.

EXCESSIVE CRYING

The crying is an expressive effort of a baby mostly in the newborn and later childhood periods. The 'wind colic' due to aerophagia is a very important cause of excessive crying in the newborn and also upto 3-4 months of age. The anal fissure mostly associated with artificial feeding and constipated stools, is also an important cause of excessive crying. The so-called 'ear ache' mostly complained is a sudden cause of excessive crying at night but there are other to be also sought for. And it is dangerous to put warm oil drops in the ears, thinking it will allay the ear ache, sometimes produces otitis externa to extend further inside and causing inflammation of tympanic membrane and extension of infection into the middle ears. Sudden insect bite, specially 'Scorpion', among infants and toddler age group is also a very important cause of excessive crying. The 'temper tantrum' in a pampered child in the age group of 9 months to one year is also a very important cause of excessive crying. The crying with screaming attack, where the baby draws up his legs and clenches the fists, should be differentiated from an organic and more vulnerable cry due to intra-abdominal emergencies by finding out associated pallor on the face from flushed and red face due to scream.

RETENTION VS. SUPPRESSION OF URINE

A careful history and general examination should be taken including details of passage of urine and meconium just after birth. One should be worried more due to no meconium passed after 24 hours instead of no urine. Because imperforate anus is much more important emergency after the birth. Moreover, only inspection of the anus may not be convincing of patent anus, instead thermometre test to detect out the patency of anus is needed. The stream of urine and bladder palpable in the abdomen are the two important signs to detect retention of urine with bladder neck obstruction. Mere presence of phimosis in case of male body is not very significant even upto the age of 5 years. The prepuce remains firmly adherent with the glans and this is physiological. Moreover, if it is associated with recurrent attack of balanitis and ascending urinary infection and more so with 'Pin hole' meatus, one should slit up the prepucial skin to look for meatal opening and then timely circumcision to be done. The obstructive uropathy with bladder neck obstruction leads to recurrent infection, renal failure and stunting of growth. The surgical correction early will be very much beneficial for relieving the obstruction, persistent infection with or without azotaemia, hypertension, hydronephrosis, etc. The screaming attack after a meatal ulcer in a male baby with napkin rash might present with retention and paediatric emergency.

References :

1. Williams, D.E. (1974) : Urology in childhood. In Encyclopaedia of Urology. Vol.15, Berlin, Springer.
2. Stanfield, I.P. (1969) : British Med. Journal, 1, 761.

CHAPTER – THIRTEEN

HAEMATOLOGY

Haemorrhagic disorders :

The clinical and haematologic picture of haemorrhage depends on the amount of loss, the rate of loss and the haemostatic adjustment after the loss. But these factors are modified in haemorrhagic disorders in the newborn period due to relative deficiency of coagulative factors except the factors I, V, VIII and also inadequate response of the bone marrow to release platelets which are normally reduced in the newborn period. The low birth weight babies specially the preterm has added hazards of increased vascular permeability and inability to effectively utilise vitamin K for synthesis of coagulation factors.

Perinatal causes of bleeding :

1. **Foetal haemorrhage :**

The bleeding may occur in a few. These are twin-to-twin transfusion, foeto-maternal haemorrhage, ante-partum haemorrhage from foetal aspect of placenta, administration of anti coagulants to mother, also taking of aspirin in the antental period.

2. **Intranatal :**

The maternal causes, such as accidental incision of placenta during caesarean section, application of ventouse on foetal scalp, may lead to subaponeurotic haemorrhage, subcapsular haemorrhage of liver due to assisted breach delivery, bad application of forceps leading to fracture of the base of the skull and fracture of the vault mainly fissure type because depressed fractures are less common. The symptoms are those of intracranial haemorrhage. Moreover bleeding may occur into the meninges, into cerebral substances, into the ventricular system and also under the pericranium, cephal haematoma in subdural space leading to subdural haematoma, which might not

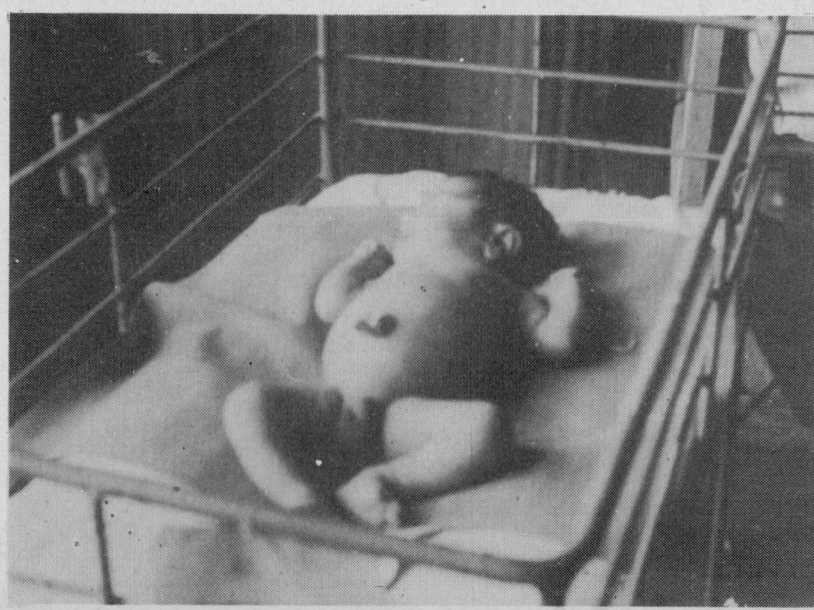

Fig 13.1 : Hypoprothrombinemic bleeding

be diagnosed initially. The condition is usually bilateral, following a subdural haemorrhage, the symptoms of a space occupying lesion develop, often after a delayed interval.

3. Neonatal haemorrhage :

The causes are defective coagulation leading on to the haemorrhagic disease of the newborn. It is characterised by haemorrhagic manifestation after 48 hours of birth upto the end of first week of life due to transient deficiency of prothrombine (factor II), also other coagulation factors might be deficient such as factor VII, IX and X. It is common in breast fed babies, more common in preterms due to inadequate intestinal flora, non-absorption of Vitamin K from the gut and also liver immaturity preventing transformation of Vitamin K to prothrombin. Bleeding occurs from gastrointestinal tract, umbilical cord, circumscision site, nose, sub aponeurotic bleeding under the scalp, subcapsular haemorrhage of liver and internal haemorrhage. The response to Vitamin K, 0.5 to 1.0 mg. I.M. is dramatic. The other neonatal causes are the hepatic insufficiency due to liver damage in hepatitis, anoxia, hypoxia, immaturity, metabolic disorders, such as galactosaemia, fructosaemia and unconjugated hyper-bilirubinaemia due to A.B.O, Rh. iso-immunization, leading to deficiency of coagulative factors, which are manufactured in liver. The hepatic causes are associated with clinical jaundice in the newborn period. Very rarely there are some inherited deficiency of coagulative factors, Haemophilia (AHG), Christmas disease (PTC or factor IX), and afibroginaemia may lead to neonatal bleeding. The maternal medications in the antenatal period specially the anti-coagulation drugs, aspirin, salicylate, barbiturates and thiazides those deplete away Vitamin K dependent coagulation factors may lead to bleeding in the neonatal period.

Then comes the deficiency of qualitative defects of platelets. It is already pointed out that definition-wise the thrombocytopenia in the new born is, if the platelet count is below 100,000 per cmm. The various causes are passively transfused from the mother as immune disorders such as idiopathic thrombocytopenic purpura and systemic thrombocytopenia -- sulfonamides, sedormid, quinine and quinidine when taken by pregnant women, they are tagged with platelets and act as an antigenic complex. Platelets antibodies from mother suffering from ITP, platelet iso-immunization like RH and ABO isoimmunisation. Intrauterine infections like rubella, cytomegalic, toxoplasma and syphilis may depress the activity of megakaryocytes in the bone marrow so that platelet deficiency and also damaging the liver cause coagulative factor inadequacy. Hence hereditary disorders like Wiskott Aldrich syndrome, a sex linked recessive disorder may present in the newborn period as thrombocytopenia besides presence of infantile eczema, recurrent viral and bacterial infections and thrombocytopenia. Hypoplasia or aplasia of bone marrow may be associated with congenial absence of radie or deformity in association with a megakaryocytic thrombocytopenia or as congenital pancytopenia. In some there are sequestration of platelets leading to thrombocytopenia in association with giant haemangioma, renal vein thrombosis and cyanotic congenital heart disease. The bleeding in preterm specially pulmonary haemorrhage on 3rd day after birth in presence of respiratory infection, is mainly due to disseminated intravascular coagulation (DIC). The bleeding in the neonatal period may be due to vascular defects specially in preterm babies with fragile vascular walls leading to bleeding from gastric vessels, intracranial vessels in presence of anoxia and hypercapnia.

The bleeding might also results from local or traumatic causes. These are from umbilical cord due to slipped ligature or laceration of the cord during delivery. Bleeding from the presenting part due to extreme degree of laceration, more of bruising type and ecchymosis or petichae in nature or may be more as in cephalhaematoma. Bleeding might result from stiff suction catheter, tubes, rectal thermometer, subconjunctival haemorrhage, may have retinal haemorrhage. Gastrointestinal bleeding as haematemesis or malena may have to be differentiated from maternal swallowed blood in case of antepartum bleeding by 'APT test'.

The Purpuras :

The pin point haemorrhage in the skin is known as purpura, it is an extra-vascular blood, to be differentiated from urticaria or wheal, which can be bleached, no change of colour as seen in purpura from pinkish, bluish and then yellowish black, takes time to fade away completely. This is a sign of many childhood disorders which can be of

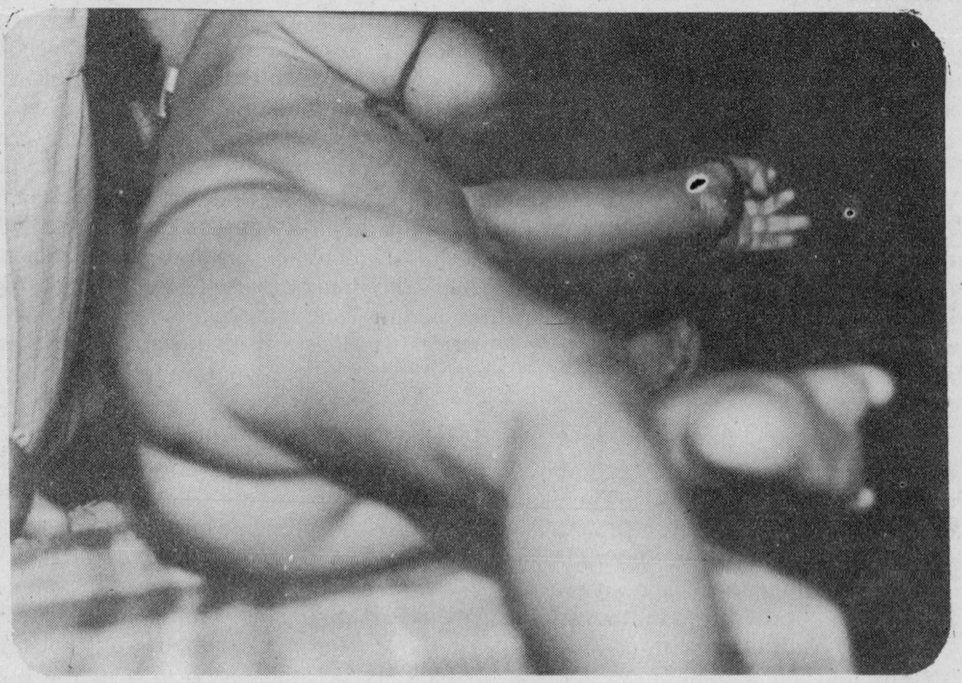

Fig.13.2 : Purpura, Pallor, Hepatospleenomegaly (Leukaemia)

two types, those are of platelet origin and those of capillary origin. This sign also helps the clinician to diagnose certain disease condition like idiopathic thrombocytopenic purpura or anaphylactoid purpura with peculiar distribution in children. The clinical and family history will help to diagnose some congenital bleeding disorders which might have platelet deficiency on-coagulation deficiency such as haemophilia. However, any bleeding disorder should be investigated with the peripheral blood film, platelet count and determination of bleeding and clotting time. Hess's tourniquet test is positive in defective haemostasis due to fragile capillary. The bleeding time is indicative of capillary contractibility and the clotting time of the integrity of the coagulation mechanisms of the blood, but both these tests have some falacies, so they should not be relied on for screening purpose. The clot retraction can be measured and is thought to reflect platelet function. The various other coagulation tests such as estimation of protbrombin time (Quick's method or thrombo-test) and fibrinogen levels should help to pin point the defects encountered in a bleeding child.

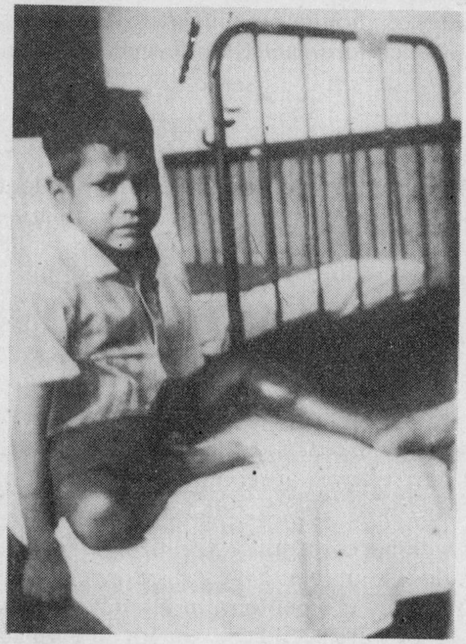

Fig.13.3(a) : Haemophilia — Haemarthrosis (Knee joint)

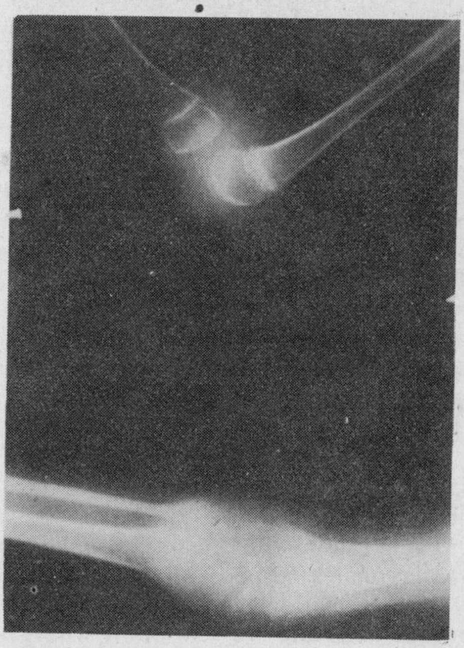

Fig.13.3(b) : Haemophilia — Haemarthrosis (Radiological findings)

Causes of purpura in elderly children :

(i) Idiopathic thrombocytopenic purpura with or without defect of megakaryocytes in the bone marrow,

(ii) Neonatal thrombocytopenic purpura (already described),

(iii) Wiskott-Aldrich syndrome,

(iv) Thrombotic thrombocytopenic purpura,

(v) Hyperspleenism factor,

(vi) Bone marrow depression by various physical or chemical agents including drugs like chloramphenicol and aspirin. The non-thrombocytopenic purpuras are :

(1) Hereditary thrombasthenia,,

(2) Henoch-Schonlein syndrome (anaphylactoid purpura),

(3) Ehler-Danlos syndrome (Cutis hyperelastica)

(4) Hereditary capillary purpura (Von Willebrand's),

(5) and other vascular purpuras such as scurvy, infection due to viral, rickettsial and bacterial diseases, snake venoms, drugs, asphyxia, septicaemia, bacterial endocarditis, mechanical trauma etc.

OBSERVATION OF 50 CASES OF PURPURA IN CHILDHOOD

Introduction :

Purpura is one of the commonest manifestations of various important diseases in childhood. Different works were done about different diseases causing purpura in children individually, but a series of all cases of purpura in this age group in general is infrequent. Cosic et al discussed the aetiology, pathogenesis and differentiation of purpura in children. The present work was undertaken with a view to find out the common responsible factors which every one of us should think in day to day practice with special reference to different age groups of children and in difference in sex and mortality figures.

Material and methods :

This study was undertaken in patients admitted in paed atric indoor of Calcutta National Medical College and Hospital for a period of last 5 years. These patients were admitted with various disease processes and purpura was observed in them during examination or on follow up, but in some cases purpura was the only presentation. In most of the cases, investigations were done according to availability and with special reference to determine the probable causes.

Results and observations :

Six thousand and five hundred patients were admitted in paediatric indoor in this centre for last 5 years. But only 50 cases of purpura was observed among them (0.76 percent).

Table I shows the age and sex incidences in the present study. Out of total 50 cases, 31 were males (62 percent) and 19 were females (38 percent). 8 cases of purpura were seen in neonatal age group, 6 cases were observed (12 percent) in infancy, 14 cases between 2nd and 3rd year of life whereas 5 cases were seen between 4th and 5th year of life, seventeen cases (34 percent) were observed from 6th to the end of 12th year of life. The sex difference was noticed particularly in males in all age groups, but both the sexes were equally affected between 2nd and 3rd year of life.

Table II shows different causes of purpura in the present series with respective mortality rates. Out of 50 patients, 21 (42 percent) expired in this series.

Purpura was observed in 5 cases of acute leukaemia, the commonest type of leukaemia encountered in children, 4 of them were in acute lymphoblastic stage and all expired. Eight cases of purpura in this series were due to Kwashiorkor, in which it is one common skin manifestation, only one of this group died due to severe malnutrition, with diarrhoea and gross electrolyte imbalance leading to heart failure.

Idiopathic thromobocytopenic purpura (ITP) was noticed in 5 patients, all of them showed platelet count ranging from 25000 to 40000/cmm. Schonlein Henoch's purpura was diagnosed in 2 cases only, where platelet count was unaltered. In one of these 2, associated with acute nephritis as a complication was encountered. Three cases of purpura were due to haemolytic anaemia, in 2 of which Hb.EF thalassemia was proved and another was a case of congenital spherocytosis. Vitamin C deficiency causing scurvy was diagnosed in a single case.

Septicaemia was seen in 4 cases of neonatal group and in 5 cases during infancy. Two out of 5 cases in infancy of haematogenous dissemination leading to miliary tuberculosis were noticed. Pyogenic meningitis was seen in a single patient. Total 5 died in this group.

Haemorrhagic measles were the responsible disease in 3 cases, systemic lupus erythematosus (SIE) was diagnosed in a patient with characteristic facial butterfly skin rash and presence of LE cells in blood.

Table — I

Age and sex incidences in the cases of purpura in childhood in the present study

Sex	Age Group 0-1 month	2nd-12th months	2nd-3rd years	4th-5th year	6th-12th year	Total
Male	5	4	7	4	11	31
Female	3	2	7	1	6	19
Total	8	6	14	5	17	50

Table - II

Different causes of purpura in childhood with mortality in the present study

Sl. No.	Cause of purpura	No. of cases (with %)	Mortality
1.	Acute leukaemia	5(10%)	4
2.	Nutritional	8 (10%)	1
3.	Idiopathic thrombocytopenic purpura	5 (10%)	
4.	Anaphylactoid purpura	2 (4%)	
5.	Scurvy	1 (2%)	
6.	Haemolytic anaemia	3 (6%)	1
7.	Haemolytic uraemic syndrome	1 (2%)	
8.	Liver disorder	4 (8%)	4
9.	Drug induced	2 (4%)	2
10.	Septicaemia	5 (10%)	3
	Pyogenic meningitis		
	Miliary tuberculosis		
11.	Viral fever (measles)	3 (6%)	
12.	Systemic lupus erythematosus	1 (2%)	
13.	Haemophilia and Christmas disease	2 (3%)	
14.	Neonatal	8 (16%)	4
	(a) Septicaemia 4		
	(b) DIC 2		2
	(c) Jaundice 2		
	Total	50	21 (42%)

In 4 out of 50 cases of purpura was seen in patients with hepatic coma and all of them died.

One interesting case of haemolytic uraemic syndrome was encountered in this series in a male child of 2 years old. The patient presented with marked pallor, scanty urination and multiple purpuric spots following an attack of acute gastroenteritis. Icterus was seen 2 days prior to admission. On investigation haemoglobin was 4.2 g. percent, reticulocyte count 9 percent, serum bilirubin 2.8 mg./dl., urine showed albuminurea, plenty of red cells with RBC cast in microscopic examination and platelet count was 38000/cmm. The child improved with countinued treatment with heparin, corticosteroid and fluid therapy.

Two cases of drug induced purpura were noticed , Stevens Johnson's Syndrome was thought in one case of 9 months old patient who was diagnosed radiologically and clinically as a case of primary complex and receiving isoniazide. The second patient was also receiving antituberculous therapy with rifampicin and isoniazide.

Apart from 4 cases of septicaemia in newborn, causes of other 4 cases of purpura were disseminated intravascular coagulopathy in 2 and jaundice in other 2 in newborn, though full investigations were not possible.

ANAEMIA

In foetal life, blood formation takes place in extra meduallary centres like liver, spleen, kidneys and some parts of the reticulo endothelial system including lvmph glands and also in the medullary cortex of bone marrow. At term these extra medullary centres have decreased and the medullary centres in the bone marrow takes up the major portion of blood cells formation not only the erythrocytes but also the granulocytes and platelets. At birth, the marrows are 'red' but gradually they become 'yellow' due to replacement of fatty tissue and the haemopoiesis is confined to limited places like the flat bones, of the skull and pelvis, end of the long bones and vertebrae. Where the remnant of marrows left but during periods of emergency the inactive marrows are restored to compensate the extra burden might have to be taken due to blood loss or destruction of red blood cells for effective erythopoiesis. The haemoglobin of foetal life differs from the haemoglobin of adult life and they are alphabetically represented as HbF and HbA. These differences are due mainly due to composition of the two pairs of polypeptide chain which makes up its globin fraction besides the haem in haemoglobin molecule which is the iron fraction. These haemoglobin F and A are normal haemoglobins both in foetal and adult life respectively and foetal haemoglobin changes to adult haemoglobin after 5-6 months of postnatal life, only about 2% of this adult haemoglobin may remain as A_2 throughout the rest of the life. Besides, these normal haemoglobins such as F, A and A_2 , there are some abnormal haemoglobins represented by alphabetical words such as C D E and S. Since these are dominantly inherited qualities it is not surprising that

FIG. 1

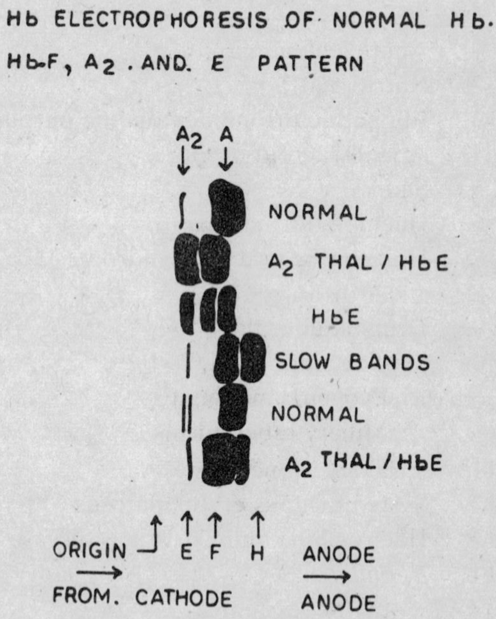

Fig.13.4 : Hb, electrophoresis of Normal Hb.

haemoglobins are double represented (homozygous) AA Moreover, the presence of a single abnormal allele is said to be represented as trait (heterozygous) for example, AS — the carrier of sickle cell trait, whereas the disease process is designated as SS. In many of these conditions in which the normal formation of haemoglobin A has been suppressed. There is a perisistence of Hb.F after the newborn period as for example in thalassaemias.

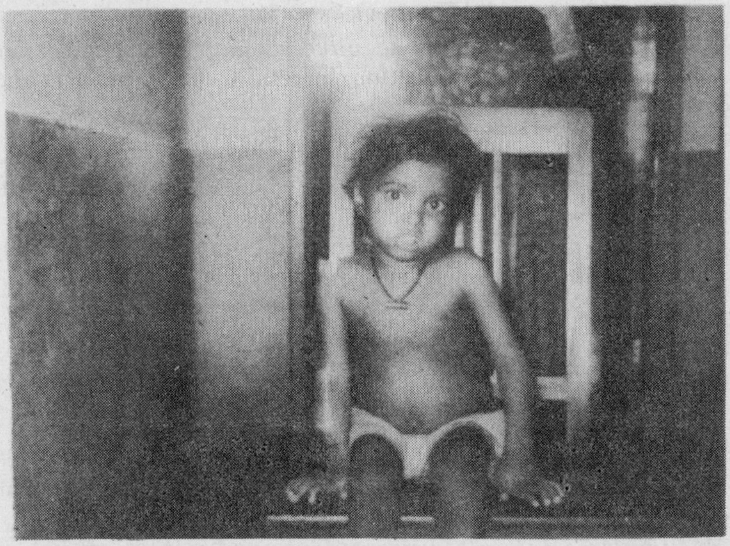

Fig.13.5(a) : Hb EF Thalassaemia

Anaemia in infancy and childhood :

When the haemoglobin concentration of an infant is less than normal level, he is considered anaemic. It has been recommended that haemoglobin levels below 11 gm/100 ml. in the infant of 6 months to children below 6 years old and levels below 12 gm/100 ml. in the older children is indication of anaemia.

Classification of anaemias :

The morphologic classification is done according to cell size and haemoglobin concentration such as —

A. Hypochromic anaemia :

(i) Iron deficiency anaemia —
during infancy — Nutritional, post haemorrhagic and in older children — Post haemorrhagic and nutritional.

(ii) Ineffective erythropoiesis — Thalassemia, pyridoxine dependant anaemia or refractory to pyridoxine, lead poisoning.

B. Normocytic normochromic anaemia :

(i) Impaired red cell production (inactive bone marrow, reticulocytes low count), physiologic anaemia of infancy, after infection, chronic renal and liver disease, hypothyroidism, pure red cell aplasia, aplastic anaemia (hereditary, idiopathic, toxic agents — physical, chemical including drugs — chloramphenicol, sulpha and nitrofurantion, infections) collagen disorders and myeloproliferative disorders.

(ii) Haemolysis — (Hypercellular bone marrow, reticulocyte count high) :

(a) Defect in RBC'S — Hereditary red cell in enzyme deficiencies, G6PD, pyruvate and mutase deficiencies, hereditary spherocytosis, haemoglobinopathies such as sickle cell and abnormal haemoglobin as C,D,E etc., paroxysmal nocturnal haemoglobinuria.

(b) Extra corpuscular defects, acquired haemolytic anaemia, anaemia due to Rh. and ABO iso-immunization, infections due to malaria and kala-azar,

C. Macrocytic anaemia :

(i) Megaloblastic erythopoiesis in bone marrow

(a) Nutritional, Vitamin B_{12} deficiency, folate deficiency in protein calorie malnutrition.

(b) Toxic — Therapy with antifolic acid compound such as methotrexate therapy with anti-convulsants — phenytoin, malabsorption, cirrhosis of liver.

(ii) Non-megaloblastic erythopoiesis— chronic haemolytic anaemia.

The aetiologic classification :

1. Anaemia in newborn :
2. Anaemia in early infancy :

   Iron deficiency anaemia, prolong breast feeding, malnutrition and malabsorption, defective absorption and diminished store of iron in preterm babies, inadequate iron in physiologic anaemia, increased demand in preterm babies, defective metabolism of iron in deficiency disease such as ricket, scurvy, hypothyroidism.
3. Megaloblastic anaemia of infancy :

   Vitamin B_{12} and folic acid deficiency.
4. Aplastic anaemia :

   Congenital type and acquired.
5. Haemolytic anaemia :

   Heriditary spherocytosis, Thalassaemias.

THALASSAEMIA

Introduction :

Thalassaemia syndromes are a heterogenous group of hereditary disorders of haemoglobin synthesis. The patients show a variable degree of hypochromic anaemia with evidences of haemolysis and ineffective erythropoiesis. In 1949, Pauling made the fundamental discovery that erythropoiesis of patients with sicke cell anaemia contain a haemoglobin with an isoelectric point which is significantly different from that of normal individuals. This provided the first depositive evidence that many adult human haemoglobins exist in more than one molecular form and it complied for the first time that many hereditary diseases of biochemical nature may be caused by genetically determined abnormalities of protein synthesis. Since then many examples of abnormal haemoglobins have been described. The incidence of abnormal haemoglobinopathies in India have been mostly described from Bengal, Punjab, Assam, Nagpur and Andhra Pradesh. The first case of thalassaemia major was reported by Mukherjee (1938) in a 2½ years old Bengalee boy from Calcutta. Broadly speaking, the thalassaemia could be due to suppression of alpha chains (alpha thalassaemia) or beta chains (beta thalassaemia). The latter is much more common in India and all over the world. In a heterozygous state, it presents as thalassaemia trait and in homozygous state, it presents as thalassaemia major. Within each clinical variant varying grades of severity are observed mentioned by O.P. Ghai et al (1980)[9]. On the basis of the amount of β -chain produced, many genes of thalassaemia such a B+-thalassaemia, B°-thalassaemia and B?-thalassaemia have been proposed[9]. In the Negroes, homozygous betathalassaemia has a relatively benign course and mild anaemia. In the Greeks, on the other hand, beta-thalassaemia runs a severe course and in the Mediterranean region considerable variation in severity is found. In the Indian population beta-thalassaemia has been reported from all parts of the country and the homozygotes generally run a severe course. In homozygotes of B°-thalassaemia, no B-chain synthesis is found, whereas in B+-thalassaemia, some B-chain synthesis can be demonstrated in the reticulocytes in vitro studies, though it is much more reduced than alpha chain synthesis (O.P. Ghai loc cit). Presumptive diagnosis of B°-thalassemia or B?thalassaemia can be made, on the basis of accurate estimation of HbA, HbF, HbE, HbA_2 amd also comprehensive family studies with the parents and the siblings of HbE thalassaemia, which is the commonest thalassaemia in Bengal (Chatterjee et al, 1956)[11]. Though for confirmation studies of globin chain synthesis should be done. In the absence of structural changes in haemoglobin and any method of directly analysing gene structure in man, the precise nature of fundamental defects and the distinction between different mutations which produce similar results is very difficult to define and often impossible (Weiseman et al, 1974)[12]. Alpha and delta-beta thalassaemia are rare in India and a few cases have been reported.

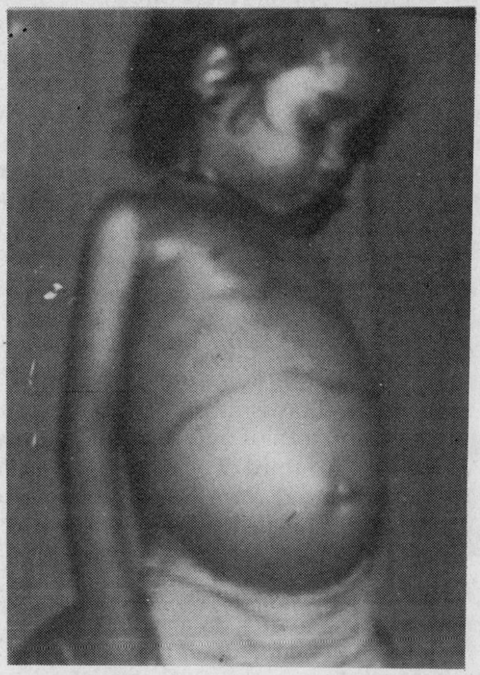

Fig.13.5(b) : Thalassaemia Major

Thalassaemia occurs world wide with an incidence of 0.01 to 11 percent in various ethnic-geographic groups[7]. In a randomly matting population, one would expect that births of subjects with homozygous beta-thalassaemia would occur at a rate of 0.25 times the square of the incidences of thalassaemia trait in the population. Thus in a population with 10% incidence of beta-thalassaemia trait, such as occurs in parts of Greece and Italy, one might expect that one fourth of 1 percent of newborns would inherit homozygous beta thalassaemia. It is usually believed that the disease was spread to the rest of the world from Mediterranean regions by the Greek traders but Lehman et al (1966)[8] feel that thalassaemia is the commonest haemoglobinopathy in Asia and should no longer be regarded as having originated in the Mediterranean region. It has been shown to be the commonest haemoglobinopathy in India[7].

Materials and Methods :

The clinical material comprised 50 cases of thalassaemia syndromes including homozygous B-thalassaemia, heterozygous thalassaemias — thalassemia trait and

HbE trait, double heterozygous like thalassaemia HbE disease. Twenty three cases of thalassaemia major and thirteen cases of thalassaemia HbE disease admitted in the Paediatrics Ward for the last three years were the main study group. The detailed family studies were done in eight families and fourteen siblings of the patients were also included in this study, which were mainly of thalassaemia trait and HbE trait. Four cases had splenectomy during this study period and also followed up after splenectomy. Among them three were thalassaemia HbE diseases and one of thalassemia major with severe protracted clinical histories, where too many transfusions were needed in the past. The severity of the disease was assessed using arbitary criteria with regard to physical growth, bony changes, hepatosplenomegaly, requirement of blood transfusions and degree of anaemia. Investigations were performed either before blood transfusions or at least four months after the last transfusion. Those splenectomized four cases were also investigated before and after splenectomy. The haematological investigations included determination of haemoglobin concentration (cyanmethaemoglobin), red cell counts (haemocytometer technique), reticulocyte count (new methylene blue) examination of a stained peripheral blood smear, staining of red cells to have an idea of counting nucleated red cells. The quantitation of HbF, HbA_2 and HbE were done by cellulose acetate elution method of Marengo-Rowe (1965)[14] screening electrophoresis for abnormal haemoglobins on cellulose acetate strip using discontinuous buffer. The age of the patients studied varied from 3 months to 12 years. This is mostly a random study, sex distribution male : female 4:3, they included children of different community settled in eastern region of India, mostly in Calcutta. Two-third of children were from Bengalee parents and some families mostly Hindus migrated from East Pakistan, now known as Bangladesh (hilly districts of Chittagong, Shillet, Kumilla, where there was prevalence of HbE trait.)

In less severly affected cases, besides pallor, irritability, fatiguability, low grade fever, listlessness and anorexia, the hepatosplenomegaly is an early sign of thalassaemic patients. The liver is enlarged early in the disease process. In fact, in two children of thalassaemia major, aged 15 months and 9 months respectively, moderately enlarged liver without palpability of the spleen but osseous changes in the way of skull bone changes were detected early. Hepatomegaly is the result of Kupffer cell hyperplasia and fibrosis stimulated by excess iron, on and off infections of bacterial and viral origin and also too many blood transfusions, more haemolysis, more iron deposition in hepatocytes leading on to cell reaction, burden of extramedullary erythopoiesis and also anaemic congestive cardiac failure, all together or sometimes singly might over burden the functions of liver and causes more hepatic damage in paripassu with spleen and bone marrow (Iancu et al. 1977)[1]. To determine the early parenchymal involvement of liver in thalassaemias besides histomorphologic studies, no suitable biochemical parameters were helpful in the past. Kattemis et al. (1977)[2] in Greece, was of the opinion to suggest serum cholinesterase (ACAH or CHE) estimation in liver parenchymatous involvement and they claimed, (ACAH) levels seems to be a sensitive index of liver impairment in thalassaemia compared with other liver function tests. Cholinesterase is an L_2-globulin synthesised in the liver. In serum, it hydrolyses acetyl choline and a variety of other esters. Because of its lack of specificity and in order to distinguish it from true cholinesterase of erythrocytic and other tissues, it is sometimes referred to as pseudocholinesterase. Serum activity of ACAH, now known as CHE (EC 3,1,1,8) varies in relation to the levels of hepatic protein synthesis. Accordingly, depressed values have been reported in malnutrition and also in the acute phase of venoocclusive disease of the liver, where they are of some prognostic value (Stuart and Bras, 1957)[10]. In disorders where hepatocellular function is abnormal, low values are characteristically present. As a prognostic index, a persistantly low level is often present in decompensated cirrhosis, thalassaemic involvement of liver, where there is deposition of pigment leading on to cell necrosis, fibrosis and cirrhosis.

The present study reports haematological picture, serum cholinesterase values with other liver functions tests and correlation wih histological changes in 50 cases of thalassaemias with mild, moderate and severely affected children to establish a correlation between the haematological picture with quantitation of abnormal haemoglobin, with presentation in the earlier age, complicated with other infection and infestations in our tropical and sub-tropical climates and also detected for the first time in elderly age group to study the clinical severity in relation to prognosis specially those cases where liver parenchyma involvement is present. The liver biopsy is also helpful in determining

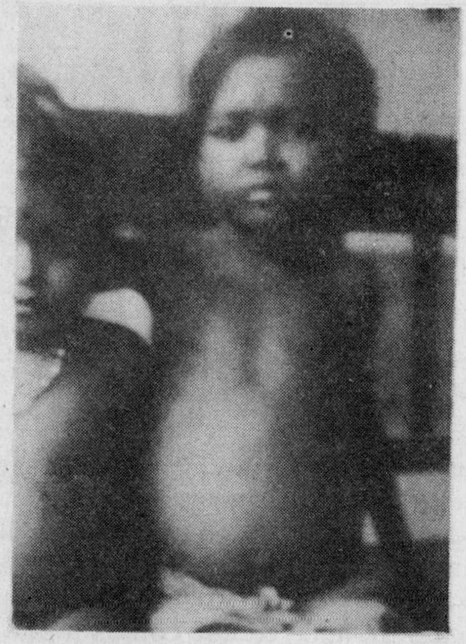

Fig.13.6(a)

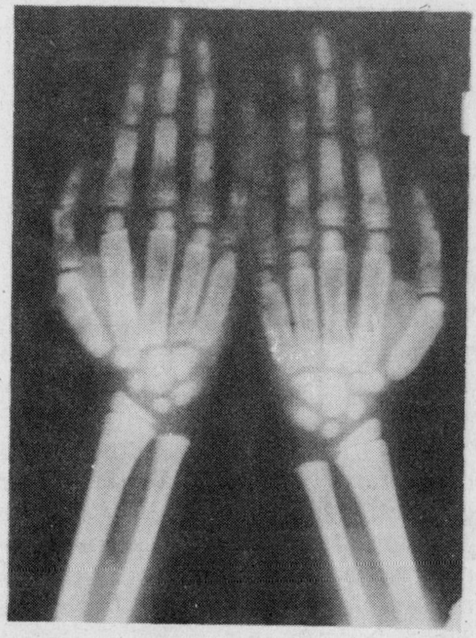

Fig.13.6(b)

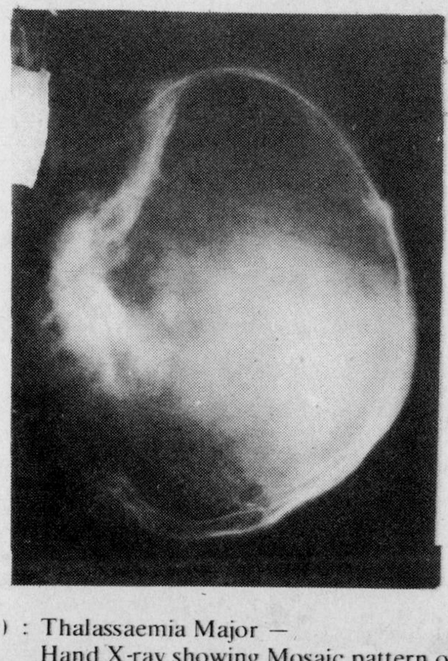

Fig.13.6(a),(b),(c) : Thalassaemia Major —
Hand X-ray showing Mosaic pattern on bones
Skull X-ray showing Hair on end appearance.

the degree of iron overload and hepatic fibrosis in B-thalassaemia major (Bary et al, 1974)[4]. Serum cholinesterase values and liver biopsy were done in all the 50 cases. Serum cholinesterase was estimated by the method suggested by La Hnegra, Yesnick and Poppar (1952)[15]. In 50 study cases and compared with age and sex matched with 25 control cases, as far as practicable, they were free from any hepatomegaly, malnutrition of gross degree, anaemia and also did not suffer from any acute infection within six weeks during the sample collection time.

Observations :

Table — 1.

Showing age and type in distribution of thalassaemia cases.

	Types of Thalassaemias				
Age	Thal.major	Thal.HbE	Thal.minor	HbE trait	Total
0 to 1 year	3	2	—	—	5
1 to 3 years	5	3	2	1	11
3 to 6 years	5	3	3	1	12
6 to 9 years	5	3	3	—	11
9 to 12 years	5	2	3	1	11
Total	23	13	11	3	50

From Table 1, it is evident that among 50 cases 23 (46%) comprised of thalassaemia major (homozygous B-thalassaemia) and double heterozygous in thalassaemia HbE disease 13 (26%). Incidence of HbE both in double heterozygous and E trait is less common 34%,than B-thalassaemia both major and minor together i.e., 66%. Most of the cases has severe anaemia, haemoglobin values raning from 3.2 to 9 G/dl. with a mean SD of 5.7 ± 1.8 G/dl. (Table 2). Haematocrit and red cell counts followed a similar pattern.

Table — 2

Haematological findings in 50 cases of thalassaemia syndromes.

	Range	Mean and S.D.
Hb (G/dl.)	3.2 — 9	5.7 ± 1.8
R.B.C. (X 10^{12} l^{-1})	1.7 — 2.69	2.2 ± 0.75
Normoblasts per 100 W.B.C.	20 — 50	37.0 ± 12.1
Reticulocyte percentage	3 — 12	6.2 ± 0.06
HBF	12 — 91	44.1 ± 16.4
HbA_2	4 — 6.5	5.5 ± 0.8
HbE	18 — 60	42.1 ± 11.9

Haemoglobin concentration was less than 6 gm./dl. or less in 60%, over one-third cases had less than 4 gm./dl. Peripheral smears showed marked hypochromia, microcytosis, severe anisopoikilocytosis, polychromasia, basophilic stippling, targetemia and normoblastimia. Varying degree of normoblastimia was present. The normoblast ranged from an occasional 1 to 5 per 100 W.B.C. Reticulocytes were elevated practically in all cases. Reticulocyte count ranged from minimum 3 percent to maximum 12%. HbF varied from 12-91%, with a mean of 44.1 ± 16.4. In fiftyfour percent of cases HbF varied from 40 — 70%. It was more than 80% in only 3 (17 percent). In one case it was 12 percent only. The percentage of HbF or its concentration showed no correlation with the age of presentation or with the clinical severity of the disease or the total level of haemoglobin present. HbA_2 varied from 4-6.6%, HbA_2 mostly elevated in thalassaemia traits. In these cases where A_2 elevated, the HbF remained less than 20 percent on an average, no correlation between HbF and HbA_2 levels could be established in the heterozygotes. For example a thalassaemia major with Hb. electrophoresis AF with 39 percent foetal haemoglobin and both the parents with slight A_2 elevation, had presence of foetal haemoglobin 6 percent in the mother and 9 percent in the father. First born, only child, no history of previous abortions or miscarriages, diagnosed at 5 months of age without palpable spleen but osseous changes showing facial changes and needed more than 8 transfusions with 10 months after diagnosis.

Thalassaemia HbE disease where E varied from 18-60% and the rest is F. The clinical severity is like thalassaemia major. In one family one male and one female among 4 children, develops clinical severity, the male child presented at the age of 4 years and subsequent investigations of whole family was done[16]. The father was HbE trait and the mother was thalassaemia trait. The rest two where the eldest daughter was HbE trait and the youngest was thalassaemia trait proved by haemoglobin electrophoresis. Both the patients had splenectomy after too many blood transfusions. The baby is still stunted in growth but not having so frequent transfusions. The girl died after one year of splenectomy, attacked with meningitis. There were 3 cases of HbE traits. It was also diagnosed by electrophoresis, showing AE pattern with more A than E.

The clinical presentation was like thalassaemia minor and the anaemia was resistant to iron therapy. But all the E conditions cause reduced erythrocyte osmotic fragility.

In 50 cases, the liver function tests i.e., albumin globulin ratio, serum bilirubin level, alkaline phosphatase and S.G.P.T. were done with serum cholinesterase estimation. The controls were done from age and sex matched 25 normal children. Table 3 shows serum cholinesterase values in normal controls and in case of thalassaemia. Normal values were found as 4.93 IU/ml. (mean) and in thalassaemia, the mean value was 2.86 ± 0.82.

Table — 3

Showing cholinesterase values in control & study group.

		Serum ACAH values IU/ml.		
		Minimum	Maximum	Mean
Control	25	2.5	5.8	4.1 ± 0.9
Thalassaemia Syndromes	50	1.5	5.6	2.86 ± 0.82*

B-Thalassaemia major	23	1.5	3.5	2.4 ± 0.57**
HbE thalassaemia	13	1.7	5.6	3.1 ± 0.76*
Thalassaemia minor	11	1.7	4.0	3.2 ± 0.81*
HbE trait	3	2.5	5.4	4.2 ± 0.68
	*P	0.01	**0.001	

Table — 4.

Showing serum cholinesterase values and other liver function tests in thalassaemia expressed in percentage of abnormal results.

Serum cholinesterase	Albumin/globulin ratio	Serum bilirubin	Alkaline Phosphatase	S.G.P.T
4.1 IU/ml. 90%	<1 65%	>1 mg% 45%	>13 KA 50%	>40 IU 42%

From Table 4, it is evident that 90% of thalassaemia showed abnormal serum cholinesterase values whereas in 65% cases albumin/globulin ratio was altered, 50% showed abnormal alkaline phosphatase values and 42% cases only showed abnormal S.G.P.T. Serum bilirubin was more than 1 mg% in 45 percent only.

Table — 5.

Showing correlation of serum cholinesterase values and histology of liver

Histology of liver	Serum cholinesterase values IU/ml. Rang	Mean
A. Normal liver parenchyma (14)	3.8 to 5.2	4.0
B. Liver tissue with hydropic (13) degeneration of hepatocytes showing early involvement of the parenchyma.	2.5 to 4.6	3.8
C. Necrosis of the liver cells in peripheral areas. Mild fibrosis with mononuclear cell infiltration in portal tract. Sinusoids dilated. Liver cells are hydropic and found in clusters. Kupffer cells are hyperplastic. Pericellular reticulin fibres are thickened. In some cellular membrane disrupted, mild pigment deposition. Chronic persistent hepatitis (6) cases and chronic active hepatitis in (4) cases.	1.9 to 4.2	3.3
D. Portal tracts are infiltrated with chronic inflammatory cells, fibroblasts, Fibroblasts from portal tract are spreading to all sides. Sinusoids are dilated with proliferation of Kupffer cells. Radicals of portal veins are dilated. Fatty changes are seen in parenchymal cells in periportal areas. Early cirrhosis in (2) cases.	1.5 to 3.9	3.1

E. Heavy deposition of iron in Kupffer cells and in hepatic cells of periportal areas. Cirrhosis due to haemosiderosis (3).	2.5 to 4.6	2.9
F. Necrosis of liver cells (1 case)	2.7	2.7

From the Table 5 above, it is evident that with more and more parenchymal involvement of liver, the serum cholinesterase values showed lowest figures.

Discussion :

In our series, among 93 total cases of anaemia (total haemoglobin varied from 9 to 3.2 gm.) which was again 1.8% of total admission in 36 months period, 50 cases were diagnosed clinically as thalassaemia syndromes including thalassaemia major, thalassaemia HbE disease, thalassaemia minor and HbE traits. Chatterjee et al (1966)[5] has reported that thalassaemia in the homozygous form in combination of haemoglobin E to be the commonest type of haemoglobinopathy in Bengal. The thalassaemias have also been reported from various parts of India. Y.R. Reddi et al (1975)[7] reported 80 cases of thalassaemia major from Andhra Pradesh. In this series thalassaemia major accounted for 11.9 percent of anaemias and 0.23 percent of total hospital admissions. Recently O.P. Ghai et al (1980)[9] presented a series of 32 cases of thalassaemia major and determination of HbF and HbA_2 in them in northern part of India. Majority of cases originally the parents or their families migrated from West Punjab now in Pakistan. Family studies revealed that cases of thalassaemia major were homozygous for B-thalassaemia and 2 cases of thalassaemia intermedia were doubly heterozygous for B-thalassaemia and a quantitative haemoglobinopathy (HbE in one case and HbG in the other). Most of the homozygous presented clinically and haematologically with a severe disease. HbF and HbA_2 determinations in these homozygotes and their families suggest that B^+ gene is the commonest thalassaemic gene present in this part of the world. Findings of heterozygous for HbS and HbE in these population in unusual. Association of G6 PD deficiency and thalassaemia trait was detected in one family. In this series of 50 cases, haematological studies revealed 23 (46%) of thalassaemia major and 13 (26%) thalassaemia HbE disease of different clinical severity. Regarding the presence of thalassaemia gene both in major and minor together 68%, which is more than double heterozygous HbE F and HbE trait i.e., 32%. So in this series, more were of homozygous B-thalassaemia or thalassaemia major than thalassaemia HbE disease, which was previously reported by Chatterjee et al (loc cit) from this part of eastern India. The family studies of 8 patients and 14 siblings showed prevalence of heterozygosity as B-thalassaemia minor with elevation of HbA_2 (4 — 6.5%) in 10 cases and HbE values, which varied from 18 — 60% both in thalassaemia HbE disease and HbE traits. As already mentioned splenectomy was done in 4 cases, where clinical severity was much more and those cases needed too many frequent blood transfusions. In all these cases pancytopenia of gradually increasing nature were detected and all of them were over the age range of 5 years, so that early hazards of splenectomy could be avoided. Yet one female child died of meningitis after 1 year of splenectomy.

The liver is enlarged early in the disease process, which is confirmed clinically by palpation but how far the parenchymatous involvement is there. One cannot ascertain by usual liver function tests. It is known that hepatomegaly in thalassaemias is the result of Kupffer cell hyperplasia and fibrosis stimulated by excess iron deposited, taken up extramedullary haemopoietic function and also anaemic heart failure. More over in our tropical and sub-tropical climates more and more infection and infestations play a great role in parenchymal damage of liver. In this study, we tried to show that a sensitive biochemical test in serum cholinesterase value is a very sensitive index to reflect the parenchymal involvement which is often missed by other biochemical test. More over, the quantitative estimation of abnormal haemoglobins showed inverse proportion with serum cholinesterase value, such as where there is high abnormal haemoglobins, the serum cholinesterase has got relatively lower values. As it was previously mentioned that even abnormal haemoglobin values is not related with clinical severity or age of presentation.

The second part of the study proved beyond doubt the efficacy and correlation of serum cholinesterase values and histologically continued more of parenchyma involement in thalassaemias. So without going for liver biopsy, one can predict prognosis of thalassaemia with more of liver parenchyma involvement by estimation of serum cholinesterase.

Reference

1. Iancu, T.C., Landing, B.H. & Neustein, H.B. (1977) : Pathogenetic mechanisms in hepatic cirrhosis of thalassaemia major, light and electron microscopic studies. Pathology Annual, 12, 171-200.
2. Kattamis, D., Papthanasion alonztu and Mata Saniotia, N. : Serum cholinesterase levels in thalassaemia — Paper presented at XVth International Congress of paediatrics, held in Delhi, India, October, 1977.
3. Bary, M., Plynn, D.M. Lersky, E.A. & Risdon, B.A. (1974) : Long term chelation Therapy in Thalassaemia major. Effects on liver iron concentration, liver histology and Clinical Progress. British Medical Journal, 2, 16, 1974.
4. Pauling : Abnormal haemoglobins — Blackwell Publications, 1969, Page 100 as quoted by J.H.P. Jonxis.
5. Chatterjee, J.B. : Bull. Org. Mond. Santo. BUll. World Health Org. 1966, 35 : 837 : 856.
6. Mukherjee, M. : India J. Paediatrics, 5, 1, 1938.
7. Y.R. Reddi, V. Sudhakar Rao, A. Nirayan and S. Laxan : 'Thalassaemia in Andhra Pradesh'. A clinical Haematologic study. Indian Paediatrics, Vol. XII, No. 2, Pp. 195-196, 1975.
8. O.P. Ghai, Priti Trehan, Nishi Madan and S.K. Sood, B-thalassaemia syndrome as seen in Northern India : Indian Paediatrics, Vol.XVII, No.3. pp-219-226, 1980.

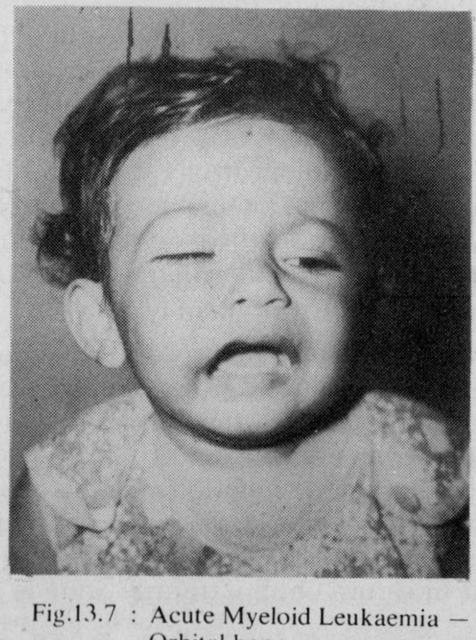

Fig.13.7 : Acute Myeloid Leukaemia — Orbital bone.

LEUKAEMIAS

Introduction :

In the last 25 years, due to progress in the basic physical and biological sciences has led to a considerable expansion in our knowledge of the blood and its various disorders including leukaemias. The advances in biochemistry, cell biology, genetics, immunology and molecular biology have contributed a great deal to our current knowledge of Leukaemias. Although the overall incidence of leukaemias in relation to other malignant neoplasm appear to be low in India. Most probably the geography, environment, racial factors are responsible. In U.K., the children with malignant disease form less than 1% of the total cancer patients in the population and some 1200 children will develop cancer every year and at the present time about 700 of them will die, although the cure rate is improving all the time. The annual incidence of all categories of malignancies is childhood (birth to 15 years) in U.K. has been given below :-

Table 1.

Tumour	Incidence %
Leukaemia	35
Hodgkin's disease	4
Non-Hodgkin Lymphoma	4
Histiocytosis	1
CNS Tumours	17
Sympathetic nervous system tumours	10
Soft tissue sarcoma	10
Nephroblastoma	5
Bone tumours (Osteogenous and Ewing's)	4
Epithelial tumours	4
Retinoblastomas	3
Miscellaneous tumours	3

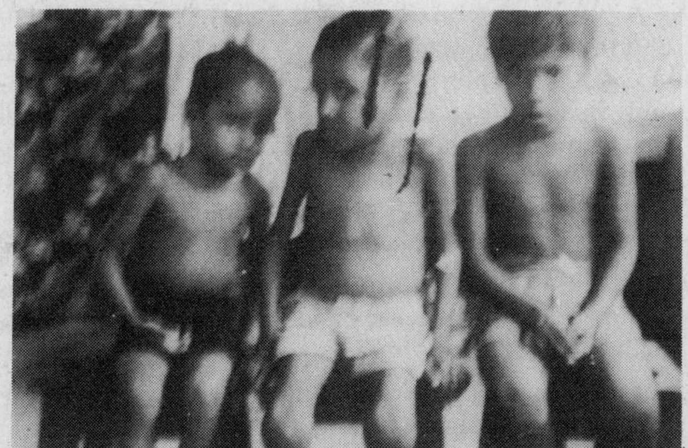

Fig.13.7(a) : Chr. lymphocytic leukaemia. Hodgkin lymphoma Non-Hodgkin lymphoma.

In India in one study (Thangan et al) of 52 cases of malignant diseases in children between 1972-77, acute leukaemia was the commonest neoplasm 38.5%, followed by lymphoma 21%. The classification of the various malignant conditions are as follows :-

Table – 2.

Sl.No.	Disease	Age (0-1)	(2-5)	(6-12)	Total	%
1.	Acute Leukaemia	1	7	10	18	38.5
2.	Acute Myeloid Leukaemia	1	1	1	2	
3.	Lymphoma		3	8	11	21.0
4.	Wilm's Tumour		5	—	5	9.6%
5.	Neuroblastoma		1	3	4	7.1
6.	Craniopharyngioma		2	—	2	11.0
7.	Medulloblastoma		—	3	3	
8.	Astrocytoma		—	1	1	
9.	Angio-fibro Sarcoma, Nose		—	1	1	
10.	Ovarian Tumour		—	2	2	
11.	Testicular Tumour	1	—	—	1	
12.	Retinoblastoma	1	1	—	2	
	Total	4	20	29	52	

Young and Miller (1975) in their series from USA found the order as Leukaemia, CNS Tumour, Lymphoma, Neuroblastoma and Wilm's tumour. In Thangan et al the leukaemia was the commonest neoplasm of childhood, 38.5% which is in agreement with that of Evans (USA) 37.5%, Victorian Cancer Registry Centre noted as 35%.

In our series the childhood malignancies formed 0.4% in our Paediatric Ward admission whereas in USA it is 168 per 1,000 upto the age of 12 years. The leukaemia in our series corresponds this of other series in India, i.e., 37.6% of which the acute lymphatic 2.5% and next comes lymphomas both Hodgkin and non-Hodgkin among the solid tumours. In this series also we have noticed 2 cases of histiocytosis 'X'. Recently Paediatric Surgery has been incorporated in the Paediatric house and we are also noticing Wilm's tumour more frequently.

However, this study of mainly clinical profile of childhood leukaemias, has been taken to the lacunae confronted in a general Paediatric department to diagnose and manage these cases, focus the paediatric clinician's approach to leukaemias to know :

(a) The mode of presentation in a general Paediatric Unit which is not backed by clinical haematological unit, radio-diagnostic and/or radio-therapy unit.

(b) The difficulties encountered specially to diagnose and also overall management of the cases without proper follow up with multi-disciplinary approach.

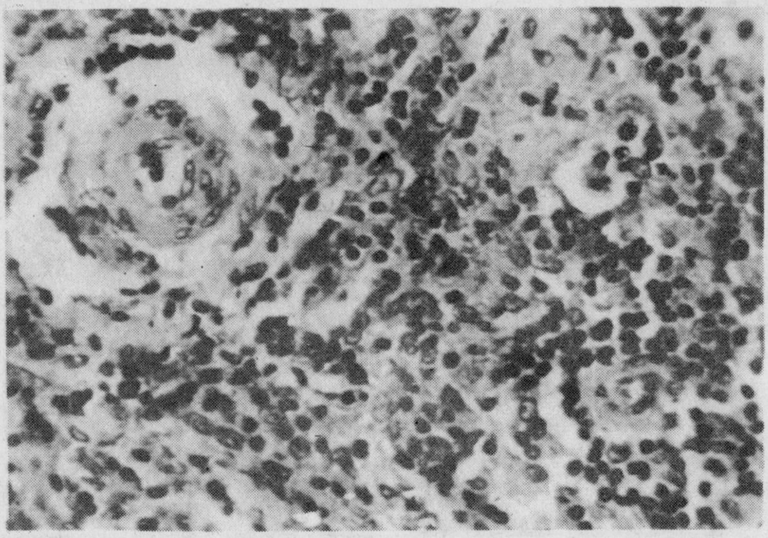

Fig.13.7(b) : Histology – Hodgkin Dorothy Reed Cells.

Table — 3.

Paediatric Department Indoor Admission, Diagnosis reference in the age group under 12 yrs. in 1981-82 (13/12) upto July, 1982.

1. All categories malignancies		—	0.4%
(USA upto 12 years)		—	(168 per 1,000)
2. Acute Leukemias and Chronic Leukaemias	both	—	37.6%
(a) ALL		—	35.0%
(b) CML + CLL		—	2.6%
(c) Lymphomas :			
	(i) Hodgkin	—	8
	(ii) Non-Hodgkin	—	4
(d) Histiocytosis		—	2
(e) Wilm's tumour		—	4
(f) Other Categories :			
	(i) Bone, ovary & testes	—	Nil in 6/12
	(ii) CNS tumour	—	18
	(iii) Retinoblastoma	—	10
	Oro-pharyngeal malignancies	—	Nil

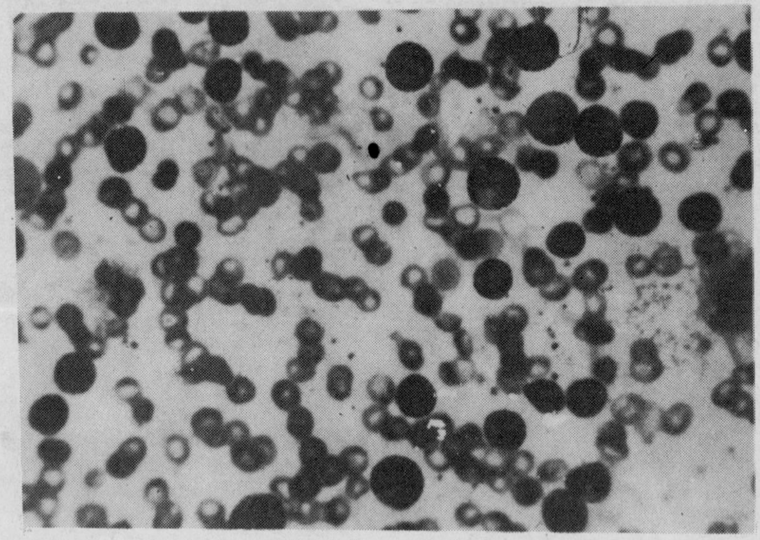

Fig.13.8 : Acute Leukaemias (blood picture)

Methods & Materials :

17 cases of leukaemia, seen in our department from April 1981 to August, 1982 were due to acute lymphatic leukaemia (ALL), 10 cases are,due to acute myeloid leukaemia (AML) 3 cases, and 4 of chronic leukaemia —3 chronic myeloid and 1 chronic lymphatic leukaemia. Among the 10 ALL, 2 presented with acute lymphoblastic crisis in non-Hodgkin lymphomas. The diagnosis of leukaemia is made with the help of haematological investigation, and radiology. But mainly the clinical features and confirmation by other haematological investigations also helped us to differentiate and confirm the original diagnosis. In this series no special study such as advanced cellular biology, immunological and chromosomal studies were done. All the cases with typical and atypical presentation reviewed in this article were noticed as initial presenting manifestations, occasionally some being accompanied by typical clinical signs and symptoms. Follow up information was available in all of them, or otherwise is made after consulting other expert opinion or standard text books and many review article on this subject.

Observation :

The type of leukaemia, the age of the patients, the atypical and typical clinical features are recorded in Table 4. It can be observed from the above that some presented with typical clinical picture and some are with atypical presentation and developed some associated complications during this study in hospital.

Table — 4

Sl. No.	Age & Sex	Types of Leukaemia	Atypical clinical manifestations	Associated symptoms	Prognosis and survival period after admission
1	2	3	4	5	6
1.	5½ yrs. M.H.	CML	Priapism	Huge splenomegaly + Hepatomegaly	Improved 3/12

2. 7 months M.H.	ALL	Pyogenic manifestations Jaundice Pyoderma	Hepato splenomegaly lymph glands + + Bleeding	2 days D
3. 4 yrs. M.C.	ALL	M.P. Detected E.S.R.	Hepato splenomegaly	7/12 RM improved with cytotoxic drug Relapsed + D
4. 9 yrs. M.M.	ALL (atypical cell)	Pallor +++ Bleeding +++ Kidneys ++	Hepato splenomegaly lymph glands +	72 hrs. D
5. 3 yrs. M.M.	AML (Mature & immature cells)	Myopathy Respiratory infection	Hepato splenomegaly Pallor	3/12
6. 6 yrs. M.H.	ALL	Pyoderma and Ecchymoses & Fracture Bone, Jaundice	Hepatomegaly Lymph glands + No spleen	10 days D
7. 5 yrs. F.M.	ALL	Jaundice ESR increased	Hepato splenomegaly Anaemia ++	20 days D
8. 5½ yrs. F.M.	ALL Cell-L,	Jaundice, Oedema face	Hepato splenomegaly Anaemia ++	20 days D
9. 5½ yrs. F.M.	ALL (atypical)	Jaundice, Oedema face	Hepato splenomegaly	2 days D
10. 9 yrs. M.H.	Non-Hodgkin Lymphoblastic crisis	Skin involvement	Cervical glands (Biopsy) Confirmed diagnosis	3/12 RM improved
11. 1 yr. 2/12 H.M.	ALL with bone (orbit)	Stomatitis Pallor ++ Proptosis	Hepato spenomegaly	18 days D
12. 1 yr. 6/12 F.M.	AML	Jaundice and heart failure	Hepato splenomegaly Pallor ++	7 days D
13. 10 yrs. F.H.	ALL	Mediastinal mass and lung ++ Oedema, Pallor, CCF, Jaundice	Hepato splenomegaly + Lymph glands ++	15 days D
14. 6½ yrs. M.M.	ALL	Oedema, Pallor, CCF, Jaundice	Lymph glands ++ Hepato splenomegaly	1/12 D
15. 8½ yrs. M.H.	CML	Jaundice ++ Skin nodules, Bone tender	Hepato splenomegaly Lymph glands +	3/12 RM with cytotoxic drug
16. 4½ yrs. M.C.	CLL	Jaundice (Haemolytic picture)	Hepato splenomegaly Lymph glands (Cervical ++)	2/12 D
17. 5½ yrs. F.H.	CML	Pallor ++ No splenomegaly	Lymph glands ++ No splenomegaly	2/12 RM with cytotoxic drug

Abbreviations :

ALL : Acute Lymphoblastic Leukaemia
AML : Acute Myeloblastic Leukaemia
CML : Chronic Myeloid Leukaemia
CLL : Chronic Lymphatic Leukaemia
D : Death
RM : Remission
RE : Relapse

In this series, the most common typical features in acute leukaemias specially all are fever, bleeding skin as purpura, ecchymosis and frank bleeding as epistaxis, haematuria, haematemesis and melena, lymphadenopathy and hepato splenomegaly. The uncommon manifestations were bone involvement — orbital, limb bone with fracture at metaphysial level, proptosis, both mediastinal glands and abdominal glands enlargement, jaundice with haemolytic feature, marked pallor and sudden death in two ALL below one year of age. Antibiotic resistant pyogenic infection, anti-tuberculous resistant mediastinal lymphadenopathy, sudden development of dyspnoea, and evidences of haemorrhagic effusion etc., will alert a good clinical man to diagnose atypical leukaemias and before starting treatment with cortisone should have an expert haematologic opinion both blood and bone marrow study and expert radiological investigation to diagnose leukaemias.

The two non-Hodgkin lymphomas diagnosed by gland biopsy presented later on as a complication of acute lymphoblastic crisis and managed in the line of ALL.

The chronic leukaemias in this series are 4. There are chronic myeloid and one a case of chronic lymphatic leukaemia, which is very rare in children and diagnosed by expert pathologist by haematological investigation.

There is a geographical bias in its incidence which has been documented by various authors and even in our own country its variations from one centre to another is striking. Many authors have mentioned about 'Chloroma' or green tumour with AML, but one of our case diagnosed as ALL, presented with orbital bone involvement. In this several haematological investigations did not show any myeloid series at any time with characteristic bone marrow and haematological findings. The other child of 4 years old presented with enlarged liver, spleen and abdominal lymphadenopathy with fracture of forearm bones but during the stay in hospital never showed any haematological and bone marrow picture of ALL but with persistence proved to be a case of ALL with complications diagnosed later on at other centre.

2 cases of ALL at the initial stage presented as aplastic anaemia and subsequently proved as and diagnosed as acute lymphoblastic leukaemia with aplastic crisis.

This atypical presentation proves that acute leukaemias with protean clinical features with aplasia of bone marrow, secondary thrombocytopenia with or without marrow-failure or marrow involvement with leukaemic tissues. Also the clinical features relating to extra medullary features such as fever, leucocytosis, liver,spleen, lymph glands involvement are present.

One case of acute myeloid leukaemia with gum-ulceration and stomatitis was noticed. In acute cases of ALL and AML presented with haemolytic features that is jaundice, dark urine, bleeding episodes and hepato splenomegaly at the onset and 2 of them simulated thalassaemia syndrome and then proved as leukaemias. The pathogenesis underlying the manifestation of jaundice explained by many as due to the infiltrating leukaemic cells in the portal tract. Another suggestion is due to reduced life span of RBC leading to haemolysis brought about by autoantigenic variation of RBC's. Alternately the changes in red cell agglutinin have been held responsible for increased destruction of RBC's, auto-immune haemolytic anaemia which is confirmed by positive coomb's test.

In 3 cases of chronic leukaemias — 2 myeloid not typed whether adult philadelphia chromosome positive or juvenile type but responded very well with myleron and 1 of chronic lymphatic which is very rare in childhood ages but again responded very well initially with cyclophosphamide therapy but relapsed with acute lymphoblastic crisis and died later on.

Discussion :

Acute Leukaemias are easily classified as lymphoblastic (ALL) or myeloblastic (AML) on morphological features following conventional stains and cytochemical methods. Recently a Franco-Americal-British (FAB) collaborator group based upon morphological features have described three sub-types of ALL (Table 5). Cell size, nuclear shape, nuclear chromatin, quality of cytoplasm and nuclear prominence have been the basis of sub-type of ALL. This classification bears no relationship to the immunological classification but it is of prognostic significance.

Table — 5.

Morphological & Immunological Classificiation of ALL.

FAB	Distinctive morphology	Immunological
L_1	Small uniform cells with little cytoplasm.	Common All
L_2	Pleomorphic cells with larger cytoplasm and nucleoli	T — All Null — All
L_3	Large basophilic and vacuolated cytoplasm.	B — All

Immunological Marking :

Immunological studies indicate the ALL is a heterogenous disease and four types of cells are recognised. Lymphoblast from majority of children with ALL lack the characters of either T or B lymphocytes but bears a surface antigen which is recognised by an anti-serum raised against non T non B cells in the rabbit. Leukaemic cells bearing this type of ALL antigen is termed as common ALL. Nearly 15-20% of children with ALL have characteristics of thymus dependent lymphocytes (T cell ALL). In 1-2% of cases of blasts cells have surface immunoglobulins of B cells (B cell ALL) B cell leukaemia is the one type of leukaemia in which prognosis is similar to cases with L_3 type. Lymphoblasts having no immunological marking on their cells are termed as Null Cell.

Enzyme :

The estimation of enzymes are helpful. Hexosaminadase iso-enzyme levels are raised in majority of children with ALL, while acid phosphatase levels are raised in T cell leukaemias. Terminal deoxynucleotidyl-transferasé 9 (TdT DNA synthetic enzyme), enzyme levels are raised in common ALL, 'T' cell ALL,Null Cell ALL but not is B cell ALL. In summary, perhaps the most useful of the increasing number of tests available are the Erosette technique or the acid phosphatase to suggest T cell lineages and the TdT to denote lymphoid origin.

Cytogenetics :

The classical leukaemia marker chromosome is the Philadelphia (Ph^1) chromosome resulting from deletion of the long arm of one of the chromosome No.22. Philadelphia (Ph^1) chromosomes resulting from reciprocal translocation with No. 9 (t 9 : 22) and also found in 1-2% of cases with ALL, in bone marrow cells but not lymphocytes or fibroblasts in patients with chronic myeloid leukaemia. Translocation (t 8 : 14) has been described in B Cell ALL, it remains to be seen whether or not this is a constant finding. A cytogenetic classification may come up with better prognostic correlation. As at present children with such chromosomal abnormalities have poor prognosis.

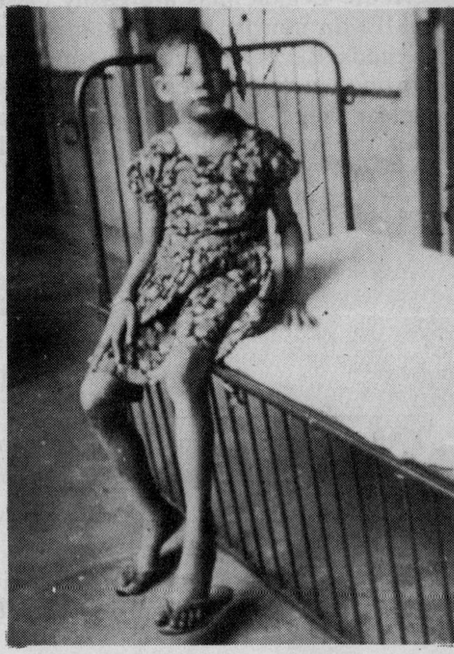

Fig.13.9 : Alopecia after cyclophosphamide therapy.

Management :

The present management of acute leukaemias specially ALL can frequently be made on the examination and the findings in the peripheral blood film. It is already pointed out that the diagnosis should, however, never be excluded on the basis of a normal peripheral blood films, as occasionally the abnormalities may be confined to the marrow at diagnosis. There can be very few suspected cases in which a bone marrow examination is contraindicated and wherever possible both an aspirate and trephine should be carried out. These are best taken from the aenterior or posterior iliac crest, but the tibia can be used in very young children. The bone marrow is usually hypercellular and the blast cell count between 70 and 100%, but occasionally there may be as few as 25% blasts. It is not uncommon for aspiration to be difficult because of a tightly packed marrow and in this case the trephine is particularly helpful. After the diagnosis is established the following investigations are also indicated; blood group, chest radiographs, plasma electrolytes, blood urea and uric acid; throat swab, urine culture and if there is any suggestion of infection, blood culture.

The immediate management in emergencies such as bleeding, blood transfusion is needed. The platelet transfusions are indicated in the presence of purpura, echymoses and some would use them prophylactically when the platelet count is less than 100,000 P.cmm (10×10^9/litre). The presence of infection often makes bleeding worse and disseminated intravascular coagulation (DIC) may complicate the bleeding tendency. If the serum uric acid is raised to levels in excess of 0.4 mml/liter (4mg%) then it is probably wise to institute treatment with allopurinol 100 mg. twice a day before beginning specific therapy as massive tissue breakdown can cause uric acid nephropathy with renal failure and uraemia. The adequate fluid intake and alkalinization of the urine are also helpful in preventing these complications.

The present management of acute lymphoblastic leukaemias can be divided into three phases; induction, consolidation and maintenance. The combination of oral prednisolone and weekly intravenous vincristine is almost mandatory in standard induction of ALL because it is non myelotoxic and induces remission in over 90% of children within four to six weeks. If the combination proves unsuccessful then addition of further drugs such as an anthracycline and/or L-asparaginase is indicated after re-examination of the original marrow to exclude AML; persistent refractoriness to therapy should prompt examination of marrow chromosomes to detect the rare Ph^1 positive ALL.

After induction therapy, the remission is defined as a bone marrow with less than 5% of blast cells and otherwise normal cellularity, a peripheral white cell count of greater than 1.5×10^9/litre (5,000 pcm) neutrophiles, 150×10^9/litre (1.5 lac) platelets and a haemoglobin of 12 G/dl. or greater. The patient clinically should be free of signs and symptoms of the disease. There appears to be sufficient evidence to warrant the routine use of at least a third drug for example 1-asparaginase in all cases of ALL. The more intensive induction therapy may well be indicated, particularly in patients with high risk of early relapse, but proper supportive facilities are essential. If prolonged intensive chemotherapy is contemplated for such patients it is advisable to start CNS prophylaxis with intrathecal methotrexate during induction.

Once remission has been achieved consolidation therapy should be started. This consists off prophylactic treatment of the central nervous system to prevent the development of leukaemic infiltration of the meninges and brain. In most instances this consists of cranial irradiation (2400 rads) combined with intrathecal methotrexate 10-12 mg./m^2 once or twice weekly for four to ten doses.

The continuing chemotherapy or maintenance therapy with greatest variety of schedules is found and an almost limitless number of protocols can be devised varying complexity from daily 6-mercaptopurine and weekly methotrexate, the main stay of many protocols, to the intermittent intensive regimens based on several factors, there are :-

(i) Availability of the drug,

(ii) various cell kinetic factors of ALL,

(iii) associated risk factors, infections, even with side effects and complication associated with treatment,

(iv) last but not the least on the centre where the follow up and treatment is going on.

However, the maintenance chemotherapy should then be given for periods between two and three years providing complete remission continues during this time. The drugs used in maintenance protocols based on the first letter of the constitute drugs for example COAP (Cyclosphamide, vincristine, cystosine arabinoside, prednisolone and POMP (Prednisolone), vincristine (oncovin). Methotrexate and purinethol (6-MP). The treatment should be given to the limits of tolerance, as indicated by the leucocyte count or other evidence of toxicity, for example mouth ulceration from methotrexate administration. The single agent chemotherapy for example with 6-MP. is associated with an unadoptble relapse rate, presumbly due to emergence of resistant leukaemic cell lines. The treatment of maintenance should therefore comprise at least two drugs, say 6-M.P. and methotrexate. In case of relapse, investigated by peripheral blood smear or confirmatory bone marrow study, the treatment or maintenance therapy is interspersed with weekly short course of prednisolone and vincristine and prevents the relapse rate.

As it is already pointed out that complications with treatment such as infections by various organisms, as for example the opportunistic organisms from bacteria, fungi, viruses and protozoa should be dealt with proper chemotherapeutic and antibiotics. The recent trend is chemo-prophlyactic treatment with co-trimoxozole (Pyrimethamine and sulphonamide) is the ideal agent.

Even with the introduction of prophylaxis to the CNS, a number of children will show evidence of the first relapse with disease in the CNS with feature of increased intracranial tension, excessive weight gain associated with a voracious appetite, due to hypothalamic involvement, a feature of encephalopathy with bizzare picture of neurological signs, so question comes of diagnosis and differential diagnosis from infection or degeneration or demyelinating diseases of CNS, should be excluded by lumbar puncture and other ancilliary investigations. There might be testicular relapse in males.

PROGNOSTIC FEATURE.

In the last 10-12 years, long term survival have greatly improved in children with ALL, based upon initial parameter. Children with good prognosis are being recognised and are treated with more intensive chemotherapy. The prognostic features which are of greater significance are as follows :-

1. **Blood leucocyte count :**

Total while cell count directly correlates with the total leukaemic mass to be the simplest. In large series it has been demonstrated that patients with white cell count less than $10 \times 10^9/L$ have better prognosis than children with a count between 10-15 $\times 10^9/L$ while children with a count of greater than $100 \times 10^9/L$ has the worst prognosis.

2. **Leukaemic cell load :**

Children with significant organomegaly and with mediastinal masses have worst prognosis as there are higher total leukaemic cell burden.

3. **CNS disease at onset :**

Initial CNS involvement is rare at first diagnosis. However, when present, it denotes a poor outcome as it almost always as fatal outcome. Approximately 5% of children have CNS disease at onset.

4. **Age :**

It has been observed that children aged between 3 and 8 years have better prognosis.

5. **Cell morphology :**

Children with T cell leukaemia occurs often over 8 years of age, have large cell count at the onset. Mediastinal mass and extra medullary infiltration are other features of T cell leukaemia. All these features suggest poor prognosis. Similarly children with B cell leukaemia have poor outcome. Children with blast cells reacting to Graves type of antiserum (C-ALL) have the better prognosis than those with Null cell ALL.

7. **Sex :**

Boys have poor prognosis. Partly they are with bigger cell mass at all ages and secondly the risk of developing testicular relapse.

8. **Karyotypes :**

These are only a few studies indicating that children with chromosomal translocation have adverse outcome.

9. **Serum Immunoglobins :**

Low serum immunoglobins at onset is associated with poor prognosis mainly because of low remission rates, early relapse and increased risk of infection.

10. **Cytoreduction :**

Reduction in bone marrow cellularity was found to be good prognostic value.

Bibliography :

1. Malignant diseases of children — (Study of 52 cases),
P. Maharatra, L. Sulochana, Chandra, Ashivathan, Tamilarasi and Thangam — Indian Paediatrics, Vol. XVI, No.8, pages 701-705, August, 1979.
2. Recent advances in Paediatrics by David Hall, Number Six, 1981.
3. Evans D'Angio and Randolph, I (1971) — Approved staging for children with Neuroblastoma Cancer 27, 374.
4. Young, J.L. (Jr.),Miller, R.W. : Incidence of malignant tumours in U.S. children, Journal Pediatr. — 1975; 86 : 254-357.

CHAPTER – FOURTEEN

THE LIVER

Anatomic, Physiologic and Clinical Consideration :

The liver develops very early in organogenesis by the third week of pregnancy and grows into a well formed hepatic diverticulum which forms a caudal cystic part, the future gall bladder and a cephalic hepatic bud, the future liver. In the fetus, the liver is proportionately large, measuring 5 percent of total body volume at the 10 mm. stage to about 10 percent in the 30 mm embryo. Subsequently, it slowly reduces in size becoming 5 percent of body weight at birth. The left lobe is larger than the right because of its oxygen-rich blood supply, coming directly from the umbilical vein.

The structural orientation of the liver, therefore reflects its diversity in specialised functions centred around synthesising storage detoxification and phagocytosis. Being an organ essential for life it is also endowed with not only a large surplus of functional tissue but also a phenomenal capacity for prompt replacement of lost tissue (Bucher, 1967). The endocrine element of the organ processes synthesis and secretes into blood a multitude of substances including proteins, lipids, carbohydrates and vitamins. The exocrine part on the other hand, puts out bile and through it a number of byproducts of detoxification. Inspite of such complexity of function, however the organ maintains a relatively simple and uniform structure, the multiplicity of work being handled by versatility and interchangeability of biochemical processes at the subcellular level.

Anatomy of the liver :

The liver in infants and young children upto the age of 6 years, is proportionately much larger, weighing approximately 5 percent of body weight during the first year of life and gradually reducing in size over the subsequent years. Also, in infancy and early childhood, the liver is an important seat of haemopoiesis, the hepatocytes replicate at a higher rate, the parenchyma consists predominantly of double cell plates and there is more glycogen as well as more fat. The size of the organ in infancy and early childhood accounts for the fullness of the abdomen which is contributed to more by the left than by the right lobe. At this age the liver is normally palpable. Particularly at the intercostal angle. The liver is situated in the upper right quadrant of the abdomen below the diaphragm, largely protected by the ribs and suspended by peritoneal folds — the falci-form ligament and triangular ligament both attached to the anterior and superior surface, and posterior and superior surface respectively. The ligament teres and falciform ligament delineated superficially by their attachment into two geographic areas, the right and the left lobe. The two other small portions are called the quadrate and the caudate lobe. The disproportionate enlargement can sometimes involve any one of these four lobes giving on palpation a resemblance to hepatic or extrahepatic tumours. At the porta-hepatis in the undersurface, which is of more irregular shape, the peritoneum folds in and is carried into the deeper hepatic parenchyma along with the vessels and ducts that enter to leave the organ. A vertical groove at the back of the organ, a little to the right to the midline, houses the inferior vena cava. The gall bladder is situated on the undersurface of the organ in a fossa extending from the middle of the inferior border to the right end of the porta hepatis. The right bend of the colon and the upper lobe of the right kidney press against and leave impressions on the undersurface of the right lobe and the stomach on the undersurface of the left lobe.

Physiology of the liver :

As mentioned above the endocrine function of liver associated with metabolism of proteins, carbohydrate and lipids, the exocrine function is to secrete the bile, now in a short descriptive way all these functions will be discussed.

Protein :

The liver is the main source of protein synthesis. The proteins for intracellular use as ferritin are synthesised on free polysomes in the liver. The proteins which are secreted as albumin are synthesised on membrane bound polysomes on rough endoplasmic reticulum. The clotting factors, haemoglobin, C-reactive protein, ceruloplasmin, transferin alpha-antitrypsin and complements C_3 and C_5 are also synthesised in the liver. Also the liver helps in utilisation of aminoacids and deamination of the excess aminoacids into ammonia which in turn forms urea.

Carbohydrate :

The carbohydrate homeostasis is maintained by liver in four major pathways. (1) storage of carbohydrate in the form of glycogen (2) the synthesis of carbohydrate chiefly glucose by gluconeogenesis (3) release of glucose from glycogen and (4) conversion of carbohydrate to fat. The liver metabolises sugars and feeds them into the glycolytic pathway. In the infant, the galactose is of major importance as a carbohydrate form, since it comprises half of the lactose molecule. The older children receive much of their dietary carbohydrate as sucrose, a disaccharide containing equal parts of glucose and fructose. In hereditary fructose intolerance and in galactosemia these inter conversion pathways are impaired, and liver disease may result.

Lipid metabolism :

The synthesis of cholesterol occurs from acetate. The esterification of cholesterol is done by serum enzyme lecithin cholesterol acyltransferase. The formation of the bile salts e.g., cholicacid and chenodioxycholic acid are formed by the liver cells. These are conjugated with taurine and glycine. The bile salts is in association with phospholipids and cholesterol form small particles called micelle. The micelles make the dietary lipids more soluble in the intestinal secretion. The solubulised lipids are absorbed in the jejunum. The bile salts are absorbed in the portal circulation at the terminal ileum. Then these salts are reexcreted through the liver. Some bile salts reach the colon, where they may be deconjugated by the bacterial action to form secondary bile salts like lithocholate and deoxycholate. These are reabsorbed and the former is believed to be hepatotoxic. The fatty acids are formed in the liver and utilised by oxidation to form Co_2 for providing energy. The phospholipids are also formed in the liver — the triglycerides are synthesised and are released into circulation as very low density lipoproteins as pre-beta lipoproteins.

Clinical consideration :

In childhood, the liver is palpable upto the age of 6 years and it does not indicate enlargement. In children the liver is palpable 1 cm. below costal margin and in infants it may be felt upto 2 cm. below the rib margin. The palpability varies according to variability of costal angle. The liver may be pushed down in lower respiratory obstructive diseases and also becomes palpable in hypotonicity of abdominal muscle. Besides the size and shape of the liver, the consistency and character of the surface and palpable margin should be evaluated for assessment of hepatomegaly. The liver should be examined for tenderness and also auscultated for any murmurs. The upper border of the liver should be defined by percussion. The abdomen should be palpated for other swellings and enlarged spleen.

Liver function Tests :

Since the liver has multiple functions, many tests have been developed to enhance the specificity, sensitivity and relability of laboratory aids to diagnosis. The short list of established tests includes total bilirubin and both unconjugated and conjugated fractions, serum aspartate transaminase (SGOT) and alanine transaminase (SGPT), alkaline phosphatase, serum protein and albumin-globulin ratio, prothrombin time before and after Vit. K. injection, and gamma globulin determinations. The antitrypsin, lipoprotein 'X' and (I^{131}) Rose Bengal excretion should be determined in the investigation of jaundice and hepatomegaly specially in newborn period. The blood ammonia should be measured in the diagnostic evaluation of Reye's syndrome, hepatocellular failure and hepatic encephalopathy. There are special as ultrasonography, as imaging procedure of non-invasive technique. Also percutaneous liver biopsy both close and open are most valuable invasive diagnostic tool in paediatric hepatopathies.

Causes of hepatomegaly :

New born :

Infections (a) 'TORCH' infections e.g., toxoplasmosis others 'O', such as syphilis, Rubella, cytomegalic inclusion disease, herpes simplex virus; neonatal septicaemia, neonatal viral hepatitis.

Haemolytic disease, Rh, and A.B.O. iso-immunisation thalassaemia, congenital spherocytosis, neonatal hepatitis-biliary atresia syndrome, congestive cardiac failure in newborn.

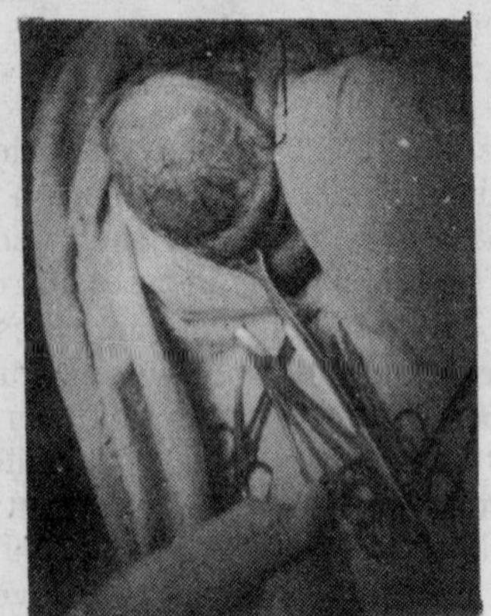

Fig.14.1 : Choledochal cyst

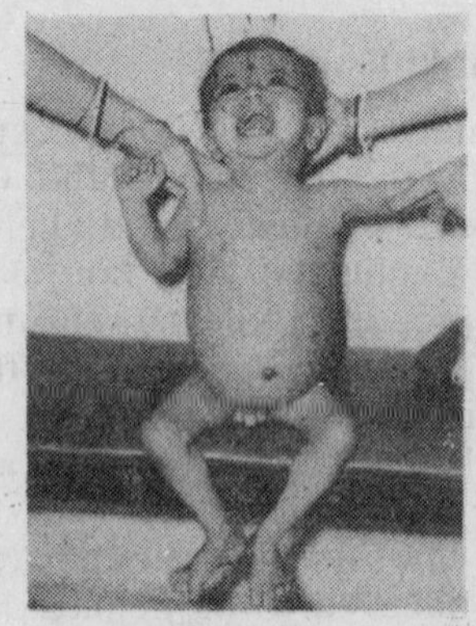

Fig.14.2 : Cong. biliary atresia cirrhosis

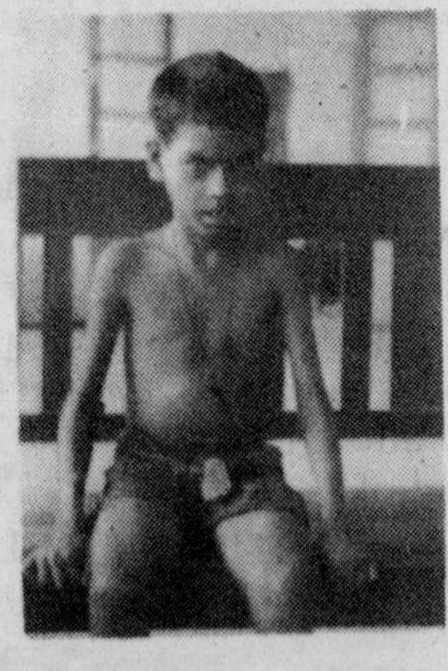

Fig.14.3(a) : Hepatic hydatid disease

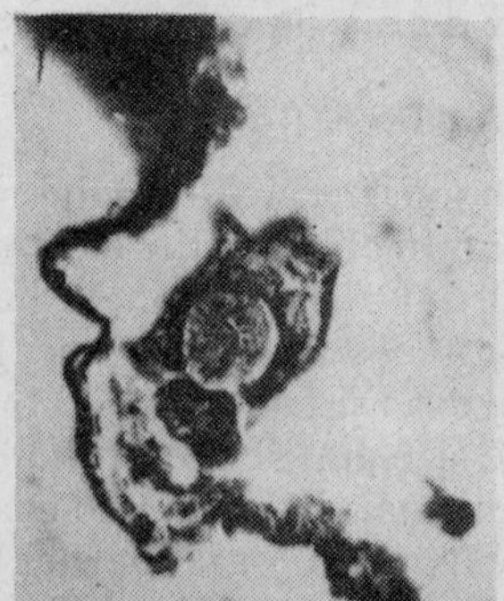

Fig.14.3(b) : Scolex of T. echinococcus of hepatic hydatid disease.

Infants and children :

1. Benign hypertrophy — after upper respiratory virus infection.
2. Fatty liver — Malnutrition, Reye syndrome, tetracycline toxicity, tuberculosis, diabetes mellitus, cystic fibrosis and galactosaemia.
3. Inflammatory processes —
   (a) Infections — intrauterine and intrapartum infections.
   (b) Hepatitis.
   (c) Infectious mononucleosis.
   (d) Parasitic infections, malaria and kala-azar, visceral larva migrans, amoebic hepatitis, hydatid disease.
   (e) Pyogenic abscess of liver, cholangitis.
   (f) Toxins — veno-occulsive disease from Bush tea.
   (g) Drugs — hepatitis and cholestatic jaundice.
4. Cellular infiltration —
   (a) Leukaemia and lymphoma.
   (b) Thalassaemias and haemoglobinopathies.
   (c) Neoplasm — primary (hepato blastoma, haemangioendothelioma).
   (d) Secondary from Wilms tumour and neuroblastoma.
   (e) Histiocytosis 'X'.
5. Metabolic — Mainly storage disorders —
   (a) Glycogen storage disease.
   (b) Galactosaemia.
   (c) Mucopolysaccharidosis..
   (d) Lipoidosis (Gaucher, Neiman Pick, gangliosidosis)
   (e) Amyloidosis.
   (f) Alpha-I-antitrypsin deficiency.
   (g) Hepatic porphyria.
   (h) Cystinnosis.
   (i) Haemosiderosis, Wilson's disease.
6. (a) Congestion.
   (b) Congestive cardiac failure.
   (c) Pericarditis.
   (d) Budd-chiari syndrome (thrombosis of hepatic vein).
7. Kupffer's cell hyperplasia —
   Granulomatous hepatitis in tuberculosis and sarcoidosis.
8. Miscellaneous —
   Cirrhosis of liver. Indian childhood cirrhosis,
   /congenital cyst. etc.

Diagnostic evaluation of liver disease :

The diagnostic investigation of liver disease in infancy and childhood years rests on the following :-

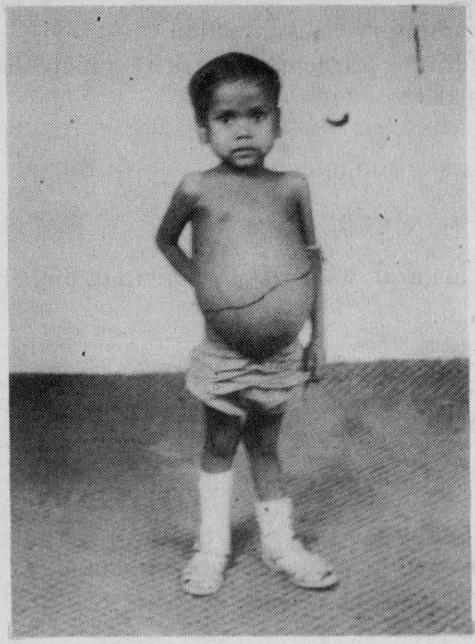

Fig.14.4 : Post-necrotic hepatitis

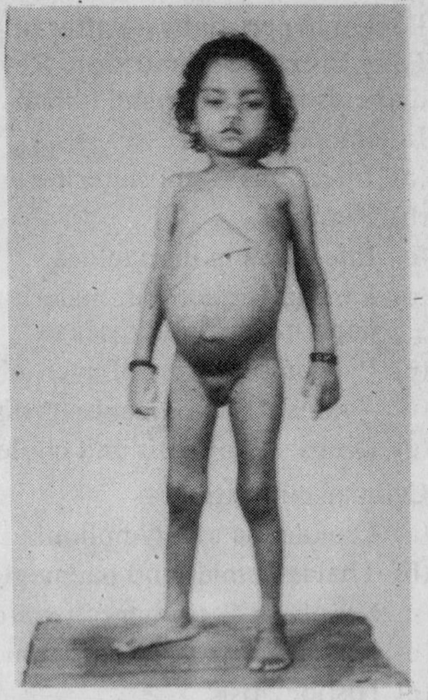

Fig.14.5 : Indian childhood cirrhosis

1. Proper assessment of symptoms and signs from the history and physical examination.
2. Judicious use of selective liver functional tests.
3. Appropriate use of modern non-invasive and invasive techniques including ultrasound, liver scan and biopsy specimens and visualisation procedures.

Assess if the liver is just palpable or is actually enlarged. It should be determined if the enlargement is due to organic causes and also the nature and severity of the illness responsible for it. A good clinical history, interpretations of the associated clinical signs and symptoms. Where necessary, the use of judicious use of laboratory investigations are helpful in arriving at a correct diagnosis in most cases of hepatopathies. The following points may be helpful :-

Age of the patient — Age of onset — 1-3 years is the age of both Indian childhood cirrhosis and Kwashiorkor liver.

Environmental factors — Indian childhood cirrhosis is common in Indian children veno-occlusive disease leading to hepatomegaly and cirrhosis common in African children due to toxication from Bush tea. Thalassaemia are much common in West Bengal than other States of India.

Associated clinical manifestations :

Malnutrition associated with fatty liver. Hepatomegaly with jaundice in newborn and young infants — Intra-uterine infections — 'TORCH' infection; E. Coli Septicaemia, metabolic disorders, haemolytic conditions, neonatal hepatitis syndrome, congenital biliary atresia, chronic hepatitis in children and adolescents. Inherited disorders — Wilson's disease. Malignancies — secondary from leukaemia and histiocytosis, parasitic infection such as malaria and kala-azar. Various hepatotoxic agents e.g., chemicals, organophosphorus, insecticides etc. Associated bowel disorders such as in ulcerative colitis, liver abscess in amoebiasis, hepatic hydatid disease.

Associated splenomegaly :

Significant splenomegaly with hepatomegaly is present with the following infections :-

(a) Malaria and kala-azar.
(b) Infectious mononucleosis.
(c) Toxoplasmosis and cytomegalo virus disease.
(d) Tuberculosis and brucellosis.

Cellular infiltration :

Leukaemia, lymphoma, thalassaemia, sickle cell disease (Spleen may be absent in advanced disease condition) and histiocytosis 'X'.

With skin rash :

Histiocytosis 'X'.

Microcephaly or hydrocephaly :

Intrauterine infections like toxoplasmosis and cytomegalic inclusion disease, Wilson's disease.

Eyes :

Cataract and mental retardation with hypatomegaly suggest galactosemia, Lowe's syndrome, presence of Kayser Fleischer rings below the corneal margin indicates Wilson's disease, corneal opacity is seen in mucopolysaccharridosis type I (Hurler syndromes).

Neurological manifestations :

Wilson's disease presents with basal ganglion involvement — ataxia, dyskinesia, extra pyramidal signs.

Skeletal changes of Rickets — may be observed in cystinosis, tyrosinosis, Wilson's disease. Lowe's syndrome, congenital biliary atrasia with cirrhosis.

Mental retardation :

Galactosemia, Wilson's disease, tyrosinosis etc.

Laboratory investigations :

Blood : Peripheral smear aids in diagnosis of leukaemia, thalassaemia, haemoglobinopathies, parasitic disease. The reticulocytosis are noted in haemolytic anaemias specially thalassaemias. High sedimentation rate in inflamatory conditions. Special liver cells with spikes of RBC's noted in anaemias with hepatomegaly of renal origin thrombocytopenia in leukaemias, infiltrative conditions etc. Proteins are low in Kwashiorkor, with altered albumin-globulin ratio.

Liver function tests :

Transaminases are increased in parenchymatous damage of hepatocytes due to necrotic lesions of the liver and hepatitis. Alkaline phosphatase level is elevated in hepatobiliary obstruction.

Special tests :

1. Ceruloplasmin is low and copper oxidase level is high in Wilson's disease.
2. Alpha-I-antitrypsin deficiency is a newly discovered metabolic error, though rare but one of the differential diagnosis with neonatal hepatitis and cong. biliary atresia syndrome.

3. Alpha fetoprotein are raised in hepatoblastoma and neonatal hepatitis syndrome.
4. Hepatitis B antigen (E) and antibody titre in the diagnosis of serum hepatitis and chronic active hepatitis.
5. Prothrombin before and after VitK injection is a very good liver function test in general hepatic dysfunction.
6. Sweat chlorides are elevated in mucovisidoses..
7. I^{131} Rose Bengal excretion in stool distinguishes biliary atresia from neonatal hepatitis syndrome, and also lipoprotein 'X' values.
8. Ultra sound scanning of upper abdomen is useful in identification of mass lesions in the liver as cysts and tumours, identification of biliary system and gall bladder and also extent of intrahepatic fibrosis.
9. Scanning with radio active isotopes such as I^{131} Rose Bengal and 99 Tc are useful to find out intrahepatic pathology.
10. Histopathological examination of the liver biopsy specimen also with chemical staining gives a definite diagnosis in most cases of hepatomegaly.

BIBLIOGRAPHY.

1. Essentials of paediatrics by O.P. Ghai, Pub : Sagar publications, First Edition : October, 1977.
2. Nelson Text Book of Paediatrics — BEHRMAN VAUAHAN — IGAKU-SHON/ SAUNDERS International Edition Tokyo, 1983.
3. The liver and biliary system in infants and children : Edited by R.K. Chandra : Churchill Livingstore, Edinburgh, London and New York, 1979.

LIVER IN KWASHIORKOR IN CHILDREN

The literature which has gathered round this subject is extensive and almost exhaustive and yet in 1986 we can truthfully state of our present knowledge of the subject, as Descartes said of the seventeenth century medicine, "all that is known, is almost nothing compared with what remain to be known". Ignorance still prevails in various domains of this subject, unexplored fields have yet to be trodden and divergent opinions have still to be unified. With a view to answer some of these questions this investigation has been undertaken, this investigation has been mainly an observation of clinical, biochemical and histological studies. Naturally many lacunae exist which shall have to be filled in by subsequent investigators.

Material and Method

This study on liver, records clinical, biochemical and histological observations on 81 cases of kwashiorkor in children.

Each patient was studied regarding the clinical enlargement of the liver with or without splenic enlargement. In most of the cases liver function tests were done on admission and before discharge. In 20 cases liver biopsy was attempted of which 8 cases failed, in 3 cases no specimen could be brought out and in 5 cases specimen was so small, that the histologist could not give any report. Among the liver biopsy specimens, apart from general studies, special studies of the liver cells for glycogen, protein and fat contents were made.

Observations

In this series of 81 cases. 33 cases were of pre-kwashiorkor and 48 cases were of florid kwashiorkor. The name pre-Kwashiorkor has been suggested for the state of sub-clinical protein deficiency in children in which a failure of growth, reduction of serum albumin and an increased liability to diarrhoea and respiratory infections are salient clinical features. There is good reason to believe that pre-kwashiorkor is extremely common in regions where the fully developed syndrome is found. The florid case of kwashiorkor is associated with failure of growth, oedema, muscle wasting, apathy, miserable, anorexia with skin and hair changes, together with enlarged liver and signs of avitaminosis.

The classical kwashiorkor cases are in the age group of 6 months to 3 years, where as the pre-kwashiorkor cases in this series are from 1-5 years. Liver may be greatly enlarged below the costal margin and might be associated with splenic enlargement too.

TABLE – 1

Showing the Degree of Liver and Spleen Enlargement

Clinical types		Liver not palpable	Liver just palpable upto 1′ below costal margin	Liver palpable more that 1′′	Liver and spleen both palpable
Kwashiorkor	(48)	6	42	—	—
Pre-kwashiorkor	(33)	3	15	12	3

Liver enlargement of more than 1′′ below the costal margin was evident in 12 cases of pre-kwashiorkor but none in kwashiorkor but liver enlargement of 1′′ below the costal margin was evident in 42 cases of kwashiorkor and 15 cases of pre-kwashiorkor. Liver and spleen were both enlarged in 3 cases of pre-kwashiorkor, group. In 5 cases of kwashiorkor and 3 cases of pre-kwashiorkor, the liver could not be felt,reason being in kwashiorkor group there was ascites and in pre-kwashiorkor group unexplained.

Choudhuri, et. al. (1960b) observed that liver enlargement of more than 1′′ below the costal margin was evident in 34 percent of cases of kwashiorkor, while the rest had less that 1′′ or no enlargement.

Gopalan and Ramlingaswami (1953) observed enlargement of liver only in their series as follows. Moderate enlargement in 10 per cent and gross enlargement in 5 percent.

Biochemical Study

Biochemical study is to explore the function of the liver. The chief modification is in the rate of drop of proteins ir the blood (Table 2). In kwashiorkor it is always lower : below 6 g. per cent and as low as 4,3 even 2 g. per cent. There is apparently no relationship between the rate of drop in the levels of proteins and the clinical features., oedema in particular.

Gopalan, et. al. (1954) studied 207 cases of nutritional oedema syndrome and analysed total plasma proteins and the albumin fraction. The total protein and the albumin level were low in all subjects. The total protein ranged from 3.0 to 6.4 per cent with a mean of 4.5 g. per cent and albumin from 0.6 g. per cent to 2.7 g. per cent with a mean of 2.1 g. per cent. In this series of 81 cases, 48 from kwashiorkor group showing total protein 4.30 g. per cent, albumin 1.84g. per cent and globulin 3.97g. per cent and whereas in pre-kwashiorkor cases total protein 4.46 g. per cent albumin 1.93 g. per cent and globulin 3.4 g. per cent.

Table – 2
Showing the Biochemical Studies

Clinical type	No. of cases	Average total protein value in g.%	Minimum to maximum total protein level in g.%	Average albumin value in g%	Average globulin value in g.%	Thymol turbidity (units)	Serum bilirubin value (mg.%)
Kwashiorkor	13	4.30	3.30 to 6.25	1.84	3.97	5.5	0.11
Pre-kwashiorkor	11	4.46	3.19 to 7.00	1.93	3.4	6.4	0.10

Histology

The liver is extremely fatty in all cases of kwashiorkor, fat accumulates first at the periphery of the lobule, later all parts of the hepatic lobule, are involved. There are also collections of cells and an increase of reticulin in the portal tracts. In the later years of childhood, adolescence and adult life varying degrees of fibrosis around the portal tracts are seen in many of livers of those living in tropical and sub-tropical countries, it is probable that these reflect the continued strain of mild malnutrition and are seldom the sequelae of an overt attack of severe kwashiorkor. Adults may develop a fatal form of cirrhosis, occasionally this occur at a younger age. It is probable that severe and fatal cirrhosis during childhood is never due to kwashiorkor, although this may occur if other injurious agents are added. such as that of infectious hepatitis.

In this series 12 cases have been studied histologically by liver biopsy. But of 20 attempted liver biopsy cases, in 8 cases failed; in 3 cases no specimen could be brought out and in 5 cases the specimen was so small, that the histologist could not give any report. Among the liver biopsy specimen, apart from general studies, special studies were made of the liver cells for glycogen, protein and fat contents. Table 3 shows an analysis of cases from pre-kwashiorkor, and 4 cases from kwashiorkor group.

Table—3 : Showing Clinical, Biochemical and Histological Findings

Sl.No.	Name	Age	Sex	Clinical type	Short clinical history	Biochemical findings	Histological findings
1.	P.D.	5	F	Pre-kwashiorkor	Gradual wasting and occasional diarrhoea suffering from malnutrition.	Total protein 5.56%, albumin 1.87%, globulin 3.69%, cholesterol 111.1 mg.% and thymol turbidity 2.9 units.	A few lobules are smaller in size, a general view shows that there are areas of comparatively healthy cells which show the staining with haematoxyline but the majority areas are eosinophilic in character, indicating poor ribonucleic acid content. Scattered inflammatory cells in the remnants of sinusoids and periportal tracts. Most of the cells show degenerative changes with vaculation look like fatty changes but are actually due to loss of nucleus. (Fig.14.6).
2.	S.	4½	F	—do—	Same history	Total protein 5.25% albumin 1.31 g.% gobulin 3.94 g.%, alkaline phosphatase 13.6% (K A units) thymol turbidity 4.0 units	picture same as above only more eosinophilic hyaline changes
3.	T.	5	F	—do—	Past history of recurrent diarrhoea on the top of malnutrition, liver and spleen enlarged, firm, not tender. Free fluid present in peritoneal cavity	Total protein 7.0%, albumin 2.25 %, globulin 4.75%, alkaline phosphatase 18.8 units (K & A). Thymol turbidity 0.8 units	Section shows extensive fibrosis, with scanty liver cells which are degenerated, mitosis of the liver cells, present in some places but regenerative healthy liver cells are few, very suggestive of cirrhosis.
4.	S.G.	1½	M	—do—	History of fever; diarrhoea, inadequate diets, one brother died of same sorts of ailments, liver and spleen palpable, firm and not tender	Alkaline phosphatase 4.84 units. Thymol turbidity 2.5 units.	Periportal area shows proliferations of fibroblasts extending from that area towards liver lobules. Kupffer cells in the affected areas show proliferation, the sinusoides are practically absent except in places. In one area partial pseudolobulation taken place. Liver cells in the included areas show enlargement, swelling and eosinophilic granules with slight pykhosis of the nuclei. It is partial pseudolobulation suggestive of early cirrhosis. Fig.14.7)

Table contd......

Sl.No.	Name	Age	Sex	Clinical type	Short clinical history	Biochemical findings	Histological findings
5.	M.S.	½	F	Kwashiorkor	History of gradual oedema, inadequate diet and skin changes. Liver palpable and tender.	Total protein 4.37%, cholesterol 210.0 mg.%, serum bilirubin 0.11 m.g%	Section shows extensive fatty degeneration of liver parenchyma.
6.	R.	2	M	—do—	History of sudden onset with oedema, typical skin changes	Total protein 4.19%. Thymol Turbidity 5.5 units, serum bilirubin 0.11 mg.%	Section shows extensive fatty changes.
7.	B.D.	5	M	Pre-kwashi-orkor	Past history of Kala-azar and measles present, duration of illness for 3 years (Fig.14.8)	Total protein 6.26g%, albumin 3.25%, globulin 3.01%, alkaline phosphatses 40.4 units. Thymol Turbidity 2.9 units.	The liver substances have come out only in bits due to its fibrotic changes. Two marked features are seen (1) necrosis of the liver cells in large sheets and columns, but the cells that are intact are fairly healthy. Inflammatory cells are present, (2) marked fibroblastic proliferation with collagen formation in places and entangling in the scar tissue proliferating bile cana-liculi. The cells that are intact fairly healthy but some of them show eosinophilic staining due to granular degneration.
8.	K.P.	2½	M	—do—	History of diarrhoea followed by odema, liver, palpable, firm and not tender.	Total protein 4.79 g.%, Albumin 1.06 g.%, globulin 3.33 g.%	Section shows, cellular degeneration, fatty changes and in some places also remnant of fibrosis.
9.	T.	5	F	Pre-kwashi-orkor	History of anorexia, swelling of abdomen, liver — palpable, free fluid present in peritoneal cavity	Total protein 6.25 g.%, bilirubin 0.1 mg.%. Icteric index 2.0 units, fasting blood sugar 68.9 mg.%	Section shows periportal fibrosis, cell cords are intact, sinusoids are patent, with Kupffer cells proliferation and cell degeneration are seen; in some cases early stage of cirrhosis.
10.	B.D.	1½	F	Kwashiorkor	History of stunted growth, oedma, skin changes and evidence of tuberculosis of the lung	Total protein 4.062 g.%	Section shows extensive fatty changes
11.	K.D.	2	F	—do—	History of stunted growth, oedema,, diarrhoea and skin changes present from 9 months of ago	Total protein 4.81 g.%. Thymol turbidity 5.0 units albumin 1.60% globulin 3.21%	Section shows extensive fatty degeneration of liver parenchyma
12.	S.B.	5	M	Pre-kwashi-orkor	Gradual loss of weight, recurrent diarrhoea, bronchitis since the age of 2 years	Albumin 2.25%, globulin 3.50%. Thymol turbidity 7.7 units, cholesterol 200 mg.%, serum bilirubin 0.1 mg.%	Section shows fatty degeneration of liver parenchyma and also fibrosis of cirrhosis.

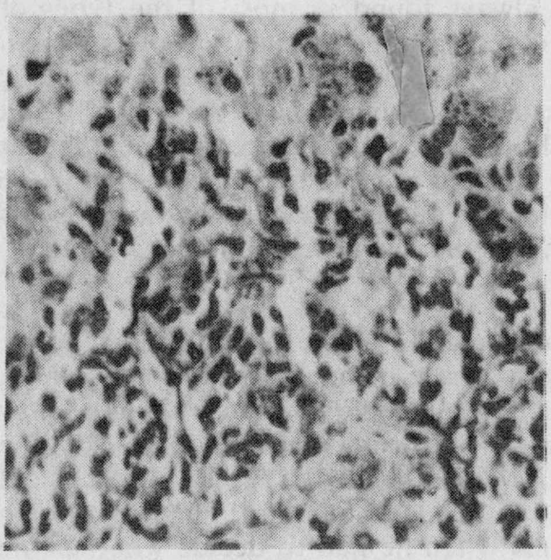

Fig.14.6 : Case of Pre-kwashiorkor

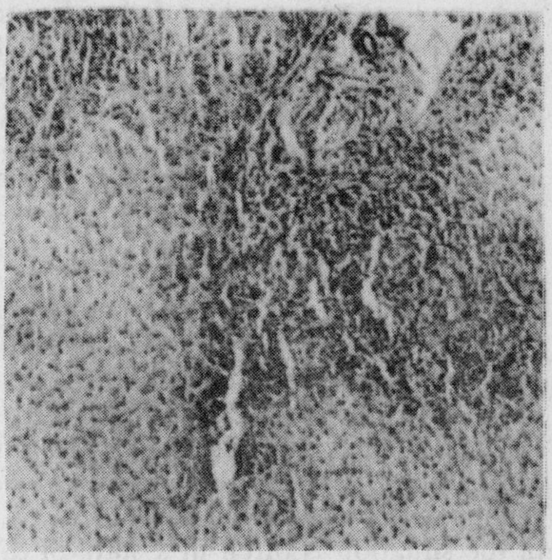

Fig.14.7 : Case of Pre-kwashiorkor with early cirrhosis.

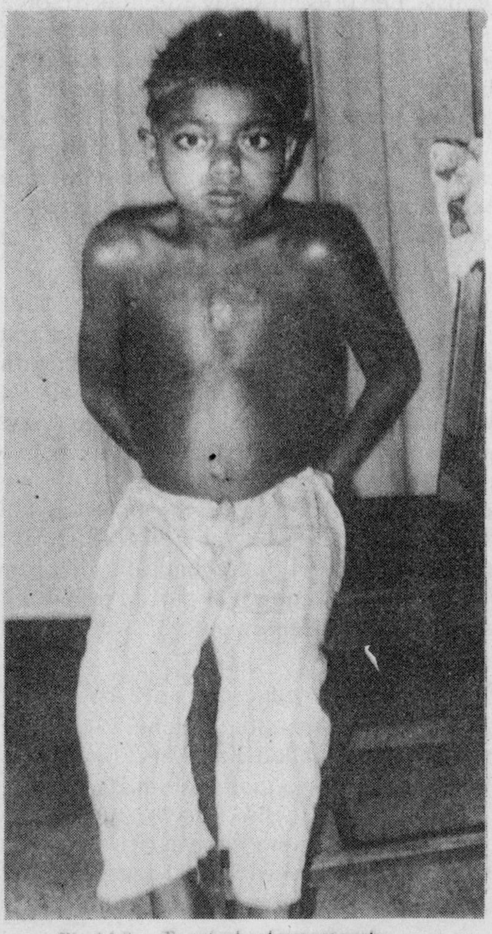

Fig.14.8 : Tropical spleenomegaly Kala-azar showing huge spleen

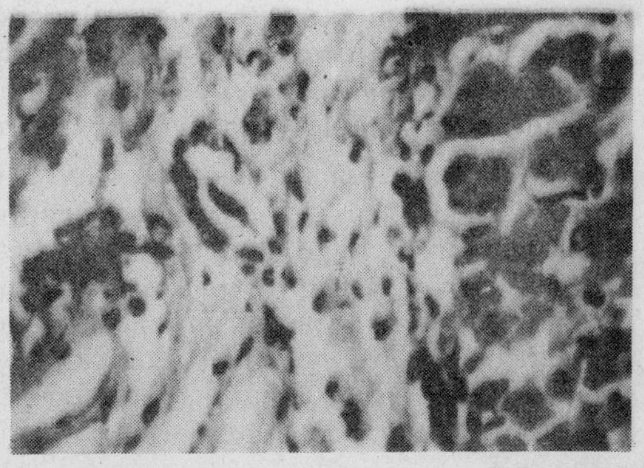

Fig.14.9 : Case of Kala azar

A moderate to marked fatty change is always found in most of the types of kwashiorkor. The fat appears first in the periportal area as small droplets, which coalesce to form large fat globules filling practically the whole cell. In florid kwashiorkor cases, the fat globules on adjoining liver cells fuse, breaking through the cell walls and look like 'Fat-cyst' which are lined by liver cell nuclei. With adequate treatment the fat disappears in the reverse order and the fatty changes are totally reversible. Although there is an increase in the numbers of lymphocytes and plasmocytes in the sinusoids during recovery the available evidence indicates that cirrhosis is not a late result.

Discussion

The child with a florid clinical picture of advanced kwashiorkor is not a diagnostic problem. However, such is not the case, with a case of pre-kwashiorkor in whom besides recurrent attacks of respiratory infections and frequent loose stools with or without demonstrable infections and infestations of the intestines a moderate degree of hepatomegaly is detected. Even here it is very difficult to co-relate the clinical finding with biochemical derangements of hepatocellular function. The pediatrician in the situation is often in a state of dilemma when he had to decide whether the hepatomegaly can be safely ignored or whether it needs further investigation to find out the histopathological changes by liver biopsy. The present study attempts to solve some of the enigmas of kwashiorkor and points to a very profitable field of study of early cases of kwashiorkor, who might progress to florid cases with repeated onslaught of infections and infestations and succumbed to the disease. Having excluded other causes of hepatomegaly by clinical and laboratory tests, the author wanted to show by histology study of liver cells that even in pre-kwashiorkor, there is also change of normal liver architecture. More so, where there are history of prolong mild, moderate and severe infections with malnutrition the liver biopsies revealed varying degrees of abnormalities including changes of early to advanced stage of cirrhosis.

In per-kwashiorkor cases where the history of repeated mild infections like recurrent attack of diarrhoea and respiratory infections were present, the histology of liver showed varying degrees of cellular degeneration, inflammatory cells infiltration and marked fibroblastic proliferation. Most of the cells show degnerative changes with vaculation look like fatty changes but are actually due to loss of nucleus. A general view shows more comparatively healthy cells which show the staining with haematoxyline but the majority are eosinophilic in character, indicating poor ribonucleic acid content. On the other hand in a few pre-kwashiorkor cases with history of long standing previous infections like measles, malaria and kala-azar the parenchynal damage of the liver shows extensive fibrosis, with scanty liver cells which are degenerated, mitosis of the liver cells present in some places but regenerative healthy liver cells are few, very suggestive of early cirrhosis. In some areas partial pseudolobulation takes place. Liver cells in the included area show enlargement, swelling and eosinophilic granules with slight pyknosis of the nuclei.

In florid cases of kwashiorkor, varying degrees of cell degeneration are associated with fatty changes. In some of the sections show extensive fatty degeneration. The cell walls are in some section given away and forming so called 'Fat-cysts'. In my own material I have found varying degrees of celullar infiltration and fibrosis in association with fatty liver. Apart from the general study of liver cells, I have studied the behaviour of glycogen and protein in fatty liver. As like others, such as Sriramachari et. al. (1953), I found that there are no gross changes with intracellular glycogen and protein content of liver cells, even with mild to moderate degree of fatty infiltration in the cells.

Summary and Conclusion

In this series of 81 cases, 48 cases of kwashiorkor and 33 cases of pre-kwashiorkor, the author has attempted to correlate the clinical hepatomegaly with biochemical derangements of hepatic functions with the histological studies. Biochemical studies reveal hypoalbuminaemia in all the cases studied by the author and previous workers also in this field observed the same features of hypoproteinaemia with hypoalbuminaemia in their series. The albumin and globulin reversal is noticed in all the patients while the flocculation test remains within normal limits with exception of high normal values observed in pre-kwashiorkor cases. The above biochemical studies raised the question of depression of liver function to explain reduction of albumin with reversal of albumin and globulin ratio but normal flocculation test with normal serum bilirubin value do not point to the impairment of hepatocellular function.

In kwashiorkor and Pre-kwashiorkor, the liver cells show degenerative changes indicated by their eosinophilic characters and poor ribonucleic acid content while extensive fibrosis with degenerated mitosis of the liver cells and occasional fatty changes were observed, which raised the question of early cirrhotic changes. Incidentally, the cirrhotic changes in varying degrees are only found in cases having history of recurrent infections of varying duration. This explains the occurrence of possible cirrhotic changes mainly in those cases of kwashiorkor and pre-kwashiorkor wtih infection in the background.

References

Chaudhuri, R.N., Basu, A.K. and Bhattacharya, A.K. Bull. Cal. Sch. Trop. Med., 8 : 95, 1960 a.

Idem—Ibid., 8:95, 1960b.

Gopalan, C. and Ramlingaswami, V — Indian. J. Med. Res. 43:751, 1953.

Gopalan, C. Venkatchalam, P.S. and Srikantia. S.S..— Indian J. Med. Resh., 42 : 4, 1954.

S. Sriramachari & V. Ramalingaswami 'Liver changes in Kwashiorkora' Indian journal of Paed. 20:77:1: 1953.

HANDLING OF GLUCOSE IN DISEASES OF THE LIVER IN CHILDREN

Introduction

The liver is the most important organ in the body for the maintenance of a normal concentration of blood glucose. The carbohydrate homeostasis is maintained by liver in four major pathways : (1) storage of carbohydrate in the form of glycogen, (2) synthesis of carbohydrate chiefly glucose by gluconeogenesis, (3) release of glucose from glycogen and (4) conversion of carbohydrate to fat. The storage of carbohydrate as glycogen requires uptake of glucose from portal venous blood into the hepatocytes and the enzyme glycogen synthetase. Regulation of this enzyme is mediated by cyclic AMP whose levels in the liver are elevated by glucagon (leading to depressed glycogen synthesis) and reduced by insulin (leading to increased glycogen synthesis). Gluconeogenesis, the synthesis of glucose from amino acids, which is of greatest importance in the late foetal and neonatal periods, is of functional significance later in life only when the amount of carbohydrate available is reduced. At this time gluconeogenesis may be increased by glucagon release.

Glucose release from glycogen is dependent on the phosphorylase enzyme (protein kinase, phosphorylase kinase and phosphorylase itself) whose activities are also mediated by cyclic AMP. In the normal adult, liver is capable of producing 8 to 16 gms. of glucose per hour, but glycogen stores for the maintenance of normal blood sugar are sufficient for only 24 hours in the absence of adequate replacement. In children, the reserve is considerably smaller, hence there is an increased susceptibility to hypoglycaemia specially with malnutrition. The conversion of carbohydrate to fat occurs only during increased carbohydrate intake and only when glycogen storage is completely saturated.

The importance of the liver for regulation of carbohydrate homeostasis is demonstrated by the occurrence of fasting hypoglycaemia in situations of mild hepatic injury. Felig et. al. (1970) noted that even in the presence to benign viral hepatitis (without massive or submassive necrosis), clinically, an apparent fasting hypoglycaemia is present in half of the subjects appropriately studied. In these patients, blood glucose responses to glucagon are lower than normal and plasma amino acid levels do not fall normally after the administration of the later hormone. Hepatocellular glycogen content, estimated histochemically, is also reduced.

However, in chronic liver disease, notably cirrhosis, hypoglycaemia is rare, whereas impairment in glucose tolerance has been reported (Hed 1958, Creutzfeld et al 1962, Megysi et al 1967). The mechanism of this "hepatogenous diabetes" has not, however, been established. In this paper, we will review briefly the characteristics of glucose intolerance in cirrhosis and discuss some of our own recent observations on hepatic glucose metabolism in normal children and compare the same in protein-calorie malnutrition (PCM), congestive cardiac failure (CCF) and nephrotic syndrome cases where long-standing parenchymatous damage of liver have been observed clinically, biochemically, histologically with histochemical studies; also assessment of carbohydrate metabolism by glucose tolerance tests and serum insulin assay.

MATERIAL AND METHODS

Forty diseased children with hepatic damage, of 1 and 12 years of age, selected from those who were admitted in the Paediatric Ward of Chittaranjan Hospital, National Medical College, Calcutta, together with 10 age and sex-matched normal children from among the children of hospital staff formed the material of this study. These 40 children were suffering from cirrhosis, protein-calorie malnutrition (PCM), nephrotic syndrome and congestive cardiac failure (CCF). The selected cases showed clinically long-standing hepatic enlargement of more than 4-6 weeks' duration with or without splenic enlargement. The liver function tests (including total protein, albumin/globulin ratio, alkaline phosphatase and SGPT) proved derangement and parenchymatous damage of chronic in nature which were again confirmed histologically in a few cases by liver biopsy. Also in a few selected cases the nature of protein, fat and glycogen studies were done by histochemical studies. Then finally metabolic studies were done by glucose tolerance test. Initially fasting blood sugar levels were done. Those who had fasting blood sugar in between 70 mg. and 100 mg. per 100 ml. were termed as normoglycaemic, those who had above 100 mg. per 100 ml. hyperglycaemic and those with value below 70 mg. per 100 ml., within 20-70 mg. per 100 ml., but who did not manifest clinical symptoms, as hypoglycaemic. They were further studied with oral and/or intravenous glucose tolerance tests. The serum insulin assay was done along with the glucose tolerance. As far as possible, the standard techniques were undertaken for estimation of blood glucose, serum insulin and liver function test.

The glucose tolerance tests and insulin assay were done in ten normal children, with comparable age, sex, and weight groups who were kept as control and who at the time of investigation were not suffering from any gross ailments or having no family history of diabetes, clinical hepatomegaly or not having drugs which might interfere with the investigations.

OBSERVATIONS

IN CONTROL SUBJECTS

The results of glucose tolerance and insulin assay in the ten control subjects are discussed below. Here, we should mention that especially in children, the duration of fasting influenced the fasting blood sugar level and also the levels reached at 1,2 and 3 hours after the glucose load, the peaking of the blood sugar at one half hour and the first hour was influenced by the concentration of the sugar solution and stomach emptying time. The blood sugar and serum insulin values during oral glucose tolerance tests (OGTT) in the age group of 1-5 years differ form those of 5-12 years. The normal value for girls and boys in the age group of 5-12 years varied, even single high blood sugar values at the first hour or second hour showed unreliable result, so assessment was done on the total interpretation of values in glucose tolerance level.

Oral glucose was given as a 25 per cent solution with flavouring agent according to the following dosages : 1-3 years of age — 2 gm. per kg. of body weight, 3-12 years — 1.75 gm. per kg. of body weight after a fasting blood sugar sample has been taken. The method followed was Peroxidase method and venous blood was taken as a sample. Blood samples were obtained at 30, 60, 90 and 120 minutes. In addition to glucose, serum insulin assay was done.

The criteria of normal OGTT showed glucose values all below 180 mg. per 100 ml. with a maximum at 60 minutes and fasting levels restored within 90-120 minutes. Elevated glucose values with a 2-hour value above 120 mg. per 100 ml. indicated diabetes mellitus (because similar curves noticed in liver disease). Flat curves with only smaller rises, less than 20 mg. per 100 ml. above the fasting level, were usually noted as flat curve associated with malnutrition and malabsorbtion. Figure 1 shows blood sugar level and serum insulin values calculated from the average figures of control cases.

IN DISEASED SUBJECTS

In 40 diseased children after clinical and biochemical confirmations, metabolic study was undertaken. The distribution of normoglycaemia, hyperglycaemia and hypoglycaemia according to fasting blood sugar samples were determined. The distribution of the cases, according to fasting blood sugar sample is shown in Table 1.

These cases may be further classified under the heading of normal, diabetic (both typical and lag curve) and flat curve according to the curves observed in OGTT. The distribution of cases according to OGTT study is shown in Table 2.

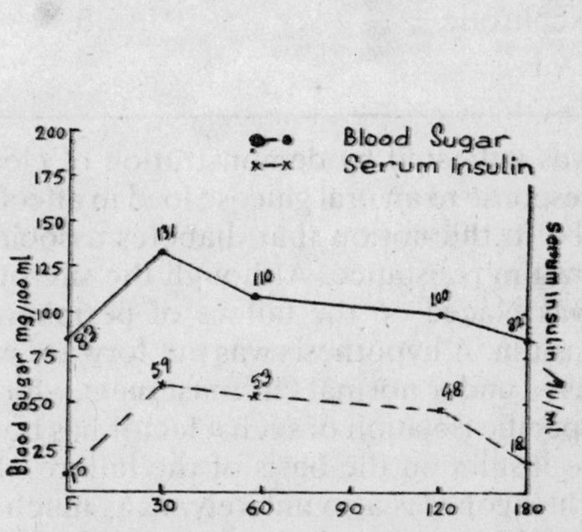

Fig.14.10 : Blood sugar and serum insulin during the standard OGTT in children.

It is evident from Table 2 that out of 40 cases typical diabetes curve was observed in 3 cases and lag curve in 4 cases. Flat curve was observed in 12 cases. Normal curve was seen in 21 cases. Only in 3 cases (30 per cent) flat curve was observed in PCM but no diabetic curve was observed. Five cases (50 per cent) of diabetic curve and 3 cases of flat curve were seen in cirrhosis. Two cases of flat curve and 1 case of lag curve were observed in CCF. Flat curve was observed in 4 cases and typical diabetic curve was observed in 1 case of nephrotic syndrome.

DISCUSSION

DIABETES IN CIRRHOSIS OF LIVER : Diabetes was noted in patients with cirrhosis with an incidence of 40 per cent. Milder impairment of glucose tolerance, as determined by OGTT as lag curve has been observed in 25 per cent and gross intolerance as typical "diabetic curve" in 15 per cent of cirrhosis cases. The insulin deficiency was not the sole or primary factor responsible for "hepatogenous diabetes"

TABLE 1

Showing the Distribution of Cases According to Fasting Blood Sugar Samples

Clinical type	Normoglycaemia (28)	Hyperglycaemia (8)	Hypoglycaemia (4)
Cirrhosis of Liver	6	4	—
PCM	5	2	3
Nephrotic	9	1	—
CCF	8	1	1

TABLE 2

Showing the Distribution of Cases According to OGTT

Clinical type	Normal	Diabetic		Flat
		Typical	Lag	
Cirrhosis of Liver	2	2	3	3
PCM	7	—	—	3
Nephrotic	5	1	—	4
CCF	7	—	1	2

was indicated by demonstration of elevated rather than diminished insulin levels in response to an oral glucose load in affected patients. The presence of hyperinsulinaemia led to the notion that diabetes associated with liver disease was a consequence of insulin resistance. Although the site of insulin resistance was not defined, emphasis was placed on the failure of peripheral tissue rather than the liver, to respond to insulin. A hypothesis was put forward which implied the production of a factor by the liver under normal circumstances which increased peripheral glucose consumption; specific isolation of such a factor has not however been reported. Peripheral resistance to insulin on the basis of the failure of the cirrhotic liver to adequately metabolize glucagon was also unlikely, in as much as a peripheral action of glucagon on glucose uptake was not demonstrated (Bondy et al 1956). More recently, an elevation in growth hormone, a factor known to decrease the effectiveness of insulin on peripheral tissues were reported in cirrhosis (Samgan et al 1969, Conn et al 1970). However, the incidence of diabetes in cirrhosis was considerably higher than that reported in acromegaly (Luft et al 1967). It was thus apparent that neither direct nor strong indirect evidence was available to implicate peripheral adipose tissue or muscle as the primary site of insulin resistance in liver disease.

From the foregoing it was apparent that (a) the liver was the principal site of action of small increments in insulin, (b) in the cirrhotics, an inadequacy of insulin was associated with altered intrahepatic processes resulting in augmented glucose production independent of peripheral supply of precursors, (c) chronic parenchymal damaged liver tissue resulted the hepatocytes to increase insulin resistance. It would appear therefore that the hepatic rather than the peripheral response to a given level of insulin was generally the key determinant of the state of glucose tolerance. This hepatic resistance to insulin might be due in part to increased glucagon level as a consequence of portal systemic shunting and/or hepatocellular injury. As compensatory mechanism, plasma insulin level was increased. In those patients who fail to achieve adequate hyperinsulinaemia, glucose intolerance developed. The postulated mechanism of glucose intolerance is shown in Fig.14.11

Fig.14.11 Showing Postulated Mechanism of Glucose Intolerance in Liver Disease.

Chronic liver disease
Hyperglucagonaemia
Hepatic resistance to insulin
Glucose intolerance
Hyperinsulinaemia
(compensatory)
Hepatogenous diabetes

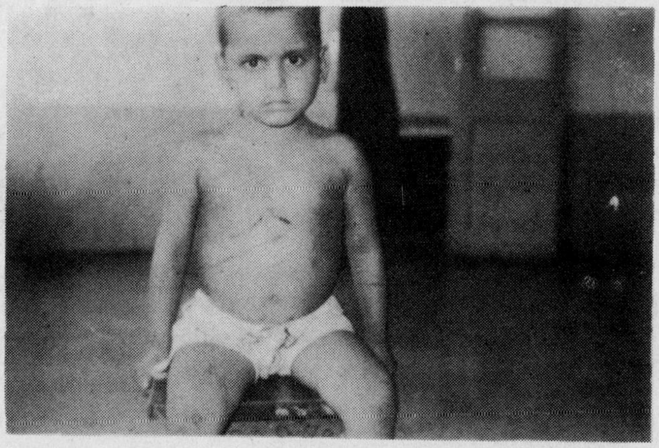

Fig.14.12 : Indian childhood cirrhosis.

Illustrative Case. A typical case, G.M., aged 4½ years with past history of infective hepatitis presented with cirrhosis, clinical hepatomegaly and splenic enlargement (Fig.14.12). Liver function tests : Total protein—4 gm. per cent, albumin : 1.5 gm. per cent, globulin : 2.5 gm. per cent, serum bilirubin—5.4 mg. per cent alkaline phosphatase — 20.7 units (K.A.), SGPT 307.5 units. Metabolic studies of OGTT and insulin values are shown in fig.14.13.

Histology — Histological study from material obtained by liver biopsy showed (Fig.14.5) : Periportal area — proliferation of fibroblasts extending from that area towards liver lobules. Kupffer cells in the affected areas show proliferation, the sinusoids are practically absent except in places. In the area partial pseudolobulation had taken place. Liver cells in the areas examined show enlargement, swelling and eosinophilic granules with slight pyknosis of the nuclei. It was partial pseudolobulation, suggestive of cirrhosis.

The illustrative case corroborated our findings in various studies on diabetic curve with high insulin values in a case of cirrhosis.

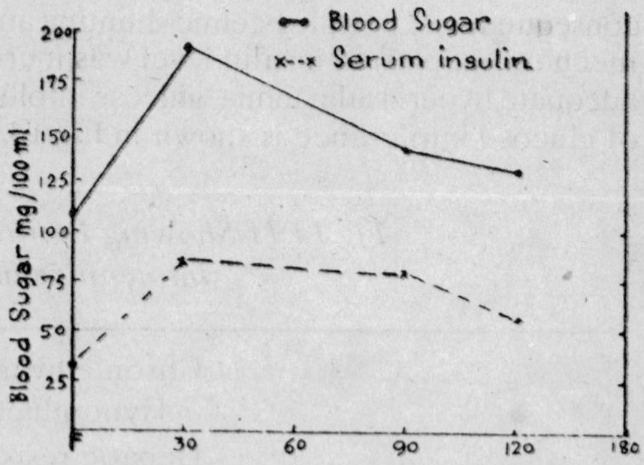

Fig.14.13 : Showing the typical diabetic curve in 8 cases of cirrhosis with insulin values.

PROTEIN-CALORIE MALNUTRITION AND DIABETES. Though abnormal oral and intra-venous glucose tolerance is very common in PCM (Baig et al 1965), Cook 1967, Heard 1966, Becker et al 1971). The precise role of insulin lack and antagonism is uncertain. There have been reports of persistence of abnormal glucose tolerance years after the acute attack of PCM (Cook 1968). This coupled with the high prevalence of non-alcoholic pancreatic diabetics in under-privileged communities (Sharper 1960, Ramaligaswami 1969) has led to the speculationn that malnutrition in childhood might predispose to adult diabetes mellitus. Our studies including OGTT and insulin values before, during and after treatment correlated with biochemical and histological studies (as illustrated below).

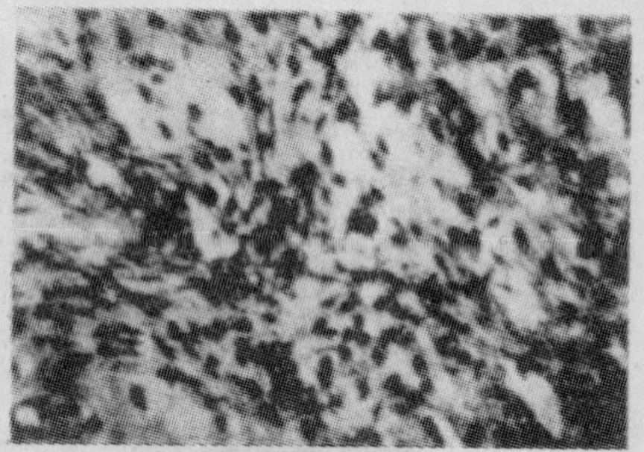

Fig.14.14 : Pseudolobular formation in cirrhosis

Illustrative Case. C.S., aged 18 months, female, coming from lower socio economic status, body weight 14 lbs. was admitted with typical features of PCM (kwashiorkor) with hepatomegaly (Fig.14.15). Liver function tests — Total protein — 2.53 gm. per cent, albumin — 1.07 gm. per cent, glubulin — 1.46 gm. per cent, cholesterol — 151.2 mg. OGTT and insulin values on admission are shown in Fig.14.16. Histological studies with special histochemical pattern of glycogen and protein are shown in Fig.14.17 and 14.18.

Histology — The changes that took place in PCM during the active stage of malnutrition are shown in Fig.14.19. The histological report reads as follows : "A few lobules are smaller in size, a general view shows that there are areas of comparatively healthy cells which takes the hematoxyline stain but the majority areas are eosinophilic in character indicating poor ribonucleic acid content. Scattering inflammatory cells in the remnants of sinusoids and periportal tracts. Most of the cells show degenerative changes with vacuolation which look like fatty changes but are actually due to loss of nucleus".

Follow-up — After 6 weeks of treatment, the case was followed up (Fig.14.20) with biochemical improvement and the repeat OGTT and insulin values are shown in Fig.14.21 which correlated again with histological study (Fig.14.22).

Insulin resistance is known to occur in PCM (K) (Alleryne et al 1972). A number of humoral antagonists to insulin are known to be elevated in PCM. Human growth hormone levels are grossly raised and fail to be suppressed adequately during an induced hyperglycaemia. Free fatty acids are elevated and plasma cortisol is raised (Primstone et al 1967, Lewis et al 1964, Alleryne 1967). Any or all of these factors may account for the insulin antagonism. It has also been suggested that enzymes of the glycolytic pathway may be deficient. Low levels of pyruvate kinase have been demonstrated (Metcoff et al 1966) and more recently the formation of lactate by musscle homogenates, taken from children with PCM, has shown to be deficient using glucose-6-phosphate and fructose—1—6-diphosphate as substrates, whereas normal responses were obtained with phosphoetanol pyruvate (Alleryne et al 1972). This suggests a block of the glycolytic pathway at the level of triose phosphate formation. It would therefore appear that both humoral antagonists and deficiency of tissue enzymes may account for insulin antagonism in PCM. In conclusion glucose tolerance was almost invariably abnormal in PCM in out studies in more than 30 per cent of cases, but after adequate dietary therapy the disturbance was of short duration only. Thus in the absence of a recurrence of severe malnutrition, PCM does not seem to predispose to pancreatic diabetes in the adult.

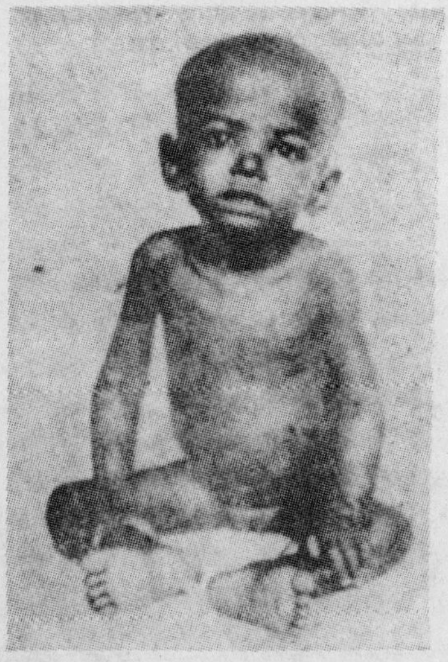

Fig.14.15 : Case of Kwashiorkor

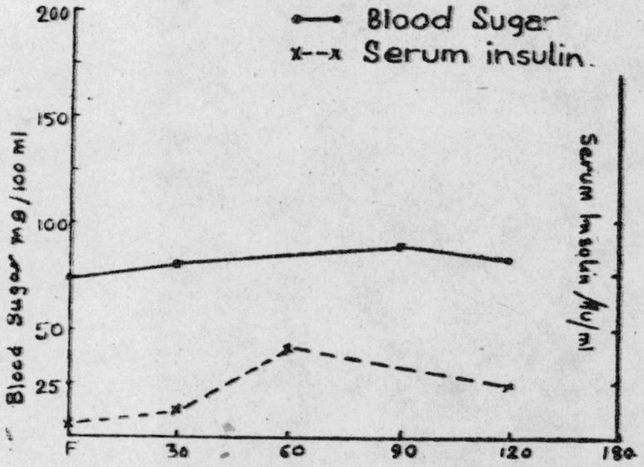

Fig.14.16 : OGTT and insulin values in PCM on admission.

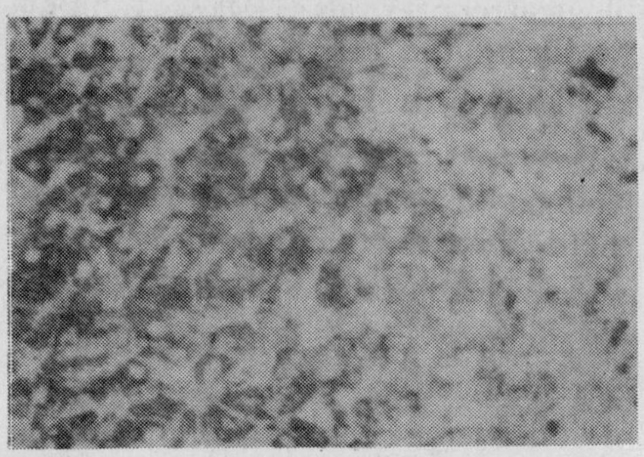

Fig.14.17 : Glycogen staining in hepatic parenchyma

Fig.14.18 : Special protein stain of hepatocytes

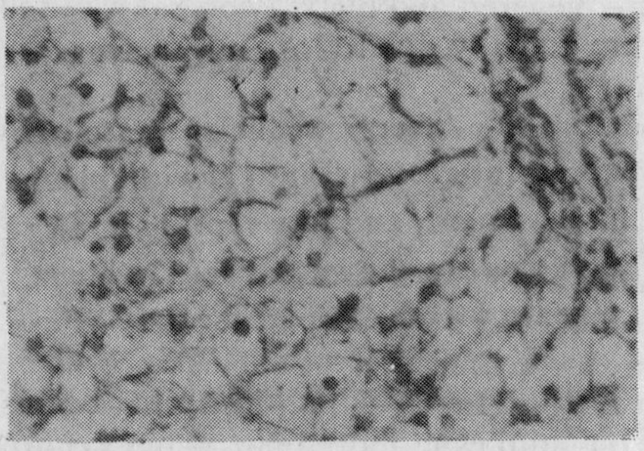

Fig.14.19 : Fatty liver

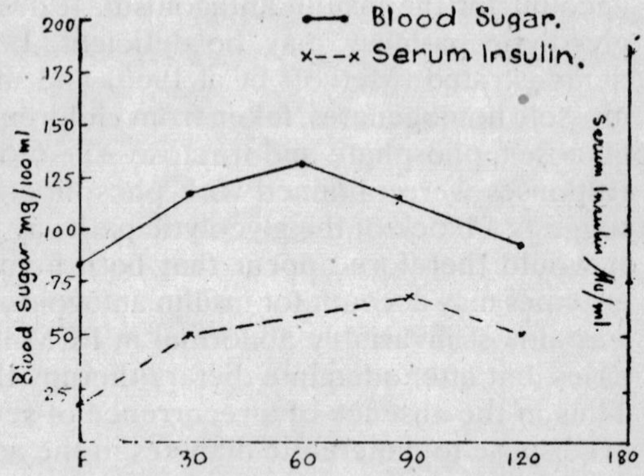

Fig.14.21 : OGTT and insulin values after 6 weeks of treatment.

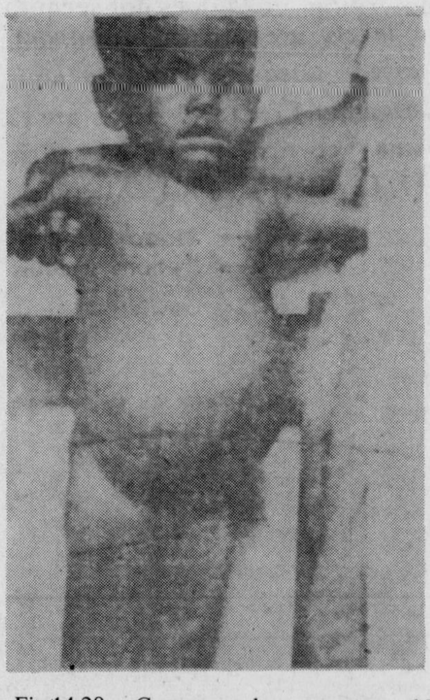

Fig.14.20 : Gomez syndrome — treated PCM

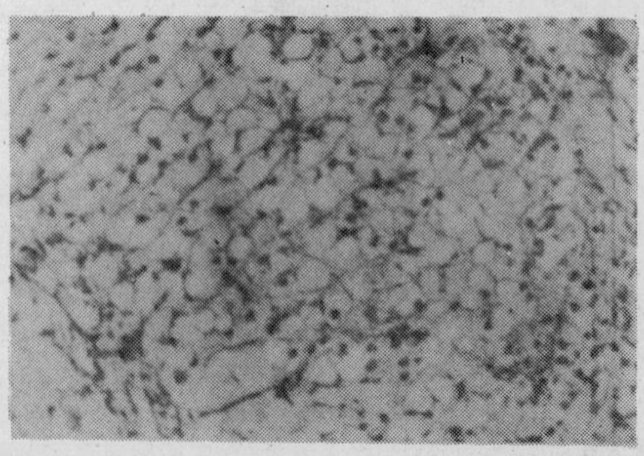

Fig.14.22 : Hepatic changes in PCM with diabetic treatment of 6 weeks.

NEPHROSIS AND CONGESTIVE CARDIAC FAILURE AND DIABETES. We have included nephrotics and CCF cases in out study to correlate the metabolic normality in spite of gross parenchymatous damage in livers in the above conditions. Here we shall review only two abnormal cases from each group of nephrotic and CCF cases. We could not conclude or put forward any hypothesis as shown in cirrhosis and PCM regarding glucose intolerance but our hope and belief are that further studies in these two categories, namely nephrotics and CCF cases of long standing, parenchymal damage of liver might have been compensated. Factors are still unknown for the maintenance of carbohydrate homeostasis in these two conditions..

Illustrative Case. R. B. aged 52 months muslim, female coming from lower socioeconomic status with poor nutrition, generalized oedema with nephrotic facies, liver enlarged moderately, no splenic enlargement. Liver function tests : Total protein — 3.23 gm. per cent, Albumin — 1.45 gm. per cent, globulin — 2.08 gm. per cent, SGPT — 130 units, cholesterol — 330.0 mg. per cent, blood urea 36.0 mg. per cent. Urine showed albumin in moderate amount, (no quantitative estimation was done). Metabolic studies OGTT and insulin values are shown in Fig.14.23

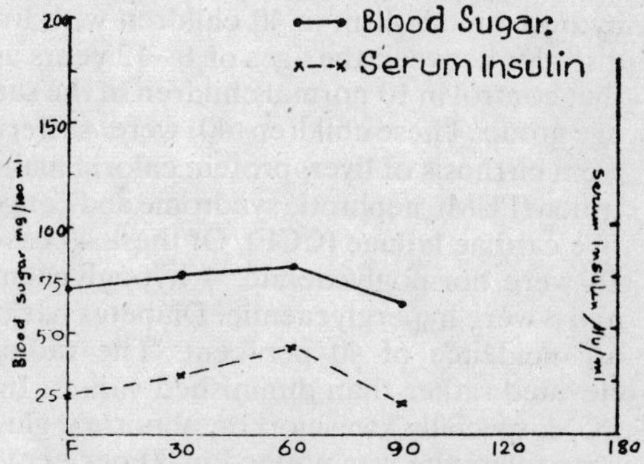

Fig.14.23 : Showing the OGTT and insulin values in a case of nephrotic syndrome.

Although in previous tables, it was shown that in nephrotics glucose intolerance was in more than 50 per cent (OGTT, 5 abnormal curves) but analysing each and individual case, the variation from the normal was negligible.

Illustrative Case. R.A., (Fig.14.24) aged 7/12 years, male nutritional status poor, coming from grade III economic status, presented with CCF of more than one month duration. Besides clinical signs of CCF, notable features were liver severely enlarged, firm, tender, with a splenic enlargement. Provisional diagnosis was CCF with VSD and respiratory infection. Liver function tests : Total protein —4.3 gm. per cent albumin —2.00 gm. per cent, globulin —2.3 gm. per cent, alkaline phosphatase —13.2 units, cholesterol —136.5 mg. per cent, SGPT —80 units, blood urea —42 mg. per cent. Urine examination — only a few pus cells without any significant accompaniment. Chest x-ray — evidence of cardiomegaly, ECG—Both left and right ventricular

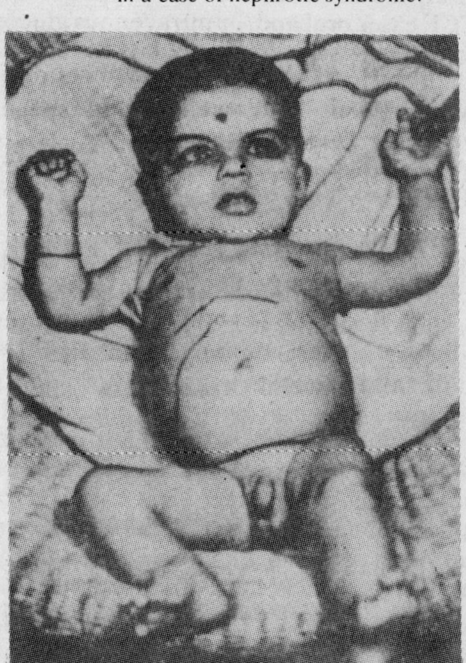

Fig.14.24 : Case of nephrosis with congestive failure and diabetes.

hypertrophy with strain pattern. Metabolic studies with OGTT and insulin values are shown in Fig.14.25

Histology—Histological study (Fig.14.26) revealed periportal fibrosis, intact cell cords, patent sinusoids with Kupffer cells proliferation and degeneration in some areas, suggestive of early stage of cirrhosis.

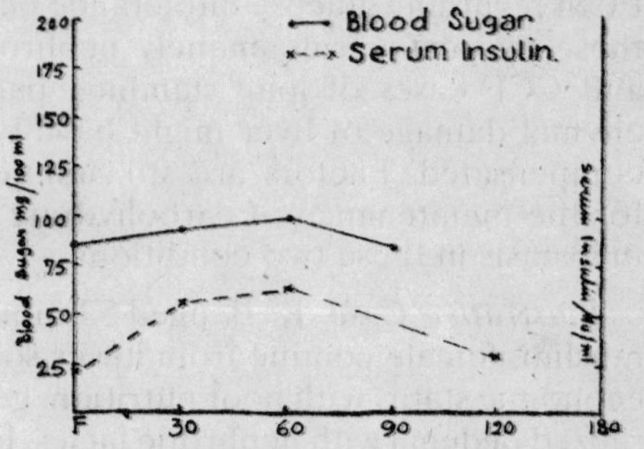

Fig.14.25 : OGTT and insulin values in a case of CCF.

SUMMARY AND CONCLUSION

This study assesses the role of liver in carbohydrate metabolism in 40 children with liver disorder between the ages of 1—12 years and that control in 10 normal children of the same age group. These children (40) were suffering from cirrhosis of liver, protein calorie malnutrition (PCM), nephrotic syndrome and congestive cardiac failuae (CCF). Of these 40 cases, 28. were normoglycaemic, 4 hypoglycaemic and 8 were hyperglycaemic. Diabetes has been noticed in patients with cirrhosis with an incidence of 40 per cent. The radioimmunoassay of serum insulin revealed elevated rather than diminished values. In PCM, specially kwashiorkor, abnormal glucose tolerance was noticed in 30 per cent, but the serum insulin levels were not precisely low in all cases. In the nephrotics and CCF cases oral and/or intravenous glucose tolerance tests were normal. It is thus concluded that hepatic rather than the peripheral response to a given level of insulin is generally the determinant of the state of glucose tolerance in chronic parenchymal damaged liver diseases.

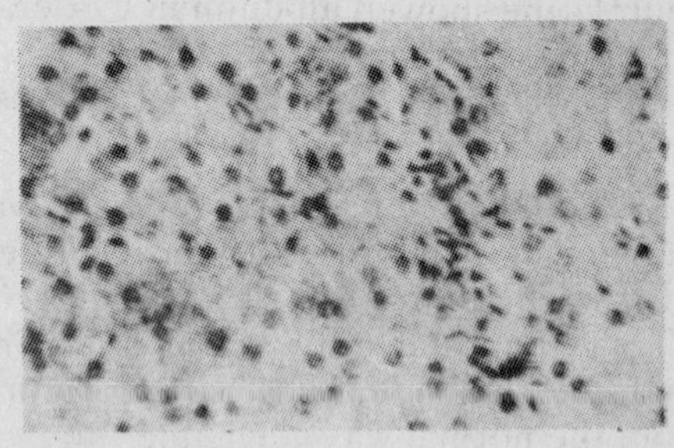
Fig.14.26 Histology of liver in CCF

In cirrhosis, the resistance to insulin might be due to increased glucagon level (not done in this study) as a consequence of portal systemic shunting and/or hepatocellular injury. As a compensatory mechanism plasma insulin level was increased. In these patients, failing to achieve hyperinsulinaemia glucose intolerance developed. In PCM cases glucose intolerance is due to both humoral antagonists as growth hormone, plasma cortisol and fatty acids and deficiency of tissue enzymes pyruvate kinase, gulcose-6-phosphate, fructose-1-6-diphosphate (not done in this study) which may account for insulin antagonism. OGTT was abnormal in more than 30 per cent of our series in PCM but after adequate dietary therapy the disturbance was of short duration. Thus in the absence of a recurrence of severe malnutrition, PCM does not seem to predispose to pancreatic diabetes in the adult. In nephrotics and CCF cases, the glucose tolerance were observed by OGTT of abnormal curves were observed, specially in nephrotics.

References

Alleryne, G. A. O., Trest, P. M., Flores, H. and Robin, H. *Pro. J. Nutnt.*, 27 : 585, 1972.

Alleryne G. A. O. and Young, V. H. -*Clin. Sci,* 33 : 189, 1976.

Bondy. P.K. and Cardillo. L. R. J. *Clin. Invest.*, 35 : 494,1956.

AETIOPATHOGENESIS OF CHRONIC LIVER DISEASE IN CHILDREN WITH SPECIAL REFERENCE TO DIFFUSE HEPATIC INVOLVEMENT

ABSTRACT

A study of aetiopathogenesis was undertaken in 58 patients suffering from chronic liver diseases in children specially with diffuse hepatic involvement. The data is lacking in children. But chronic diseases occur in considerable fewer than 5 percent. Incidence in this study is 1.7%. The total number of cases studied includes clinical, biochemical, bacteriological, histological and in three cases autopsy studies to find out the aetiological background of these various chronic liver disease conditions. The aetiological classification were based on (1) congenital (2) posthepatitic (3) malnutrition with infection and infestation (4) Indian childhood cirrhosis (5) infiltrative, metabolic and/or neoplastic and undetermined aetiology. The post-hepatic was 13.79%, then malnutrition with protozoal infection and infestation 12.06%. Thalassaemia syndromes 10.34% and Indian Childhood cirrhosis 8.62% respectively. The mortality was 13.73%.

INTRODUCTION

In chronic hepatopathies in many cases of chronic childhood liver disease, if not the majority, there are no recognisable preceeding acute episodes. Commonly the acute attack is superimposed on a chronic malady in primary malnutrition. Various tropical infections and infestations, moreover genetically predisposed (Indian Childhood Cirrhosis) conditions. From a practical point of view, the majority of chronic cases result in overlapping clinical and laboratory manifestations with or without clinical jaundice. Except for the large variety of tropical infections and infestations (Malaria, Kalaazar, amoebic hepatitis, hepatic hydatidosis) with chronic liver involvement and the focal disorders (Hepatic tuberculosis), there is little specificity and the pathogenesis is often ill understood in some cases of hepato-portal fibrosis leading on to non-cirrhotic portal hypertension in older children, mentioned in undetermined (more than 10%) in this study. Histological features vary from mild focal hepatocellular degeneration or portal triad cellular infiltration to extensive fibrosis and regenerative nodules. Liver biopsy particularly of the percutaneous variety, may not mirror the severity of the clinical course and more than 15% of needle biopsy show some degree of sampling errors. In many cases there are no diagnostic or pathognomic lesions that can be used to make exact reports as to etiology.

METHODS AND MATERIALS

The clinical material comprised of 58 cases of hepatopathies in the age group of 3 months to 12 years of age who were admitted in the Paediatric ward of Chittaranjan Hospital, National Medical College Calcutta during the past 2 years. The total admission during this period were 3,400 in the indoor, so the percentage of hepatopathies was 1.7%. There were 32 male children (55%) and 26(44.8%) female children. The cases showed clinically long standing hepatic enlargement from 6 weeks to 6 months standing with or without splenic enlargement with or without ascites and repeated history of upper gastrointestinal bleeding. The hepatocellular function studies include besides clinical evidences of hepatocellular degeneration, the biochemical parameters such as liver function tests corroborated with histological and in some cases histochemical studies. In some cases with evidences of portal hypertension, the radiological studies include besides demonstration of oesophageal varices, splenoportography to demonstrate the splenic pulp pressure and site of obstruction in portobiliary system. In a few children with younger age group with severe jaundice and hepatocellular damage upper abdominal sonogram and as an excretory test with 131 Iodine, rose bengal was employed. Above all in 3 cases only, the autopsy studies were done to know the clinicopathological correlation of the aetiological background of these various hepatopathies in different stages of chronic diffuse parenchymatous changes leading on to various degrees of hepato-cellular failure.

AIMS AND OBJECTIVES

There are (1) to evaluate the aetiological diagnosis of chronic parenchymatous liver changes in childhood years (2) to corroborate the biochemical changes with histological studies and also (3) to determine the risk factors involve in these cases to evaluate the prognosis and management of these cases.

OBSERVATIONS

Table — 1 :

Showing the distribution of age and sex
in those cases studied

Sex	Age group			Total
	3—12 months	1 yrs — 5 yrs	5 yrs — 12 yrs	
Male	3	8	21	32(33.17%
Female	3	6	17	26(44.85%
Total	6	14	38	58(

Table — 1 shows the distribution of age and sex, the maximum cases are from 5-12 years of age and mostly the ailments of the disease process started and continued for more than 2-3 years on an average in these cases with spikes of activity (inflammation, degeneration and regeneration of the hepatic parenchyma) in clinical presentation. The six cases noted from 3-12 months of age group were mostly with congenital hepatopathies as neonatal hepatitis and congenital biliary atresia.

The sex difference in this study was not very significant.

The socio-economic status of these children was from lower socio-economic group mostly and so in more than 75% of cases were associated with various degrees of protein energy malnutrition.

The geographical background of these children to highlight the incidence of aetiological background was stated. The children were mostly from eastern part of India, more than 90% were of Bengalies. The dietetic and feeding practices and nutritional calories derived from mixed vegetable protein sources, with a background of prolong breast feeding, the poor supplements of weaning foods,minerals and Vitamins in their early years.

The immunization status was very poor, less than 15% were immunized against small pox, tuberculosis, whooping-cough, diphtheria — Tetanus, poliomyelitis, measles and Typhoid cholera.

Table 1-A

Showing clinical picture

Signs	No. of cases	Percentage
1. Malnutrition	43	75
2. Pallor	28	48
3. Clubbing	6	10.5
4. Ascites	23	40
5. Anasarca	12	21.5
6. Hepatomegaly	31	54
7. Hepatosplenomegaly	26	45
8. Portal Hypertension	8	13.7
9. Hepato-cellular failure -CNS, Oestrogen	10	16.6
Symptoms		
1. Fever	32	55
2. Wasted extremities abdominal distension	29	50
3. Failure to thrive, anorexia, weakness, abdominal pain, Nausea-vomiting, diarrhoea	20	35
4. Jaundice	18	32
5. Gastrointestinal bleeding haematemesis, melena	7	12.8

The children with chronic hepatopathies presented with similar clinical manifestations regardless of their specific aetiology they are malnourished with 75% having wasted extremities, protuberant abdomen in more than 50% of cases. Some of them complain as general symptoms such as anorexia, weakness, abdominal pain (35%) nausea vomiting, loose motions and fever in (40%) of cases. The fever was often present with other signs of infections and infestations in (60%) of cases but in 15% cases as a sign of hepatocellular failure. The clinical jaundice was present in (32%) of cases. The oedema as generalised or only as puffy face and dependent pitting oedema in the lower limbs was present in (40%) of cases. Marked pallor was noticed in (48%) of cases, specially those with detectable anemia and history of recurrent gastrointestinal bleeding with mild to severe blood loss in (15%) of cases. In some clubbing was present with associated evidences of tuberculosis disseminated type and malabsorptive diarrhoeas.

Among the clinical signs, the hepatomegaly was present in more than (65%) of cases, in some left lobe (30%) much more enlarged than the right. The spleen was enlarged in (45%). There were two cases where splenectomy was done previously in one for hypersplenism in Thalassaemia syndrome, and the other congestive splenomegaly — due to huge splenic size presented with further evidences of portal hypertension with ascites and gastrointestinal bleeding. The venous collateral anastomosis between portal and systemic was noted only in 10% of cases.

The extrahepatic features of hepato-cellular failure such as spider-naevi, gynaecomastia, testicular atrophy or small size testis, central nervous system features as flapping tremor or brisk jerks were noticed in less than (12%) of cases either with a few signs on all together respectively. The special noticeable features of haematemesis and melena more of haematemesis than melena (not from Piles, which is rare in children) from swallowed blood was noticed in 32% of cases.

In this group, the clinical evidences of portal hypertension was present as splenomegaly with or without ascites, venous collateral anastomosis or upper abdominal venous engorgements and upper gastrointestinal bleeding.

Laboratory Investigations : It included routine blood examination — hemoglobin, total W.B.C., R.B.C., peripheral smear for demonstration of abnormal cells both in W.B.C. and R.B.C. series, platelets, reticulocyte counts, ESR besides demonstration of malarial parasites. The haemoglobin electrophoresis were done in thalassaemia syndrome. The bone-marrow study was done for demonstration of L.D. bodies, tissue histiocytes in **Histiocytosis 'X'**, leukaemias etc.

The liver function tests included routine serum Bilirubin — both direct and indirect fractions, albumin/globulin ratio transaminase (APT). The routine prothrombine time estimation was done in a few cases with risk of haemorrhages before liver biopsy was done. The serum protein electrophoresis separation was done in two cases with features of obstructive jaundice to rule out α-1-antitrypsin (PIZ) deficiency which is associated with absence of α 1-globulin fraction. Moreover to assess the prognostic value of hepatic dysfunction, the albumin level was assessed in few cases.

Table 2

Showing the abnormalities of LFT in 58 cases

LFT	No. of cases	percentage
Sr. Bilirubin	8	12%
Albumin/globulin ratio	18	32%
Alkaline phosphatase (ALP) in KA Units	18	32%
Transaminase (ATP)	14	24%
Total :	58	100%

Radiological examination : It included routine chest, skull, X-ray of hands, and moreover demonstration of oesophageal varices by Barium swallow. In 8 cases splenoportography was done to demonstrate the site of obstruction on spleno-portal tract. In one case, the combined liver scan, plain chest X-ray helped to diagnose hepatic abscess when other investigations failed to diagnose this condition. Besides the typical 'hair on end' appearance in thalassaemia, one case also showed typical osteolytic lesion with rarefaction in some places in case of histiocytosis. In some disseminated tuberculosis cases with suspicion of hepatic tuberculosis, the chest X-ray showed associated tuberculous pathology. One case of congenital syphilis with liver involvement as secondary stage of pericellular cirrhosis also showed associated osteochondritis in upper end of humerus and lower end of femur.

The special investigations included the demonstration of Australia antigen in 2 cases of posthepatitis. The ultra sound sonogram of upper abdomen was done in 2 cases of intermittant obstructive jaundice and one case of advanced cirrhosis with failure just to avoid invasive technique.

Histology : The histological studies were done in all the cases to determine the aetiopathogenesis and it was a closed needle biopsy. But in more than 15% of cases there were failure of definitive diagnosis from one criteria alone so comprehensive attitude was undertaken in this study to diagnose. In some cases of histological studies besides routine haematoxyline and eosin stain, special stains were used such as PAS, Pearl and reticulin stains to diagnose cell inclusion bodies and/or parenchymatous structures.

Broadly speaking, all the cases have been decided into three broad groups : such as (1) diffuse involvement (2) Hepato-portal sclerosis (3) obstructive features with canalicular dilatation and giant cell hepatitis. The diffuse variety is again sub classified as (a) early hydropic degeneration of hepatocytes showing early involvement of parenchyma (b) the necrosis of the liver cells in peripheral areas of the lobule and mild fibrosis with cellular infiltration in portal tract. The sinusoids have dilated. The liver cells are hydropic and found in clusters : Kupffer cells are hyperplastic. The pericellular reticulin fibers are thickened. (c) The above picture and also in some cellular membrane disrupted, mild cellular deposition of materials (d) the next stage is portal tract in filtrated with chronic inflammatory cells, and the fibroblasts. The fibroblasts from the portal tracts are spreading to all sides. The sinusoids are dilated with proliferation of Kupffer cells. The fatty changes are seen in parenchymal cells in periportal areas. The picture is of early cirrhosis (e) the lobular structure are distorted with pseudolobular formation and more of fibrosis a picture of aggressive fibrosis with peripassue regenerative nodules — suggestive of cirrhosis.

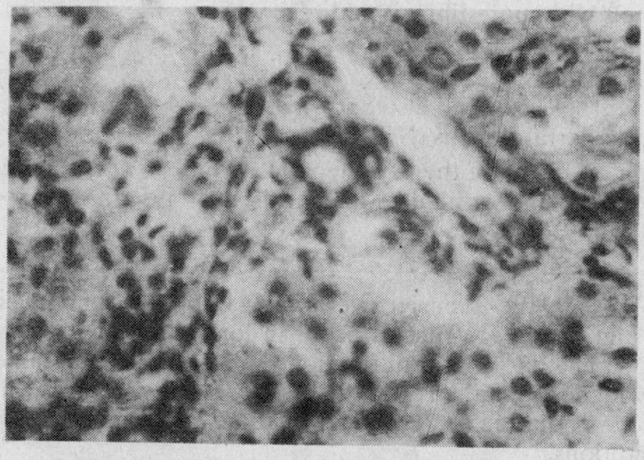

Fig.14.27 : Histology of non-cirrhotic portal fibrosis

The next big group is Hepato-portal sclerosis also known as non cirrhotic portal fibrosis (NCPF)- the central histologic features are of portal obstruction with fibrosis, intimal thickening of medium and large sized intra-hepatic portal veins and multiplicity and reduced size of veins in smaller portal tracts. Focal necrosis and signs of regeneration may be present. In some cases recanalised thrombi are seen in the large intraphepatic portal vein branches. The fibrosis are prominent in the subcapsular area. The last group is with obstruction or atresia of the extrahepatic bile ducts EHO are not associated with gaint cell transformation of the liver parenchyma only restricted to biliary channels. The canalicular ductules and ducts are dilated with inspissated bile. In early and mild cases, the canalicule in the central zonal area of the liver lobule only may be dilated.

Table 3

Showing Histological distribution

Histology of liver	No. of Cases	Percentage
A. Ch. parenchymatous disease		
(i) Early hydropic degeneration	3	5.1%
(ii) Peripheral cell necrosis, mild fibrosis, portal tract with inflammatory cells infiltration, kupffer cells hyperplasia, pericellular reticulin thickening.	10	16.6%
(iii) the above picture with cellular membrane, disruption, deposition of materials in cells.	10	16.6%
(iv) Portal tract involvement with centrizonal approach with fibrosis : early cirrhosis.	12	21.5%
(v) More advance cirrhosis with pseudolobular formation and involvement to both afferent and efferent vascular channels with more fibrosis and regenerative nodules.	8	13.7%
B. Hepato-portal sclerosis and also known as non-cirrhotic portal fibrosis (NCPF).	8	13.7%
C. Obstruction or atresia of the extrahepatic bile ducts (EHO) and/or neonatal hepatitis (giant cells) morphology.	7	12.8%

Histopathologically the extensive overlapping of findings in both congenital atresia of bile ducts and neonatal hepatitis occur in long standing cases of more than six weeks duration. The bile duct proliferation was not infrequent in neonatal hepatitis and patients with congenital atresias of bile duct some times show marked giant cell transformation — pointing to the theory of some common causative factor in both these two conditions.

In two cases laparotomy were done to diagnose hepatic hydatid disease, where the excision of cysts were needed. Also one case of choledochal cyst leading to extrahepatic obstructive jaundice in a 4 year old female child presented with a lump in right hypochondrium complaining of colicky pain and intermittent obstructive jaundice was operated.

In this study the mortality was 13.7%. Two cases were from neonatal hepatitis, one each from malnutrition with Kala-azar and malnutrition with bacterial septicaemia respectively. One died from malnutrition with tuberculosis one each from Hodgkin and Histiocytosis 'X' and the later on autopsy examination revealed it to be malnutrition with extensive tuberculosis involving all the internal organs. So total eight cases died in this study.

The two other autopsies were from 2 cases of neonatal hepatitis, here also before hand the etiology could not be determined.

DISCUSSION

The chronic hepatopathies may be defined as clinical or biochemical evidences of hepatic involvement continuing beyond 6 weeks to 6 months of the onset of the acute infection, superimposed on primary parenchymal liver involvement with malnutrition, metabolic, congenital infection, drug induced and last but not the least an unknown aetiology.

However with the clinical history, past, present and family background, particularly the neonatal histories and thorough clinical examinations, relevant laboratory investigations with liver function tests, histological studies were done to find out the aetiology. Beyond the above mentioned investigations, in more than 30 cases, relevant special investigations were done to corroborate with the other investigative findings.

Table — 4

Shows the etiology, total number of cases in each group with percentages

Cause	No. of case in each group	Percentage
1. Congenital Neonatal Hepatitis	1	8.6
Cong. Biliary atresia	1	1.7
Choledochal cyst	1	1.7
2. Post-hepatic Infective hepatitis	8	13.7
Serum hepatitis	1	1.7
3. Malnutrition		
(a) Malnutrition with toxins	2	3.4
(b) Mal.with protozoal infection malaria, Kala-azar, Ent. Hysto	7	12.8
(c) Mal.with helminthiasis	2	3.4
(d) Mal.with Non-specific bacterial infection	1	1.7
(e) Mal.with tuberculosis (Hepatic tuberculosis)	3	5.17
4. Indian childhood cirrhosis	5	8.6
5. Infiltrative		
(a) Hodgkin disease Non-hodgkin's lymphoma	2	3.2
(b) Histiocytosis 'X'	1	1.7
(c) Thalassaemia syndromes	6	10.3
6. Misc :		
(a) Cardiac	4	6.8
(b) Drug induced	3	5.1
(c) Undiagnosed	6	10.3

In this study of 7 cases neonatal hepatitis and cong biliary atresia 2 cases died from hepatitis group. One case of extra hepatic obstruction due to choledochal cyst was operated and the other one with both intra and extrahepatic obstruction, planned surgery was done after laparotomy and with reconstructive surgery pt was improved.

In the post hepatic group, 2 cases of persistant hepatitis and one case of chronic active hepatitis were diagnosed histologically. The big group was with malnutrition, associated with infection and infestations (15) cases. Two were hepatic hydatidosis besides one bacterial pyaemic abscess. The mortality in this group was 3. The cases with Indian childhood cirrhosis, the age did not belong to typical age of onset that is — 1-3 years, but even elderly children upto 8 years — with histologically proved cases were studied. And from one case A antigen was positive. These cases were managed with recent immunomodulation therapy and till the date of reporting, no mortality was detected. In the infiltrative group, most were from the thalassaemia syndrome. These are long standing cases. Some developed haemachromatosis with pigment cirrhosis and also with various degrees of hepatocellular failure. The above aetiological diagnosis were possible more or less with available investigative procedures. But in 8 cases from the miscellaneous group in elderly children, the age from 6-12 years, presented with hepatomegaly with or without ascites, also with upper gastrointestinal bleeding. The relevant investigations with splenoportography and histological studies proved that clinically they presented like cirrhosis with portal hypertension but histologically 'Hepato-portal fibrosis' was detected with minimal parenchymal damage, mostly involving the intrahepatic portal vein tributaries with intimal thickening, sparing the arteries, in some there were ductular dilatation of bile canaliculi. Due to absence of wide spread hepatocytic damage, the biochemical disturbances were minimum. The obstructive nature was more of presinusoidal nature — extending in some cases to proximal portal veins. The causes postulated as were chronic congestion due to congestive cardiac failure, in some associated tuberculosis, in 2 cases with big spleen, malarial parasites were demonstrated — suggestive autoimmunity with malarial antibodies and also in a few cases of associated intestinal helminthasis particularly ascariasis were thought.

SUMMARY AND CONCLUSION

A study of aetiopathogenesis of chronic liver disease in children with special reference to diffuse hepatic involvement was undertaken in 58 cases of children with age group of 3 months to 12 years. Though it is a selected study of hospital admissions in 2 years yet from the nature of aetiological background one can guess the main causes of these chronic liver disease with diffuse parenchymatous involvement.

Among 58 cases of diffuse hepatic involvement noticed in neonatal hepatitis/biliary atresia, post-hepatitis, persistent hepatitis and ch.active hepatitis, malnutrition with nonspecific bacterial infection, Indian childhood cirrhosis in advanced stages, various infiltrations with hepatocyctic infiltrations with iron, glycogen, mucopolysaccharides, etc.

The focal fibrosis were noticed in malaria, Kala-azar, tuberculosis, amoebiasis, hepatitic hydatidosis, eight cases in the miscellaneous group histologically proved hepatoportal Sclerosis-also called non-cirrhotic portal fibrosis (NCPF) (Nayak and Ramalingaswami, 1969) in older age group. In this group portal hypertension was presented as either gross splenomegaly or repeated upper gastrointestinal bleeding. Altogether 8 cases (13.77%) died in this study.

Bibliography

1. Chandra R.K. : "The liver and Biliary system in infants and children" Churchill Livingstone, Edinburgh, London, New York, 1979.
2. Ghai O.P. "Essentials of Paediatrics" 1st Edition October, 1977.

3. Nayak, N.C. and Ramalignaswami V (1969) "Obliterative portal venopathy of the liver". Archives of pathology, 87, 359-369.
4. Guha Mazumdar, D.N. et al "etio pathogenesis of non-cirrhotic portal fibrosis (NCPF) with special reference to gut etiology" — Institute of Post-graduate Medical Education and Research, monthly bulletin, 1982.
5. Chakraborty Bijan Kumar, et al "Clinico-pathological study and estimation of serum cholinesterase levels in thalassaemias — Indian Paediatrics, Volume XII no. 10. October, 1979.
6. Chakraborty. B.K., Handling of glucose in diseases of the liver in children — Archives of child health, Vol. 20 no 1, January, 1978. Paper read at XV International Congress of Paediatrics, New Delhi, October, 1977.
7. Chakraborty, Bijon Kumar et al — "Cholinesterase and haemoglobin pattern in thalassaemia syndromes" — paper read at XVI International Congress of Paediatrics, Barcelona, Spain, September, 1980.
8. Basu, A. K. and Guha B. N. (1976) : Profile of portal hypertension in India with and without — cirrhosis of liver. In progress in clinical medicine. Ed. Aluya, M.M.S.CH. 18,p. 373, New Delhi,
9. Basu. A.K. and Guha B.N. (1976) : Profile or portal hypertension in India with and without — cirrhosis of liver. In progress in clinical medicine. Ed. Aluya, M.M.S.CH. 18,p. 373, New Delhi, Heinemann.

CHAPTER – FIFTEEN

ANNEXURE-1

Population of India as on 1-12-1985	730 millions
Decennial growth rate (1971–81)	24.75%
Total area	3.3 million Sq. kms.
Density of population	221 Sq. km.
Distribution of population – Below 15 years of age	39.3%
Sex ratio	935 females to 1000 males
Proportion of Urban population to Rural	24 : 76
Per capital National income at current prices	Rs.1378–00
People below poverty line	48.4%
Handicapped children per 1,00,000 children between 0–6 years of age :	
Totally Dumb	10
Totally Blind	29
Totally Crippled	43
No. of hospitals	6670
No. of Primary Health Centres	5532
Doctor population ratio	1 : 3600
No. of Medical Colleges having P.G. Courses in pediatrics	58
P.G. Seats in Pediatrics –	
M.D.	255
D.C.H.	304

Targets of Health for all by 2000 A.D.

Index	National Average	
	Present	2000 A.D.
Crude birth rate (per 1000)	33.3	21.0
Crude death rate (per 1000)	14.2	9.0
Natural growth rate	1.91	1.20
Perinatal mortality rate	60–109	30–35
Infant mortality rate	125	Below 60
Pre-school (0–5 years) death rate	35–40	10

Maternal mortality rate (MMR)	5.8	Below 2
Effective couples protection	22.0	60.0
Net reproduction rate	1.67	1.0
Family size	4.3	2.3
Birth weight below 2500 g.(%)	30%	10%
Life expectancy at birth (Yrs.)	52.6—M, 51.6—F	64 years
Pregnant mothers receiving ante-natal care (%) :		
Rural	56.3 (estimated)	100
Urban	43.5 (estimated)	100
Deliveries by trained birth attendants (%)	10—15% (estimated	100
Maternal Mortality	4.8	Below 2
Population with sound excreta disposal (%) :		
Rural	— —	50
Urban	34	100
Population with protected water supply (%) :		
Rural	10	100
Urban	80	100
Immunisation status (%) :		
(a) T.T. (Pregnant mothers)	21	100
(b) D.P.T. (Infants)	51	100
(c) Polio (Infants)	18	100
(d) B.C.G. (Infants)	65	85
% coverage by Vit.'A' prophylaxis (0—5 yrs)	25%	Maintenance (50%)
% coverage of nutritional supplement (Iron-Folic acid)	25—30%	Maintenance (50%)
Tuberculosis :		
Total number of cases detected as percentage of total estimated case load	30%	100%
Diarrhoeal Disease (Reduction mortality)	— —	Above 95%
Respiratory disease other than TB (% reduction)	25%	Maintenance (70%)
Dental Health	—	Above 95%
School Health (population coverage)	—	100%

Facts about children in India

1. Out of every 1,000 babies born alive in the country, 120 die in the first year of life.

2. Forty percent of all deaths in the country are among children below five years of age.
3. With a baby born every one and a half second, there are 21 million births a year.
4. There are about 60 million malnourished children in India.
5. Every month about 1,00,000 children die due to effects of malnutrition.
6. About 2.5 million children in India are threatened by blindness in early childhood (1—5 years) because of lack of Vitamin A. About 12,000 — 14,000 go blind every year of this deficiency.
7. Out of every 100 children who enter Class I, less than half complete Class V and only 24 complete Class VIII.
8. Out of every 100 girls who enter Class I, only 30 complete Class V, i.e., about 70 percent of the girls drop out from school even before they acquire functional literacy.
9. Five to ten percent of all children are working, giving India the largest child labour force in the world.
10. Children workers constitute about six percent of the labour force in the country.
11. Juvenile crime accounts for about five percent of all congnizable crimes in the country.

IMMUNISATION SCHEDULE

	First Course	Reference
B.C.G.	0 to 1 month	0 to 1 year
Triple Antigen	3 injections × 6 to 8 weeks apart commencing 2 or 3 months	First course completed within first year
Or		
Double Antigen	3 injections × 6 to 8 weeks apart commencing at 3 months	First course to be completed within first year.
Polio (Oral)	4 to 5 doses × 6 to 8 weeks apart from the 2 or 3 months onward	First course to be completed within first year
Measles	After 9 months and before 15 months one injection only	
T.A.B.	2 injections 1 to 3 weeks apart at the end of first year (Each of 0.1 ml. intradermal)	
Cholera	1 injection only advised for cover during epidemics as dependable immunity is very short.	

BOOSTERS

B.C.G.	After 5 to 10 years if tuberculin is negative.
Triple Antigen	At 8 to 24 months and again at 4 to 5 years.
Tetanus Toxoid	When injury requires a Booster cover, i.e., when last D.P.T. or D.A. injection has been given more than 6/12 before the injury.
Polio	At 18 to 24 months and again at 4 to 5 years and every 3 years till 15 years.
T.A.B.	One injection every year within 1 year of first course.

NORMAL GROWTH OF INFANTS

Weight :

(a) (Age + 3) × 5 = Wt. in lbs.

Or

(b) Age × 5 + 17 = Wt. in lbs. (under 6 years)

Birth — 3 Kgs.

Then ½ kg. per month upto 1 year.

Then 3 kg. every year.

Height :

2½ (Age in years) + 30 = Ht. in inches

Birth	= 50 cm.
1 year = 50 + 25 cm.	= 75 cm.
2 year = 75 = 12 cm.	= 87 cm.
3 years = 87 + 6 cm.	= 93 cm.
4 years = 93 + 6 cm.	= 99 cm.

and then 4 cm. a year thereafter.

Skull circumference :

Birth	= 14″
3/12	= 16″
6/12	= 17″
9/12	= 18″
1½ year	= 19″
2½ years	= 19.5″
5 years	= 20″
By 18 years	= 21″ plus.

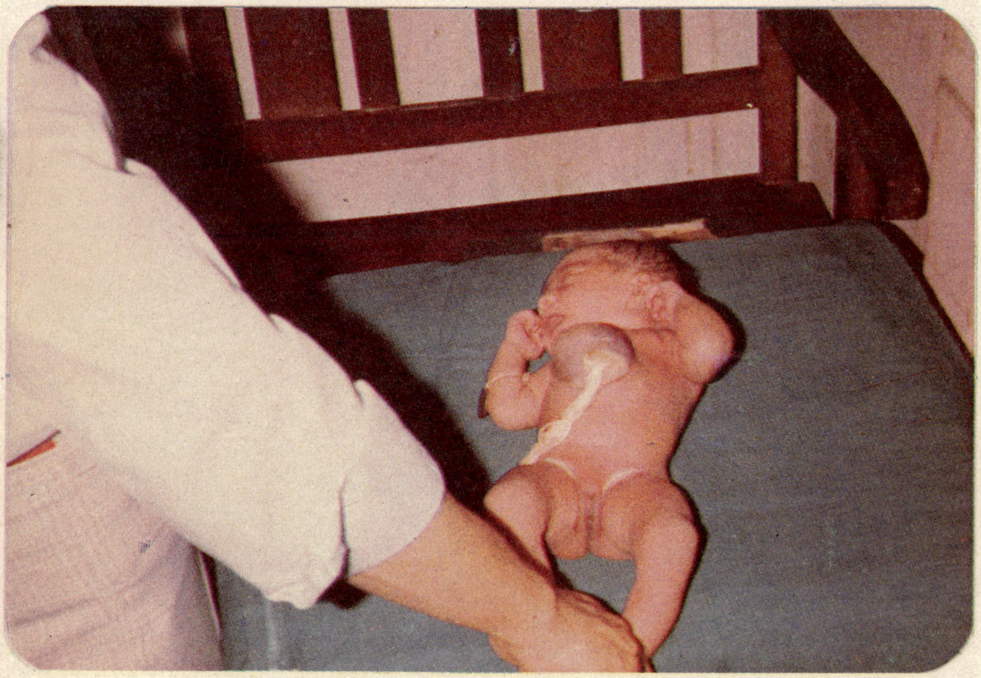

Fig.1.2 : Congenital malformation – Omphalocele.
For fig. 1.2 refer to Chapter 1, Page 7.

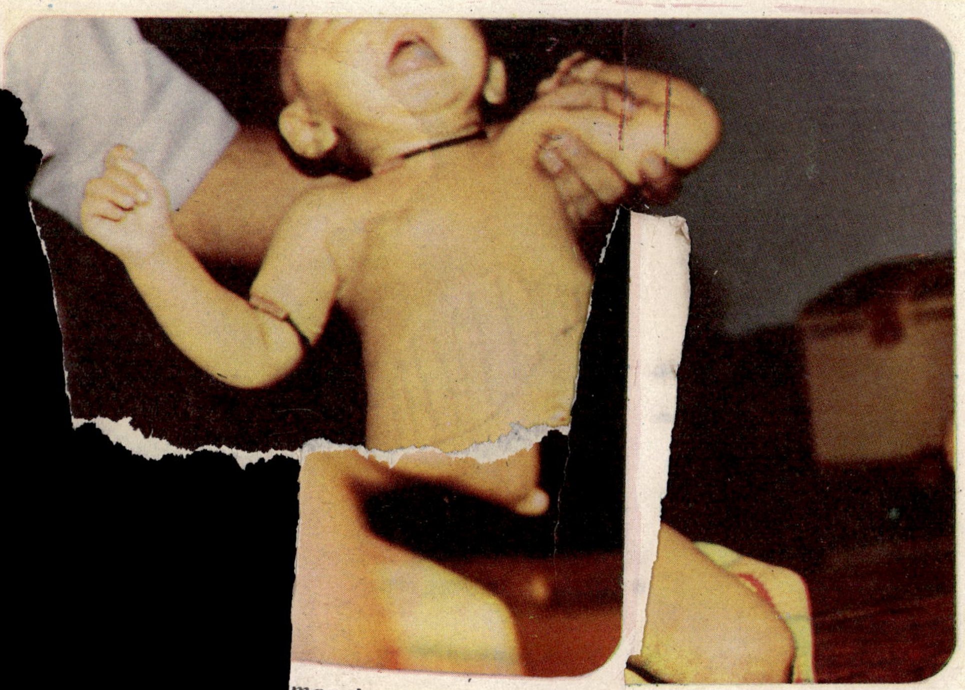

megaly.

in

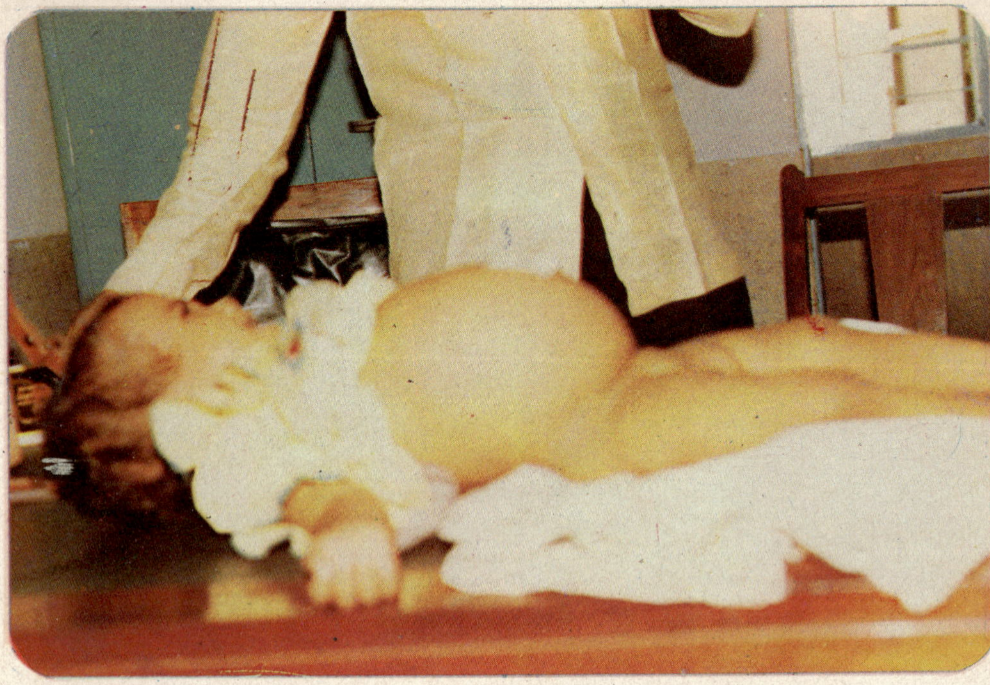

Fig.12.2 : Acute abdomen — Intestinal obstruction
For fig. 12.2 refer to Chapter 12, page 119.

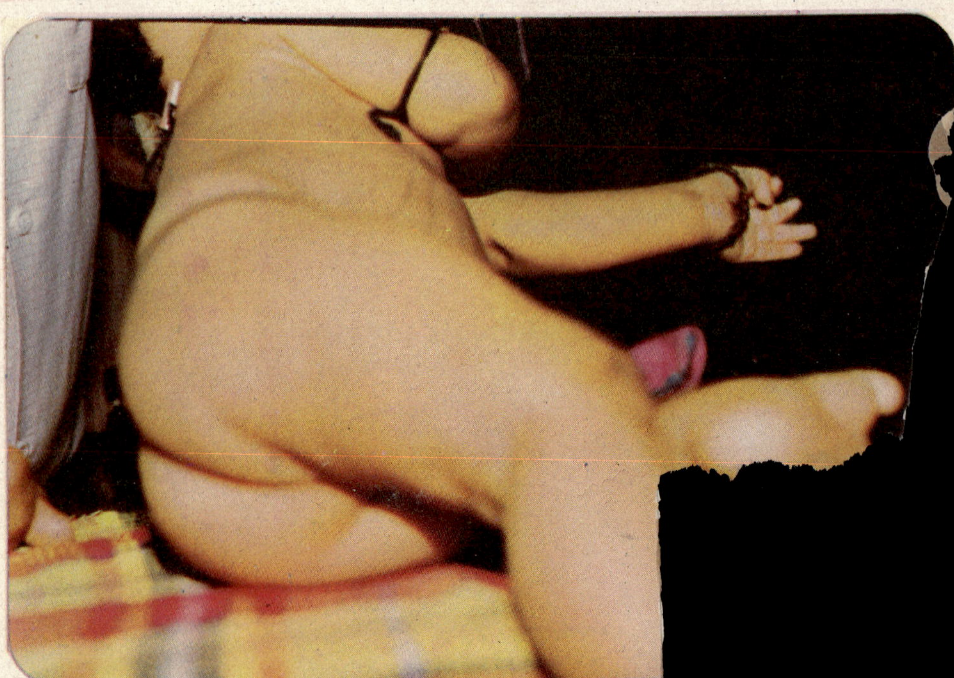

Fig.13.2 : Purpura, Pallor, Hepatospleeno
For fig. 13.2. refer to Chapter 13, page 124

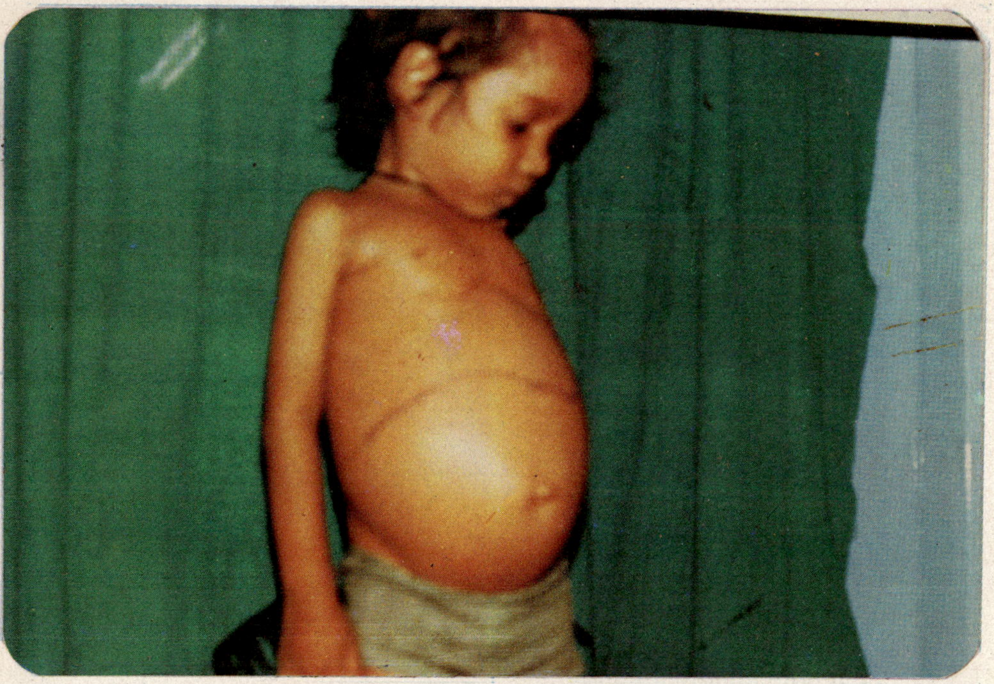

Fig.13.5(b) : Thalassaemia Major.*

For fig. 13.5(b) refer to Chapter 13, page 131.

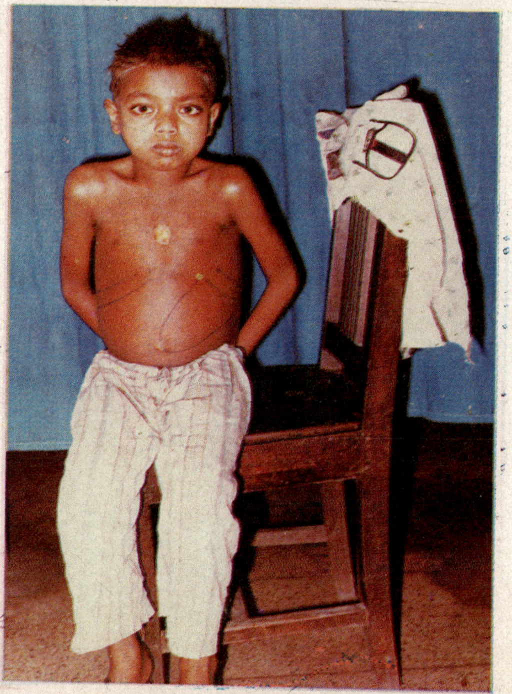

Fig.14.8 : Tropical Splenomegaly
— Kala azar, showing huge enlarged spleen.

For fig. 14.8, refer to Chapter 14, page 161.

Baby's Weight Chart

If child requires special care, state why :

*To complete the chart, fill in the months in the boxes provided for each year. Start by filling in baby's birth month in the boxes marked with an asterisk. During the first year, weight will be recorded once every fortnight. Therefore, 24 boxes have been provided for the first year — two boxes for each month.

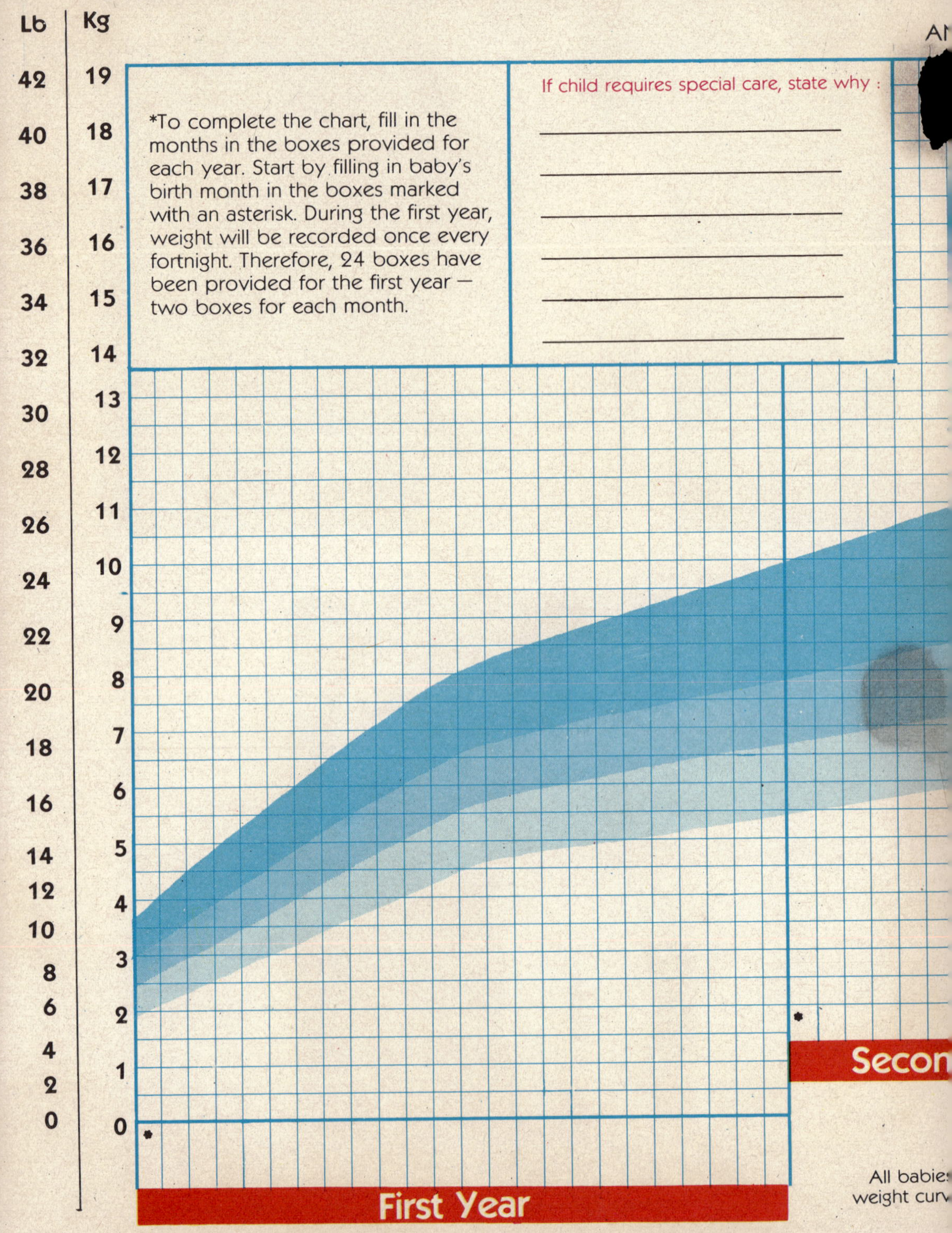

All babie
weight curv

from birth to five years

XURE — 4 (Baby's Weight Chart)

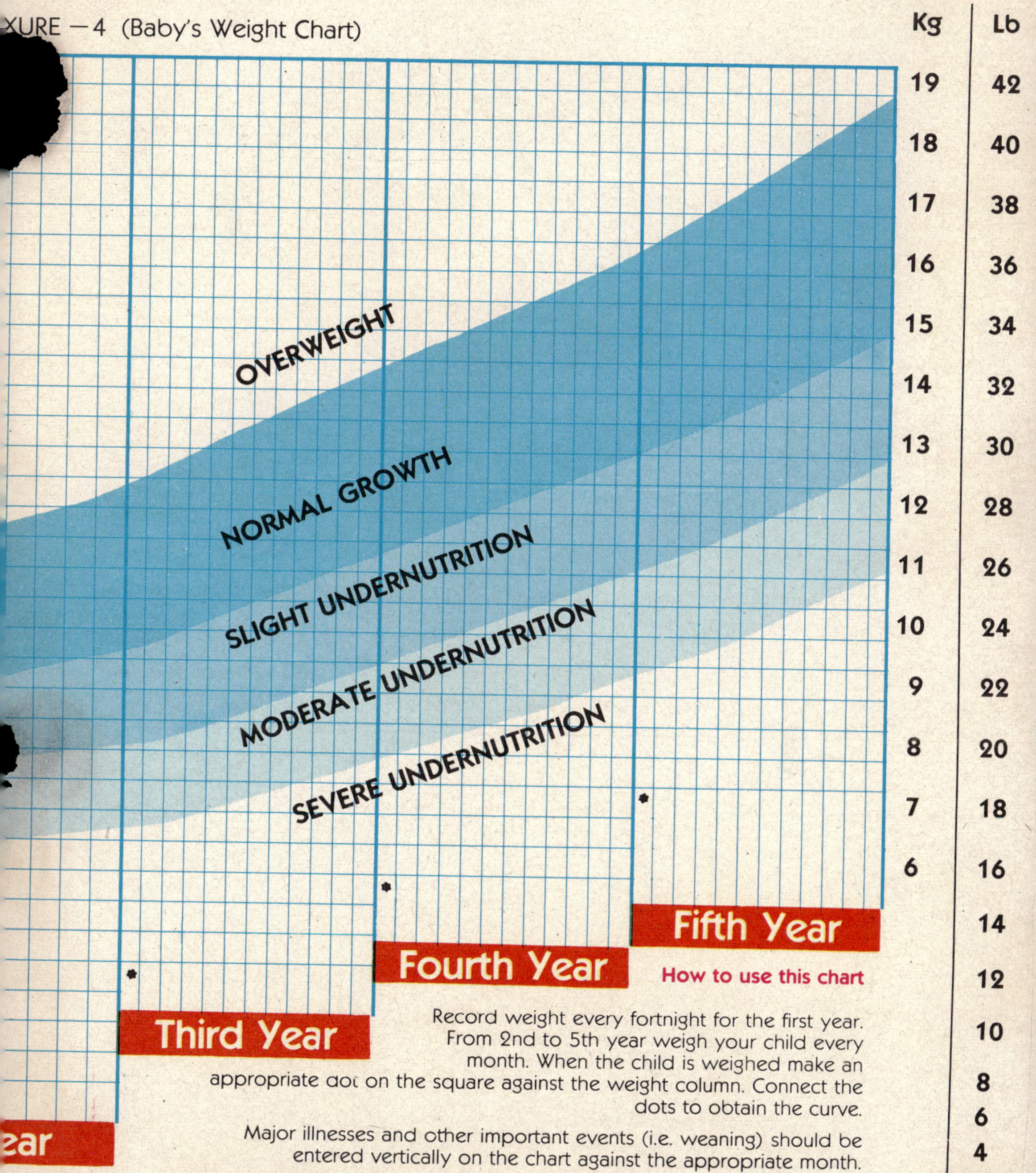

How to use this chart

Record weight every fortnight for the first year. From 2nd to 5th year weigh your child every month. When the child is weighed make an appropriate dot on the square against the weight column. Connect the dots to obtain the curve.

Major illnesses and other important events (i.e. weaning) should be entered vertically on the chart against the appropriate month.

The average weight curve indicated on the chart is based on the standard weight tables for Indian children from birth to 5 years issued by Indian Academy of Paediatrics.

erent, especially in the rate of growth. So, if your baby's weight increase does not follow the chart, there is no cause for alarm. As long as his monthly weight increase is to your Doctor's satisfaction, he is perfectly healthy.

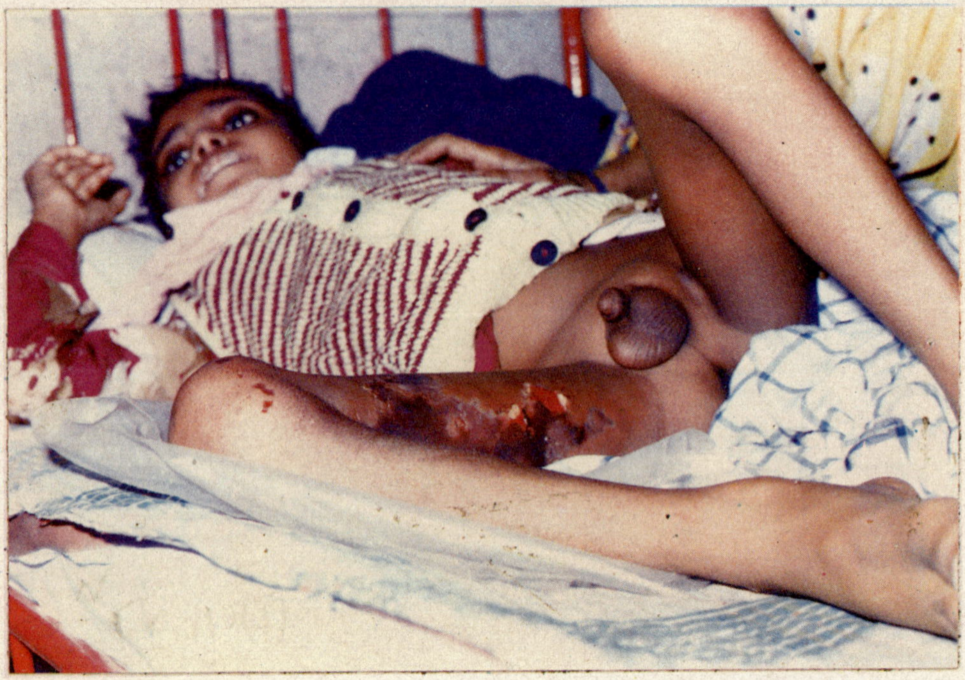

Fig. 10.1 : Nephrotic Syndrome, frequent relapses of chronic nephritis and renal failure.
For fig. 10.1 refer to Chapter 10, Pg. 100.

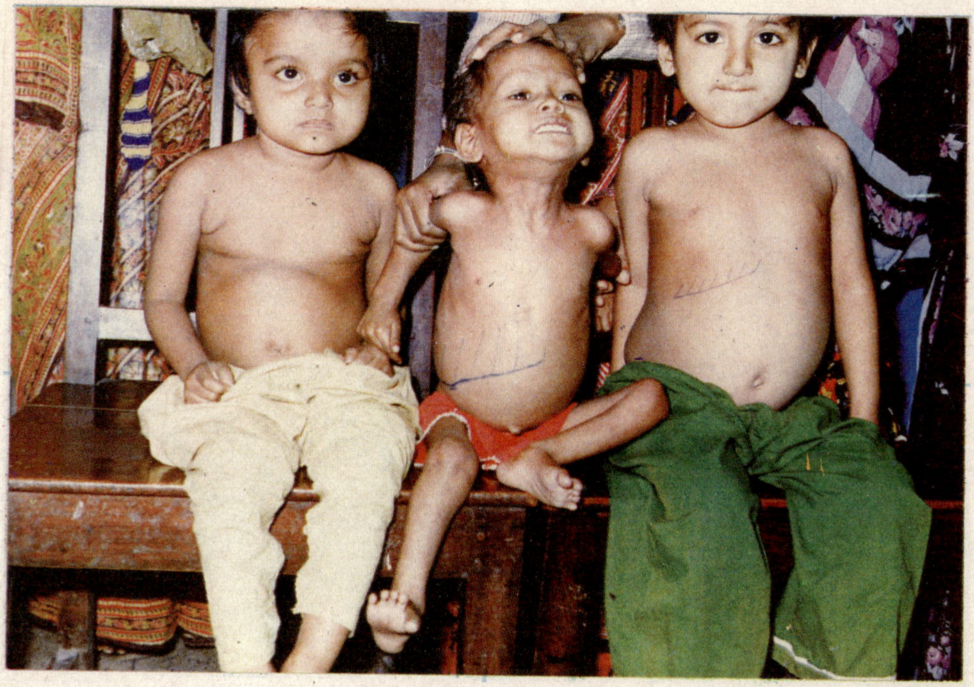

Fig.13.8(a) : Hepatospleenomegaly, Pallor
Left — aplastic anaemia.
Middle — Indian childhood cirrhosis with T.B.
Right — Treated case of ALL.

Fig.13.8(a) is connected with the matter depicted on page 142.

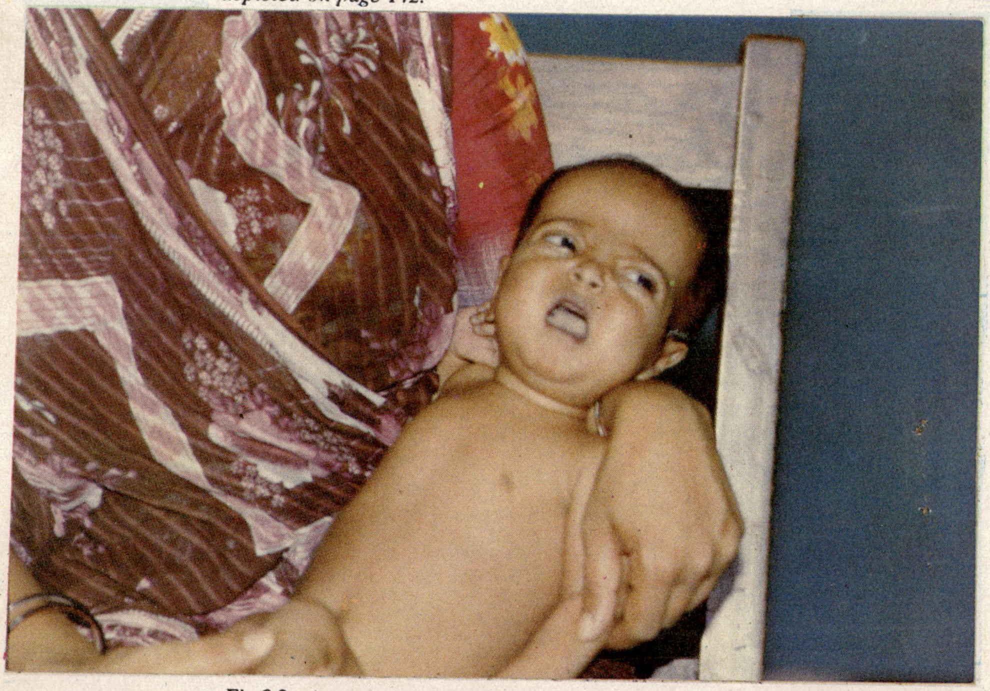

Fig.9.3 : A case of congenital cyanotic heart disease.

Fig.9.3 is connected with the matter depicted on page 84.

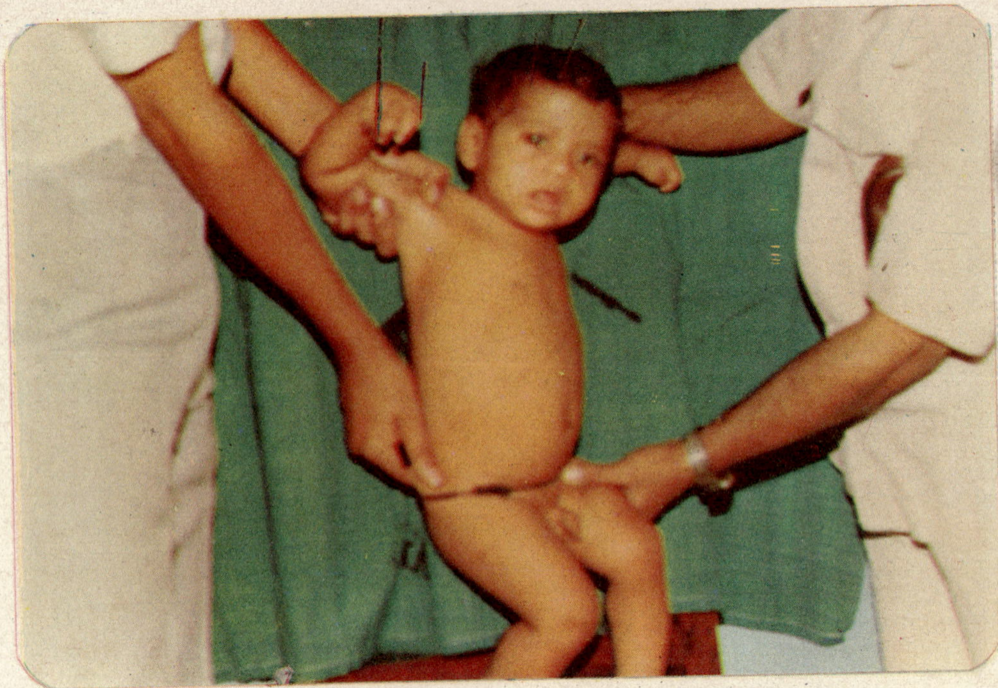

Fig.13.0 : Jaundice, Hepatospleenomegaly, Haemolytic anaemia,
Fig.13.0 is connected with the matter depicted on page 128,